The process of
PATIENT TEACHING IN NURSING

The process of
PATIENT TEACHING
IN NURSING

BARBARA KLUG REDMAN
R.N., B.S.N., M.Ed., Ph.D.

Professor of Nursing (on leave), University of Colorado
Medical Center, Denver, Colorado

FOURTH EDITION

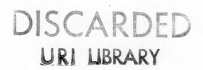

The C. V. Mosby Company

ST. LOUIS • TORONTO • LONDON   1980

FOURTH EDITION

The C. V. Mosby Company
11830 Westline Industrial Drive, St. Louis, Missouri 63141

Library of Congress Cataloging in Publication Data

Redman, Barbara Klug.
   The process of patient teaching in nursing.

   Includes bibliographies and index.
   1.   Patient education.   2.   Nurse and patient.
[DNLM: 1.   Nurse—Patient relations.   2.   Nursing
care.   3.   Patient education.   WY87 R318p]
RT90.R43   1980   613'.07   80-15310
ISBN 0-8016-4100-4

AC/M/M   9   8   7   6   5   4   3   2   03/C/319

Preface

This book is written for all nurses who want to know more about how to teach patients and families. Students of nursing should be ready to use the book when they recognize the need for learning in their patients and when they are sufficiently knowledgeable in the subject matter to be taught and competent in their interactions with patients.

The impetus to write the book began with students, by way of their interest in the excitement of directing learning in their patients. It came also from frustration on the part of student and teacher alike over the lack of materials specific to the patient-teaching process in nursing.

After a beginning statement about the relevance of teaching to nursing, the chapters are organized around elements of the teaching-learning process. Examples given are not meant to be exhaustive; they are only illustrative of the process. It will be advantageous if the student already has a basic understanding of the psychology of learning, because this complex subject must be abbreviated in a book of this size.

Barbara Klug Redman

Contents

The process of
PATIENT TEACHING IN NURSING

CHAPTER 1

The place of teaching in nursing

■ Almost everyone will agree that the nurse ought to explain many things to the patient. This statement leads to questions: Does the patient want to learn? How important is it for him to learn? What should he know? What is the best way to teach? Does the nurse need the physician's permission to teach? How does the nurse know whether or not the patient has learned? Also of importance is an understanding of how teaching came to be a tool of nursing, of what it is expected to accomplish, and of the ways in which nurses now function as teachers. Such a perspective helps to delineate what the role of teaching in nursing can be. The present chapter develops this perspective in preparation for the following chapters, which focus on the process of teaching-learning.

HISTORIC, PHILOSOPHIC, AND LEGAL BACKGROUND

Early English leaders in nursing in the middle and late nineteenth century saw the importance of teaching families about sanitation, cleanliness, and care of the sick. Since much of the care of the sick at that time was done by the family, the efforts of nurses to teach represented a way of extending their services. This same reason no doubt motivated the early visiting nurses in the United States, who fought together with other workers against disease and poverty among immigrants. Also basic to these health education efforts was the realization that health could not be legislated or mandated suc-

cessfully. These tenets remain important today.

A number of factors have converged to bring health teaching into prominence. The greater effort in this century to maintain health rather than just treat disease has enlarged the sphere of knowledge a person needs and has demanded a change in attitudes about health. World War II emphasized the need for teaching in rehabilitation, perhaps because of the return of so many servicemen in need of this service. Shortened hospital stays with early ambulation require preparation for the convalescence the patient will undergo at home. There has also been an increase in long-term illnesses and disabilities, and both the patient and his family should possess a high degree of understanding of the illness and its treatment.

Statements by the National League of Nursing Education reflect the concern during this century with preparing nurses for their teaching tasks. The following comment shows such a concern as early as 1918:

Another limitation of the ordinary training is that it deals only or mainly with disease, neglecting almost entirely the preventive and educational factors which are such an essential element in the many new branches of public health work, such as school and visiting nursing, infant welfare, industrial welfare, and hospital social service.*

---

*National League of Nursing Education: Standard curriculum for schools of nursing, Baltimore, 1918, The Waverly Press, p. 6.

1

The 1937 curriculum guide commented, ''The nurse is essentially a teacher and an agent of health in whatever field she may be working. . . .''[67] In 1950 some of the areas common to all nursing curricula were identified as ''teaching, contributing subject matter, psychology (especially principles of learning) . . . knowledge of principles of learning and teaching . . . [and] teaching skills.''[68] Note the extension of the place of teaching in nursing and the increasing interest in knowledge of the scientific bases of the teaching-learning process, which are characteristic of each of these statements of nursing thought at different times in this century. These recommendations represent the thinking of the nursing leaders; actual translation of these thoughts into schools of nursing and then into nursing practice seems to have occurred much more slowly.

The centrality of patient teaching varies with formal philosophies of nursing. Kreuter identifies teaching of self-care and counseling on health matters as nursing operations needed to provide care.[48] Sister Olivia views teaching as one of the tools of the nurse with the objective of promoting spiritual, mental, and physical health.[71] Some authors imply that nursing involves teaching. So it is with Henderson, who says that nursing assists the sick or well to do health activities they would do unaided if they possessed the necessary strength, will, or knowledge, with a goal of increasing independence.[34] Other authors view the teaching-learning process as more central to nursing. Lambertsen characterizes nursing as an ''educative process,''[50] and Peplau describes nursing as a maturing force, an educative instrument.[75] Hall views some of the tenets of teaching as central to her philosophy of nurse-patient interaction— the nurse facilitating the patient's verbal expressions by reflecting them so that the patient will hear what he is saying. Hall believes that through this process the patient comes to grips with himself and will learn to be well.[33] Travelbee indicates that both the patient and the nurse

learn as a result of the interactive process and that if changes do not occur in either or both of the participants, a relationship has not been established.[100]

Major changes in conception of the teaching function in nursing seem to have been occurring. Peplau sees a shift in emphasis from traditional mother-surrogate activities to more educative-nurturing ones.[76] Kinlein's description of her practice, based on Orem's theory, provides a view of a truly nursing focus for patient education. Kinlein proposes a health care system in which the person is the primary giver of care to himself—by virtue of choosing the health professional who the person thinks would be most helpful to him at the time.[43] Nursing is assisting the person in self-care practices with regard to his state of health. Instead of a practice focused on support of medical goals, the nursing focus in practice involves the use of nursing knowledge to help achieve the patient's health goals.[44] Indeed, the patient's knowledge, skills, and problem-solving ability form a self-care asset worth developing in and of itself.

Many of these expressions of philosophy emphasize the similarity of teaching and nursing; each involves a helping relationship that has as its objective development of independence in the subject. Teaching is seen as one means toward the goal of nursing, with both the nurse and the patient assuming responsibility for movement toward that goal.

Recent additions to social thought on patient education reflect more strident themes, such as control and patients' rights. Some see that medicine has become a major institution of social control by making the labels ''healthy'' and ''ill'' relevant to an ever increasing part of human existence. The new definitions of these terms appear to be that anything shown to negatively affect the workings of the body in some way and to a lesser extent the mind can be labeled an ''illness'' and jurisdictionally a ''medical problem.'' Further, the patient's moral character is not demonstrated in having the disease but in what he does about it.[108] It follows from this point of view that patient education would be one means of effecting control.

In elucidating the character of the professional functioning in medicine, Freidson concludes that "professional" is a way of organizing work rather than an orientation toward work or a body of knowledge. In contrast to the general notion that patient welfare is protected by professionals, one finds no generally accepted notion of due process for the client in professional work, including medicine.[26] In the same vein, Myra Levine has charged that, in fact, a large percentage of what is called "teaching" is actually communication of the rules of behavior dictated by the rituals that the nurse has been taught to value. The intransigent patient is one who either rejects or fails to understand the rules in the same way that the nurse understands them.[53]

The legal base for medicine has long included the patient education area of practice. As

---

A PATIENT'S BILL OF RIGHTS*

The American Hospital Association presents a Patient's Bill of Rights with the expectation that observance of these rights will contribute to more effective patient care and greater satisfaction for the patient, his physician, and the hospital organization. Further, the Association presents these rights in the expectation that they will be supported by the hospital on behalf of its patients, as an integral part of the healing process. It is recognized that a personal relationship between the physician and the patient is essential for the provision of proper medical care. The traditional physician-patient relationship takes on a new dimension when care is rendered within an organizational structure. Legal precedent has established that the institution itself also has a responsibility to the patient. It is in recognition of these factors that these rights are affirmed.

1. The patient has the right to considerate and respectful care.
2. The patient has the right to obtain from his physician complete current information concerning his diagnosis, treatment, and prognosis in terms the patient can be reasonably expected to understand. When it is not medically advisable to give such information to the patient, the information should be made available to an appropriate person in his behalf. He has the right to know, by name, the physician responsible for coordinating his care.
3. The patient has the right to receive from his physician information necessary to give informed consent prior to the start of any procedure and/or treatment. Except in emergencies, such information for informed consent should include but not necessarily be limited to the specific procedure and/or treatment, the medically significant risks involved, and the probable duration of incapacitation. Where medically significant alternatives for care or treatment exist, or when the patient requests information concerning medical alternatives, the patient has the right to such information. The patient also has the right to know the name of the person responsible for the procedures and/or treatment.
4. The patient has the right to refuse treatment to the extent permitted by law and to be informed of the medical consequences of his action.
5. The patient has the right to every consideration of his privacy concerning his own medical care program. Case discussion, consultation, examination, and treatment are confidential and should be conducted discreetly. Those not directly involved in his care must have the permission of the patient to be present.

*Reprinted with the permission of the American Hospital Association, copyright 1975.

Continued.

A PATIENT'S BILL OF RIGHTS—cont'd

6. The patient has the right to expect that all communications and records pertaining to his care should be treated as confidential.

7. The patient has the right to expect that within its capacity a hospital must make reasonable response to the request of a patient for services. The hospital must provide evaluation, service, and/or referral as indicated by the urgency of the case. When medically permissible, a patient may be transferred to another facility only after he has received complete information and explanation concerning the needs for and alternatives to such a transfer. The institution to which the patient is to be transferred must first have accepted the patient for transfer.

8. The patient has the right to obtain information as to any relationship of his hospital to other health care and educational institutions insofar as his care is concerned. The patient has the right to obtain information as to the existence of any professional relationships among individuals, by name, who are treating him.

9. The patient has the right to be advised if the hospital proposes to engage in or perform human experimentation affecting his care or treatment. The patient has the right to refuse to participate in such research projects.

10. The patient has the right to expect reasonable continuity of care. He has the right to know in advance what appointment times and physicians are available and where. The patient has the right to expect that the hospital will provide a mechanism whereby he is informed by his physician or a delegate of the physician of the patient's continuing health care requirements following discharge.

11. The patient has the right to examine and receive an explanation of his bill regardless of source of payment.

12. The patient has the right to know what hospital rules and regulations apply to his conduct as a patient.

No catalog of rights can guarantee for the patient the kind of treatment he has a right to expect. A hospital has many functions to perform, including the prevention and treatment of disease, the education of both health professionals and patients, and the conduct of clinical research. All these activities must be conducted with an overriding concern for the patient, and, above all, the recognition of his dignity as a human being. Success in achieving this recognition assures success in the defense of the rights of the patient.

early as 1898, giving proper instructions to a diabetic patient in relation to care of his injured limb was found to be a duty, and failure to supply these instructions was abandonment. Today, other duties include explicit instruction in the use of prescribed medication, follow-up care, and informing the patient he or she has a condition requiring continual treatment.[41]

In regard to disclosure, in the Canterbury versus Spence case and others following it, the trend is to disregard the local community or national standards of disclosure and to substitute in their place the needs of a reasonably prudent patient. Such a rule is likely to lead to either greater disclosure or greater liability. It is permissible to withhold information if the disclosure will cause physiological or psychological harm to the extent that the effectiveness of the procedure will be impaired, but it is not permissible to withhold information merely to negate the possibility of the patient's refusal of treatment or his making a "wrong" decision.[46]

Finally, revision of some nurse practice acts has made explicit the inclusion of patient education, in addition to increasing the independence of the nurse. No body of legal opinion regarding standards of practice in this area appears to exist, although several professional associations have issued statements regarding the nurse's practice in patient education.

The Patient's Bill of Rights, developed and approved by the American Hospital Association, appears on pp. 3 and 4. A modified version of this Bill became state law in Minnesota. It has been suggested that once a hospital adopts the Bill of Rights as policy, the provisions can be the basis for legal action in the same manner as the hospital's bylaws and rules of nursing practice.[73] Courts may use the Bill as a higher standard of hospital conduct than was previously the case. The position of nursing regarding the compliance of physicians with the Patient's Bill of Rights is not yet clear[35] but may well include involvement in upholding the hospital's policy.

OBJECTIVES OF HEALTH TEACHING
General goals

What health teaching can accomplish is a key question. In general, health education is concerned with learning to live life in the healthiest way possible.[97] Alternative approaches to change in health behavior, such as legislation and environmental controls, ultimately depend on education for acceptance by people. In addition, many actions seen as important for improved health and welfare, such as family planning and seeking early diagnosis, are privately controlled and are not completely open to other approaches to effect behavioral change.[82] It is possible to prevent, to promote, to maintain, or to modify a number of health-related behaviors by means of teaching.

Several global objectives have been suggested. "An objective when dealing with illness is for the patient to fully participate in and integrate the illness in his life experience in order to prevent regression or dissociation of the event."[75] Closely related is the view that instruction should help the individual to find meaning in illness as well as in measures he must take to conserve health and control symptoms of illness.[100] Teaching plays a part in the general goal of nursing to help patients strengthen themselves through strengthening role performance. This includes support during role change initiated by growth and development, movement into a new geographic or social environment, or transition between health, sick, and handicapped roles. To this end, the nurse in the outpatient department helps the diabetic patient reconcile his sick role with that of worker role, and a public health nurse gives prenatal counseling to parents.[102] Other more specific goals fit within the general framework of carrying out one's role as a patient. Included are follow-through on treatment and rehabilitation; self-direction, including participation in decision making; and self-care.[28,63] Closely related to carrying out one's role as a patient is the objective of relieving the tensions of illness by means of learning.[42,94] It is believed that a patient is reassured when someone he trusts gives him authentic information when he needs it.[31]

It has been said that a general characteristic of psychosocial nursing treatment, of which patient teaching is a part, is that the goals are usually short-term and palliative rather than curative. For example, the nurse may discuss a patient's fears with him preoperatively with the intention of decreasing the probability of postoperative complications, but the goal does not involve altering the patient's psychologic reaction to operations in general.[107] To the extent that this statement is true, it demands reflection on the value of such goals, on our ability to attain them, and on ways in which accomplishment of numerous short-term goals affects attainment of the long-term goals.

These views about objectives are the basis of the comment that every person who receives health care has some need to learn; at least he is likely to need orientation to the environment and perhaps to his diagnosis, and he may need an interpretation of how to be sick or well. This information gives him an opportunity to assess his rights as a patient.[94] For the families of these individuals there is need to learn how to support the sick and how to maintain and promote good health for the family unit.

Major objectives of teaching are often classified by phases of health care. Nurses teach about health care facilities, growth and development, nutrition and hygiene, safety, first aid, preparation for childbearing, and other such topics so that people will maintain health and prevent disease. During the phase of diagnosis and treatment, the patient and family learn about the disease, the need for care and treatment, and hospital or clinic environment. During the follow-through phase there is need for an understanding of care at home, including medications and diet, activity, continuing rehabilitation, and prevention of recurrence or complications. Nurses in public health, schools, and industry center their teaching activities in the phases of promotion of health, prevention of illness, and follow-through. Examples include classes about parenthood and health classes, counseling in day centers for the elderly,[5] and prenatal counseling done by the occupational health nurse.[51] Nurses working in hospitals deal primarily with teaching during the diagnosis and treatment phases and the beginning of the follow-through phase. The nurse in the outpatient clinic or nursing home may have the opportunity to teach during all phases.

A number of strong forces in the health care field, including widespread and growing dissatisfaction with the results of enormous expenditures on therapeutic medicine and the consumer movement, have thrust health education forward into a position of higher priority than it has held before. These forces have brought with them goals for patient behavior change. One area for such change is in the individual's responsibility for his own health, which is seen by some as a moral obligation. This means doing things that require special effort: exercising regularly, improving nutrition, going to the dentist, practicing contraception, ensuring harmonious family life, submitting to screening examinations. The individual then has the "right" to expect help with information, accessible services of good quality, and minimal financial barriers.[47] Such responsibility is seen as essential to financial savings from reduction of demand for health care. Although the elements that will be effective in reducing this demand are often not known with certainty, to change consumer expectations and behavior is one such strategy.

The self-care movement, if properly managed, is seen as supporting the goal of the individual's responsibility for his own health and goals of cost containment. There is a strong "antiestablishment" thrust within the self-care movement. It began outside the traditional, or formal, medical delivery system. Its goals include helping the public protect itself against the abuses of medical services provided by institutions, determining one's own risk mix, and assisting toward restoring a more appropriate control over professional and technological domination. Estimates show that perhaps 85% of all health care may now be self-provided; purposeful self-care is necessary as a part of the health care system to avoid the flooding of certain services.[52] Educational support is obviously a necessary part of the self-care movement. The model promotes an organizational approach and philosophy that nurture self-reliance, responsibility, and initiative, rather than ones that decrease utilization by creating barriers, for example, by allowing extended waiting times.

Evidence of effectiveness

Empirical evidence of the effects of patient teaching in reaching a variety of goals is beginning to accumulate. From one study it was found that patients who were given more thorough explanations participated somewhat more effectively with the physician in planning care and in accepting the plan.[78] After an educational experience carried out with 40 families whose children were seen at a mental retardation clinic, parents tended to assume goals for the child that the staff considered more realistic than those they held before the experience.[61] A study of patients with long-term congestive heart failure has shown that it is possible to achieve improved adherence to regimen, higher levels of functioning, and a reduction in hospital readmissions for congestive heart failure, by means of a continuing educational program.[92] Nurses functioning as family health management specialists with families of patients in a pediatric clinic for the care of the acutely ill were able to increase compliance with medications and procedures, appointment keeping, and understanding of the illness, in comparison with a control group that received the usual clinic care. The family health management specialist was concerned with the task of implementing the diagnosis and treatment plan, involving the family and physician in its development and interpretation, and assuming responsibility for follow-up.[23,24]

Determination of the effect of teaching on the operative course of patients has been a goal of a number of studies. Several of these show positive effects associated with teaching, as well as apparent limitations. Patients were judged best prepared for surgery with both administration of pentobarbital sodium (Nembutal) and a preoperative explanatory visit by the anesthetist, but better prepared with the visit alone than with the pentobarbital sodium alone.[20] A nurse who gave an experimental group of surgical patients special encouragement and instruction about how to deal with postoperative discomfort found that these patients were discharged earlier than those receiving routine care but found no difference between them and a control group in regard to vomiting and nausea, body temperature, pulse rate, amount of narcotic adminis-

tered, patients' estimate of pain severity, and the patients' satisfaction with the first postoperative night's sleep.[39] This is in contrast to the findings of two other studies. In one study done on 51 patients who had gynecologic surgery, the nurse was the instructor, whose goal was to help patients attain a suitable psychologic state (primarily, relief of distress), through a process of interaction. The patients who received this teaching-counseling had a significantly lower ($p < .01$) rate of postoperative vomiting than did similar patients who received the usual preoperative preparation from the hospital staff.[19] In another study, patients provided with preoperative and postoperative instruction about postoperative pain—where they would feel it, how long it would last, how they could handle pain—requested significantly less ($p < .01$) narcotic after the immediate postoperative period than did those without such instruction. An independent observer rated the instructed patients as more comfortable and in better physical and emotional condition than the patients in the control group. The instructed patients were also allowed to go home an average of 2.7 days earlier than the control group ($p < .01$), even though neither the observer nor the surgeons who discharged them were aware of who had been instructed.

More recent studies have shown a decrease in anxiety across coping styles, from preoperative teaching,[45] and a decrease in anxiety and increased psychological well-being but no differences in ventilatory function, as compared with a control group.[22] Another study shows significantly better physical functional capacity in patients receiving instruction (both physical activities while at the hospital in the immediate postoperative period and activities of daily living at home) that was still evident at 33 days. Comparisons with a control group showed no differences in length of hospitalizations or readmissions.[25]

Male patients who had surgery for inguinal hernia and had received "individualized" or "informative" nursing care had a significantly lower mean analgesic index and shorter hospitalization than patients with no such treatment, but no differences were found in other criteria, such as nonesterified fatty acids in the plasma or eosinophils in the blood.[10] In a small study of relief of pain in surgical patients, it was found that, as opposed to the view that the complaint is primarily a request for pain medications, the nursing approach that focused on accessing what the patient meant by "pain," ascertaining his needs, and then giving whatever nursing intervention was indicated gave greater relief, particularly initially.[56] Two studies of children who were to have tonsillectomies focused on interaction with the parent that was aimed at listening to parental feelings and beliefs regarding the child's hospitalization, identifying the basis for those feelings, and giving information. In contrast to similar groups that did not receive this special interaction, the children of parents in the experimental groups experienced significantly smoother postoperative courses, in terms of physiologic variables and behavior patterns.[59,94] Subsequent studies have found a combination of systematic preparation, rehearsal, and supportive care conducted before each stressful procedure to be superior to a single-session preparation conducted after admission or consistent supportive care given by one nurse at the same stages but including no systematic preparation or rehearsal.[104]

A study by Janis provided additional direction, although still tentative, in the determination of goals for preoperative teaching. The study relates the level of anticipatory fear to probable postoperative behavior and suggests the direction that psychologic preparation should take. Worrying in moderation before surgery was seen as necessary for coping successfully with the stresses of the postoperative period. Patients who worried moderately sought information and built up defenses that were usually adequate, unless there was a gap in their knowledge about postoperative occurrences.

Those with low anticipatory fear did not build up these defenses, and Janis suggests that the angry resentment they showed afterward might have been reduced by decreasing internal resistances to the point at which such patients would have begun thinking over the threatening situation. Patients with high anticipatory fear tended to show this same fear postoperatively. For them it is suggested that preparation would have reduced the excitement so that the work of worrying could be carried out effectively.[37] However, a subsequent study did not support Janis' findings for patients with low anticipatory fear; rather, the relationship between preoperative fear and postoperative emotional disturbance was found to be linear.[40]

Teaching related to several procedures has also been successful. Patients before delivery were more accepting of and had better results from an enema if the nurse focused her interaction on the patient's reaction to the procedure, instead of limiting remarks to the procedure itself.[101] In another study, patients who were taught to give their own perineal care after delivery were believed to be as successful as those to whom the nurse gave the care.[69]

Alterations in diet by means of educational programs have had varying degrees of success. A teaching program aimed at increasing intake of vitamin C and thiamine among a group of well-educated patients after delivery (85% had education beyond high school) showed that there was a significant difference in choice of appropriate foods compared with a group with no such treatment.[72] On the other hand, a teaching program was not able to effect change in compliance with a weight-controlling diet among black primigravidae.[54]

Descriptions of other studies of the effect of teaching on patient behavior may be found in Chapter 10.

Several questions are raised by these and related investigations. First, two similar studies contained more than one experimental group in which an instructional, or informational, approach was predominant, and another study focused on "supportive," or "individualized," care.[10,80] It was reported to be difficult to distinguish between these two approaches, and in another study such a distinction was dropped because it became too difficult to keep the two approaches separate in practice.[21] Generally, either approach was more successful than the regular care patients were receiving, but no differences in results could be found between the two experimental approaches. Good teaching has long been known to include both information and support, and it seems that additional efforts will have to be made to determine differential effects of elements of the two approaches.

Second, it is not at all clear who can best do teaching to achieve desired effects or what kind of preparation is most effective. The nurses acting as family health management specialists estimated that 62% of their clients could have been helped as effectively by a nonprofessional health aide and an additional 27% by an aide with nursing consultation.[23] Perhaps there are some instances in which the nurse's role does not provide the person with enough authority to teach effectively. For example, is part of the effectiveness of preoperative teaching by anesthetists related to their supposed ability to modify the danger of surgery? In several studies, the investigator carried out the experimental teaching programs, and control care was given by regular staff. To what extent were the effects altered by what patients might have interpreted as special attention by a special person and by better developed skills of investigators?

Finally, as studies continue, the general boundaries of effectiveness of teaching as an approach to behavior change should be outlined. Although Fink's studies show that the family health management specialist is capable of having a positive effect, the overall level of compliance and understanding was still discouragingly low.[23] One could speculate that the lack of effect in the Lowe study, aimed at control of weight gain among black primigravidae, was related to difficulty in effecting diet change by any means, particularly in a group that might have been of low socioeconomic status and therefore less susceptible to educational approaches that are commonly middle class in their design.

There are multiple factors that can cause such a lack of effect. Two very important ones are limitations of the subject matter used to produce the desired effect and deficiencies in knowledge about how to produce the behavioral change desired. It has been charged that a severe limitation of mental hygiene education is that, although there is agreement on the fallacies regarding mental health, there is no set of practical positive actions to recommend to the public for personal adjustment and the prevention of mental illness.[17] Similarly, parent education must be accommodated to the fact that the effects of parental acts on childhood and on later personality and the permanence of these effects appear to be largely unknown. Since there is a vast amount of unintegrated and conflicting data about the influence of parents on children's character development, parent educators have the difficult job of deciding what information they will use and what they will discard.[57] The current, generally accepted view that enough is known about diabetes mellitus and its treatment to allow physicians, through guidance and education, to help patients achieve good control in most instances, has been questioned. A study of adult diabetic patients drawn from several medical practices indicated that the more the patients knew about their disease, the better they carried out the recommended therapy, but there was no significant correlation between performance and day-to-day control. Seventy percent of the patients studied were judged to be in poor control, and the author cites as supporting evidence other studies that show 45% to 66% of the patients in poor control.[106]

Much also remains to be known about how

to effectively change behavior through teaching. The degree to which health attitudes are related to behavioral change seems to be small. It has been charged that views on teaching methodology in health education remain largely subjective and that measurement studies have concentrated more on the status of what people know, feel, or do about health than on change.[103] If, as Woolridge and associates indicate, very little social practice theory can be unambiguously deduced from existing theories in the behavioral sciences,[107] considerable work remains to be done to accomplish an adequate research base for patient teaching practice.

CURRENT NURSING PRACTICE IN TEACHING
Definitions of teaching

The definition of teaching as "activities by which the teacher helps the student to learn" is broad yet useful, for it emphasizes active learning by the student as the primary goal. Equally broad is the view of teaching as any interpersonal influence aimed at changing the way in which other persons can or will behave. The centrality of control is evident in these two definitions of education. Activities are used in which the learning of one or more persons is being deliberately controlled by others,[6] and there is a controlled introduction of discontinuities in the form of new or novel objects, events, or information into the learner's environment.[74]

Teaching is a special form of communication and so encompasses what is known about that subject. Again very broadly, teaching has been seen as communication specially structured and sequenced to produce learning. Some authors view teaching as limited to activities designed to change behavior in the learner; they feel that other interaction is outside the realm of teaching. Although it is true that a change of behavior should occur, it is not always easy to obtain evidence of the change immediately. Therefore, teaching is seen by many as involving the intention to produce learning and not necessarily success in doing so. This is consistent with the fact that we do not know exactly how and to what extent teaching contributes to or causes learning.

Perhaps it is most useful to nursing practitioners to view all interaction with patients as contributing to the broad process and objectives of teaching-learning. For example, each time nurses are with patients, they are assessing patient needs, some of which can be met by providing patients with information, clarifying their thinking, reflecting their feelings, or teaching them a skill. Nurses also communicate nonverbally and by example about such topics as health and good hygiene practices.

Differentiation from related interpersonal skills

Other functions such as counseling, guidance, and support are related to teaching, as are skills used in crisis intervention and psychiatric nursing. Counseling may be regarded as emotional, intellectual, and psychologic support.[81] One author views the teacher role in nursing situations as a combination of roles including counselor,[75] implying that teaching is the more general of the two. Thus these definitions are confusing at present. Teaching, guidance, counseling, and support all have the common goal of development of the individual or group, although support may not involve active development on the part of the patient. Guidance, counseling, and support focus on development of attitudes and feelings, whereas the most traditional focus of teaching has been intellectual growth, and training has been thought of as concerned with psychomotor growth; however, these distinctions are by no means clear-cut.

The boundary between education and psychotherapy has been variously defined. It is believed that significant learning is facilitated by psychotherapy, aimed at such goals as accepting oneself and one's feelings and those of others, becoming self-confident and self-directing, and adopting realistic goals for oneself.[83] The function of psychiatric nursing, as defined by Travelbee, is to create a therapeutic milieu in which the ill person can develop as a human being, to assist the person in respecting himself and others, and to help the patient derive enjoyment and pleasure from socializing and becoming a part of the human community. The nurse helps the ill person cope with present problems, conceptualize problems realistically, perceive participation in an experience, face emerging problems, envisage alternatives, and test new patterns of behavior, as well as communicate, socialize, and find meaning in illness.[100] These goals seem to overlap with those of patient teaching. There are those who argue that much that is regarded as intrapsychic dynamics can fruitfully be seen from a skills-ability perspective. Rehabilitation programs with mental health patients need to pay attention to information, skills, and abilities that an individual needs to satisfactorily adapt to community life. Indeed, problems of living, on which community mental health is based, may not be part of the same continuum as chronic psychoses.[62]

Education is seen as the use of techniques directed toward the healthier conscious and near-conscious aspects of the individual personality to effect change.[57] Its limitations in the attaining of important goals have been pointed out in the area of parent education. Educational programs are generally of little help to parents whose anxiety pervades all aspects of their functioning or whose anxiety is so intense in the area of their parent-child relationships that it paralyzes them. For these parents, treatment services are indicated. For people without such a degree of difficulty, the following question remains: What content is teachable through the use of educational methods alone? It has been suggested that the assumption that much of parents' behavior toward their children is under conscious and volitional control is erroneous and that as parents become aware of a "better"

method that they cannot pursue, their guilt may increase.[57] There has been no adequate resolution of this issue, but it is clear that education is but one of several kinds of activities necessary to help parents achieve full effectiveness in their parental roles.

A therapy in which teaching skills are a component is crisis intervention, which is carried out during the time when the person in crisis is establishing a coping pattern. Crisis intervention is seen by Aguilera and Messick as being on a continuum with psychoanalysis, psychoanalytic psychotherapy, and brief psychotherapy. Crisis intervention does not require the practitioner to have mastery of knowledge of the intrapsychic and interpersonal processes of an individual in crisis. This therapy includes direct encouragement of adaptive behavior, general support, environmental manipulation, and anticipatory guidance, but the nature of intervention technique is highly dependent on the preexisting skills, creativity, and flexibility of the therapist. More specifically, helping individuals to gain an intellectual understanding of their crises, helping them bring into the open their present feelings to which they may not have access, exploring coping mechanisms, and reopening the social world can be part of crisis intervention.[1] Stated in another but complementary way, part of the therapist's procedure is to state the problem in terms that the patient can assimilate in the available time, to help the patient see the problem in a new light, and to show the patient where previous coping mechanisms have failed; all these processes are aimed at crisis resolution, which involves solving the problem that is novel to the individual.[15] Nurses work daily with patients who are undergoing some degree of maturational or situational crisis, and nurses do help patients and their families solve daily living problems affecting their health. If the nurse's efforts are not working and the patient or family shows signs of increased anxiety, it is suggested that the nurse obtain the help of someone trained in crisis intervention or a mental health worker.[1]

It can be seen that within the general goal of effecting behavior changes, there are a number of interpersonal techniques. Teaching has general but imprecise boundaries in terms of kinds of behavior change that can be accomplished and kinds of intervention techniques to effect it. Teaching also seems to be part of a combination therapy described as useful when patients have problems they cannot solve. It is very difficult to determine how the various therapies interrelate on a theoretic level and at the level of nursing practice. Each has grown up from diverse, partially developed theories, so that there is little in terms of a common point of view. There is little evidence of the areas of effectiveness for each of the therapies, nor has there been much study of comparative effectiveness of each for particular goals, given certain characteristics in the patient. Without this knowledge, the following lines of thinking are possible:

1. For a particular patient at a particular time, one of these therapies is most likely to produce the desired change.
2. A particular patient at a particular time displays a variety of behavior that can best be dealt with by an integration of, or successive use of, several of these therapies.
3. Because of the commonality of an underlying theory of interpersonal relationships, such as development of a relationship that is warm and honest, it does not matter which therapy is used.

There are no clear answers to the questions raised by these lines of thinking. Nursing has tended to adopt the first approach, but often without clear definition of behavioral clues that signal more appropriate use of one or two other therapies. The task of accomplishing the integration suggested in the second approach is considerable, and lack of guidelines to accomplish it no doubt contributes to lack of patient teaching as well as to other effects.

A point of view that is rising in importance is that there are basic ingredients of therapeutic change. Therapists create and maintain helping relationships, characterized by respect, interest, understanding, tact, maturity, and a firm belief in their ability to help. This provides a power base from which therapists may influence patients through persuasion, encouragement for openness, interpretations of patients' behavior into conceptual schemes that enable patients to reconceptualize their problems, provision of a model, and manipulation of rewards. The patient does need to have the capacity and willingness to profit from the experience.[99]

There also is beginning evidence that the strategies caretakers use toward clients are partly dependent on the time frame in which their contact occurs. In emergency rooms, where the time perspective is very short, giving of orders (a kind of overt coercion) is more predominant than is the progressive socialization that occurs in settings with longer time perspectives.[85] It is an open question whether all such activity can be characterized as "helping" (helping includes ethical standards for the protection of the patient), but its purpose is always the same—change of behavior in the client.

As theory development continues in nursing, more comprehensive explanatory systems may incorporate a number of interpersonal skills. A general principle such as "tension prevention through interaction" has been cited as an example of a nursing theory of practice that would utilize a wide variety of specific means.[107]

The educational model in health

The disease model has been found to be far too limited a perspective, particularly for several areas of health-illness in which the psychosocial component has been seen as a major factor influencing the outcome. The disease model is too limited not only for defining the situation but also for treating it; the addition of the educational model is seen as imperative.

This perspective regarding a model has been identified in the area of mental health with the view that most mental disorders may primarily be learned patterns of socially deviant behavior that are inappropriately conceptualized in the disease model. Calling these problems "diseases" leads to inappropriate actions for treatment.[13] One definition of what the altered treatment might be is reality therapy, which differs from conventional psychotherapy in its emphasis on the therapist's role as a teacher. The goal is to accomplish in a relatively short, intense period what should have been established during normal growing up. In conventional therapy, teaching is limited to helping the patient gain insight into the causes of his behavior, whereas in reality therapy the aim is to fulfill the goal by teaching patients better ways to fulfill their needs.[30] Another definition of altered treatment of mental disorders based on the educational model includes training of new mental health professionals and new institutions for giving care more closely related to schoolteachers and schools than psychiatrists and hospitals.[13] Indeed, it is said that the line between education and therapy is becoming much thinner than it was perceived to be 20 years ago.[75]

The field of rehabilitation, although evolving from medical roots, represents a significant departure in concept from the traditional medical model. Several of these differences are as follows:

1. There is no cure.
2. The patient is not a passive recipient; maximum success depends on client initiative.
3. Rehabilitation does not focus on the pathologic processes but on modification of patient behavior to increase functional capacities and performance in the presence of infrequently modifiable pathologic processes.

Rehabilitation teams have for some time included a variety of disciplines that contribute to altering patient behavior in a number of ways, one of which is patient teaching.

Mental retardation, viewed as a complexity of human existence often physiologic in origin but essentially a matter of decelerated and/or impaired cognitive functioning, is quite responsive to certain educational models.[74] Indeed, the rationale of referring to retardation that resists cure as a sickness can be dehumanizing and detrimental to retarded individuals.

As nursing evolves into an independent profession concerned with individuals and groups in the full range of health and illness, it must include in its view a number of models that focus on human development. The educational model is one of these, and others will be concerned with learning.

Nurses' perceptions of teaching

The perceptions of nursing practitioners as to what teaching is have been studied most extensively by Pohl in a study completed 15 years ago. The group completing her questionnaire consisted of 1,500 nurses, members of the American Nurses' Association from throughout the United States, working in private duty, general duty, public health, occupational health, or office nursing. Of significance is the fact that 37.2% (107 cases) of those refusing to answer the questionnaire indicated on follow-up that they gave direct nursing care but did not teach. Pohl found that the concepts of teaching held by a large proportion of the practitioners were unclear.[77] This was so in spite of the fact that American Nurses' Association statements of Functions, Standards, and Qualifications included teaching as a function of all these workers,[3] as do the 1973 Standards of Practice.[4] Monteiro notes that in her experience bedside nurses often viewed teaching narrowly as formal instruction and that opportunity for informal teaching was missed.[64]

Many authors have been dissatisfied with the teaching done by nurses. Brown notes that although large numbers of persons are employed in doing something for the patient, an examination of ward care reveals that systematic plans for teaching patients how to care for themselves after leaving the hospital are rare indeed.[7] A small study of public health nurses in Seattle showed opportunity for teaching about nutrition in 66% of the studied home visits; the investigator found that 38% of the teaching opportunities were missed.[96] In 1953 an investigator interviewed 19 nurses in medical-surgical units of eight general hospitals in a metropolitan area. The investigator found no teaching programs organized in any of these hospitals. None of the nurses thought that all her patients received enough teaching regarding prevention of disease and promotion of health, and teaching by nurses about disease was often completely lacking. The area of teaching found to be most neglected was rehabilitation; in six of the eight hospitals studied, no organized program existed.[98] Other authors have written of aspects of health teaching by various groups of nurses as being inadequate.[55,70,93] Of the five categories of nursing care identified as essential in one study, teaching and preparation for home care were consistently evaluated by patients, physicians, and members of the nursing team as being less well accomplished than physical care, emotional care, nurse-physician relationships, and administration.[87] Indeed, there is evidence that nurses are not as effective as they could be in their use of sociopsychologic means in general.[107] Is the basis for these suggested inadequacies wholly due to lack of clarity as to what teaching is?

Many of these studies are old. Programs for teaching patients have increased considerably. Yet many of the limitations identified in these early studies seem to still be with us.

Preparation of nurses for teaching

A major factor affecting quality of professional practice is the preparation for it. Pohl found in her 1965 study of a random selection of American Nurses' Association members from five job areas a significant lack of preparation for the teaching role. The mode (average) nurse was a diploma graduate with no college work and no courses in principles or methods of teaching. One third of the respondents reported that they had no preparation for the teaching they were doing, and only one fifth felt they were ready for the task. There were indications that nurses who had had courses in teaching had clearer concepts about it than did those who had not.[77] Hospital nurses in a large metropolitan area identified seven reasons why nurses did not teach. Some of the major ones were lack of knowledge about content, inadequate knowledge of teaching skills and lack of skill in using them, and lack of responsibility in assuming the functions of a health teacher. Formal course work in teaching and in-service preparation were suggested by these practitioners as means of overcoming deficiencies in preparation.[98]

Any such program must be cognizant of the very real change in orientation necessary for some nurses to utilize the teaching approach. One must be very secure to give up the satisfaction that comes from giving services and begin to derive it from teaching. The latter, which involves guiding patients through slow, fumbling, half-hearted efforts to do something for themselves can be trying and fatiguing to the nurse. In addition, nurses who undertake teaching programs with patients must be willing to be concerned about them and to work through their learning problems with them. Again, this is a kind of nursing very different from just giving essential physical care and following a physician's orders.

Typical public health nurses in Pohl's study differed from typical nurses in that they had had college work and one or more courses in teaching.[77] This reflects the wide gap between preventive and curative health services in the United States. Health education as a field has given little attention to how health teachers might function where illness has commenced or recovery is under way. Health educators have infrequently functioned in the curative health field; educational functions have to some extent been carried out by physicians, nurses, and social workers.[91] Therefore, there is a special need for investigation of the role of health teaching during the curative phases of illness and of how being in this phase affects the patient's receptiveness to teaching.

Although there should be some nurse specialists who develop high-level teaching skills, it would seem essential for every nurse to obtain some degree of proficiency. The opportunity and necessity are too great to be left to a few specialists. Indeed, auxiliary helpers also should learn very basic teaching skills, for they are in contact with patients when their need to learn is expressed or can be observed.

Confusion about nurse's role in health teaching

The role of nurses in health teaching does not seem to be clearly defined, particularly in regard to the degree of independence with which they should function. Lack of clear allocation of responsibility for teaching among personnel and poor communication between members of the health team have been suggested as contributing factors.

There has been some study of subject areas that nurses feel are or are not a part of their teaching role. A questionnaire study of 103 medical-surgical staff nurses in four Seattle hospitals revealed that the majority did accept teaching about toxic symptoms of medications to be used after dismissal from the hospital, mechanical devices to be used at home, and symptoms that might indicate recurrence or complication of illness as a nursing responsibility. The majority thought that nurses could not be responsible for teaching the purpose of medications to be used after dismissal from the hospital, foods allowed or limited on a diet, and when to see the physician after discharge.[38] A study of hospital nurses in one metropolitan area identified teaching in the subject of rehabilitation as weak, partly, it was felt, because nurses thought this was the physician's or social worker's area.[98] These investigations are only

suggestive, but description of such a line of demarcation can be useful in understanding teaching behavior.

Some programs with a teaching emphasis represent somewhat recent reorientation or a new orientation to an area of care. For example, orientation to the patient as a member of a family and a community redefined the role of the nurse in pediatrics from that of "substitute mother" to that of a person who assists the mother and father in helping and supporting the child through the hospital experience.[86] Programs in hospital units following this philosophy have been described,[58] including those in which parents are taught to give their children care and to prepare them for events, as well as those in which general health teaching and anticipatory guidance are used.[12] A description of the well-known Loeb Center program interprets the importance of teaching in a caring situation, done by nurses who are helping patients during the rehabilitative stages of hospitalization. The aim is to develop an environment of permissiveness and nurturing where patients can learn about themselves and evaluate both the resources and liabilities with which they must cope. Rehabilitation is seen as something achieved by patients through a learning process.[8]

Much confusion about the teaching role of nurses seems to stem from either lack of clarity about the physician's role in teaching or poor performance of that role. It has been found that many patients, particularly those from lower socioeconomic classes, feel that they are imposing on the physician by asking questions; they therefore secure information about their condition from acquaintances rather than from their physician.[91] Among a group of hospitalized medical-surgical patients, giving a "poor explanation" was the single most criticized aspect of medical care.[93] Indeed, this information about breakdown of physician-patient communication supports the notion that another person, who serves as intermediary, is needed to help the patient formulate questions and interpret in simpler language what the physician says. However, because the nurse's relationship with the physician used to be dependent, even service as an intermediary may seem to some nurses to be too independent or by others too subservient an action. It has been considered ethical for a nurse to refer questions back to the physician; however, in these days when some patients are quite enlightened, it is difficult for the nurse to parry the questions without seeming to know less than the patient.[9] Teaching under a physician's direct order would seem to remove hesitancy because of feelings in regard to appropriateness of teaching; yet only 2 out of 90 nurses in one outpatient department thought the physician would ask them to teach the patient.[60] Although medical education is beginning to address issues of competency in psychosocial skills, more rapid resolution of these turf questions seems to be occurring by means of agency policy aimed at improving care and protecting agency liability. Nurses functioning in more independent roles often assume responsibility for full patient care, including teaching.

Although the consequences of confusion about patient teaching are difficult to assess, some study has been done of two areas commonly rated as important for teaching: posthospitalization care at home and preoperative preparation of patients. Although there appears to be a need for more systematic information about what happens when patients go home, some studies already outline deficiencies either in patients' will to follow health teaching or in their lack of understanding.[79] Studies of medication-taking behavior of elderly patients at home have shown a startling lack of carry-over from the physician's and the nurse's teaching to actual taking of medications.[14,90] Regarding preoperative teaching, Kutner's study suggests that the lack of unanimity among medical house officers, nurses, and surgical patients concerning who should teach what produces the effect of decreased communication between all three

groups, so that patients come to the operating table emotionally unprepared for surgery and its aftermath.[49]

The birth of a defective child is an example of the kind of situation that may cause a communication trap into which health workers and their patients can fall. If physicians do not tell mothers when a child is defective, nurses cannot usurp physicians' prerogative, but neither can they escape from the situation since their caregiving and comforting functions demand their presence. Nurses are faced with producing evasive answers with which they are uncomfortable, and so they stay with the patient only long enough to give necessary care. This is possible because care involving social and psychologic matters is not assured by accountability and is consequently left to chance occurrence. The patient, who has just endured the stress of delivery, is isolated, probably is alarmed about her baby, and perhaps becomes mistrustful of physicians and nurses from whom she will need help to make long-term adjustments.[105]

Lack of expectations by employers

Limited studies show that nurses perceive obstacles to patient teaching as lack of emphasis by nursing service administrative personnel,[98] lack of time, heavy work load, and inadequate staffing.[77] Part of this complaint may reflect rationalization for professional inadequacies in knowing how and when to teach. However, the confusion about this role, linked to a possible shortage of professional personnel and to the confusion about their proper use, may well result in lack of expectation. Indeed, the lack of preparation for teaching in basic nursing education may have produced administrators who have risen through the ranks without developing sophistication in this area of care themselves and are therefore unable to provide enlightened supervision to practitioners. It has been suggested that some past means of assignment contributed to an orientation toward getting routine work done, reporting observations to the physician, and shifting responsibility for difficult situations rather than developing a therapeutic nursing relationship.[32] Primary nursing, as a system of nursing activities, tries to support conditions necessary for a therapeutic relationship.

A study of 90 nurses in Boston outpatient departments yielded interesting information about the complexity of reasons why patient teaching may not occur. It was found that nursing supervisors did not expect the staff nurses to teach; rather, they saw them as assistants to the physician and administrator of the clinic. Administrative duties were therefore defined as having high priority and teaching duties low priority. If the patient was not taught, few persons knew. This administrative view of the nurse's function affected the relationship between the nurse and the patient. When they talked, their conversation was about those things that would inconvenience the department, such as not keeping an x-ray appointment, rather than about the "what" or "why" of the treatment or illness.[60] Teaching, it would appear from this study, was not rewarded and was not encouraged by staffing patterns—another item in the complex of factors affecting teaching behavior by nurses.

I agree with the view that health care agencies need to make their personnel accountable for many social and psychologic actions that currently are left to personal discretion.[28] It is also clear that this orientation requires considerably more than a statement of expectation to personnel.

Reasons for ignorance in patients

Another factor affecting teaching behavior relates to the use of information as controlling power. Knowledge about a patient's disease and treatment is a commodity useful in controlling the health practitioner–patient relationship. Giving this knowledge to patients may help them to dispute the physician's or nurse's authority[27] or take over their own treatment.[65] This has been suggested as the reason for the secrecy ritual in nursing.[89] Sarosi charges that such patient reaction may have contributed to nursing's clinging to a role that limited client participation; the author sees nursing clinging to mother surrogation, in which it is assumed that the patient is not really a person but a child—regressive, dependent, egocentric, helpless, anxious, lacking in understanding, withdrawn from adult responsibilities, unable to make decisions, and preoccupied with symptoms and illness.[88]

Patients have been observed to hesitate to ask questions, complain, or ask for services because they feared negative reaction, particularly from nurses.[93] It has been suggested that uncertainty on the part of medical personnel about diagnosis and treatment contributes to failure to inform patients.[16] This restriction can be self-protecting for the professional because, if patients are not informed about their care and treatment, they are hampered in evaluating whether nurses are performing their duties adequately.

There is a range of opinion about the most effective level of enlightenment. On one hand, there is the belief that patients must be taught the technical and cultural language of the hospital; that treatment can be viewed as the temporary sharing of a common definition of a situation by persons of such diverse backgrounds as patient, nurse, physician, and dietician; and that patients should be taught how to evaluate the care they receive from each of the health team members.[11] On the other hand, the lack of socialization of patients into the short-term hospital can be seen as functional for the institution, in that the organizational system need not depend very heavily on patients' voluntary contribution to the system, nor can the unsocialized play much of a disruptive role in moments of crisis. It is recognized that lack of socialization may be fear provoking for patients since they are isolated from sharing their experience with each other, and the staff ensures conformity by making the deviant patient feel shame and guilt.[84] Since there is no doubt truth in both positions, one would hope for an elaboration of the relationships between individuals and the system that serves both better.

Also affecting the teaching-learning process is the patient's wish to remain ignorant and thereby maintain a sense of security.

It is not to be presumed that the goal of health education is abolishment of all ignorance, for its presence is inevitable and sometimes functional.

There is no comprehensive survey of the quality of care that includes patient teaching. There are published studies that are descriptive of this area of care, but there is no way to know how typical the findings are. Two studies have portrayed very grim pictures of this quality, and although the analysis of causative factors is limited, the descriptions are valuable in and of themselves.

A study of medical and surgical patients in a teaching hospital showed very limited and faulty communication between members of the health team. Orientation to hospital routines was left by physicians to nurses, who were usually so rushed that they took little time to do this. The chief communication link between physicians and nurses was the physician's order book, which was a one-way message, usually limited to what was required in the staff's technical performance in diagnosis and treatment of disease. The nurse-patient relationship was judged to be technical, administrative, and task oriented, not person oriented. Registered nurses perceived partially or correctly the mental status of only one third of the patients; licensed practical nurses perceived partially or correctly the status of 80%. A similar situation existed between physicians and the patients. Patients did not expect physicians to diagnose and treat their psychosocial disturbances; indeed, the study staff found that only 2% of the patients reported that they talked with their physicians about their

disturbed feelings while they were in the hospital; an additional 35% did communicate the ways they felt about themselves; and 63% did not talk with physicians regarding their feelings. In the face of a poor prognosis, the personal and social realities for the patient and his family were usually discounted or ignored, as all parties concentrated on the treatment of the physical disease. Everyone guessed at what was being said. Isolation, suspicion, and distrust were common. Of the 155 study patients discharged alive, 14% were not disabled, 24% were disabled from physical disease, 44% were disabled from psychosocial disturbances, and 18% were disabled from a combination of these causes, as judged by the study staff.[18]

A study of children in the hospital for tonsillectomy indicated that typically, the staff approached the patient as a work object on which to perform a set of tasks rather than as a participant in the process or as an individual who needs help in adjusting to a new environment. The attending surgeon's interaction with the child was limited primarily to the performance of the operation and the release from the hospital. The nursing staff tended to initiate interaction only when they needed some data for their charts or had to perform an instrumental act. They offered very little information and were usually evasive if questioned directly. If the mother displayed stress, the staff tried to ignore it or to get her to leave the ward.[94] A subsequent study by the same authors showed that the mothers' anxiety levels could be reduced through interaction with an authoritative person, in this case a nurse, who provided information and emotional support.[95]

SUMMARY AND DIRECTIONS FOR CHANGE

In summary, although the usefulness of teaching as a tool of nursing practice has been known and patient teaching has been approved for years, this teaching appears to have been irregularly practiced. A complex of factors, including questionable preparation and confusion about the teaching roles of various members of the health team, appears to have contributed to this pattern of practice. The effects on patients are difficult to determine but have aroused dissatisfaction.

Suggestions for improvement of the practice of patient teaching include using assignment methods that promote teaching, strengthening the teaching components of nursing care plans,[36,98] providing in-service preparation for the teaching function, preparing teaching guides and visual materials, instituting better charting about teaching, and constructing a climate supportive of learning for the patient.

In light of the evidence cited, it would seem that these recommendations could be successful in reaching the goal of more enlightened patient education by dealing first with discrepancies in the acceptance of teaching in the nurse's role. It is agreed that no one profession expects to accomplish all the objectives of health education, but a clearer delineation of goals and the division of labor would likely yield more effective care. Some of this initiative must come from nursing.

STUDY QUESTIONS

1. What would be a reasonable response to a head nurse who tells her staff that they should check with her before doing any patient teaching?
2. What does the following statement mean for patient teaching: ". . . there are no disease conditions of which we know the cause in which human behavior is not a critical element in the control of that disease''?[97]

REFERENCES

1. Aguilera, D. C., and Messick, J. M.: Crisis intervention; theory and methodology, ed. 3, St. Louis, 1978, The C. V. Mosby Co.
2. American Hospital Association: A patient's bill of rights, Chicago, 1972, The Association.
3. American Nurses' Association: Functions, standards and qualifications for practice, revised, New York, 1963, The Association.
4. American Nurses' Association: Standards of nursing practice, Kansas City, 1973, The Association.
5. Anderson, H. C.: Newton's geriatric nursing, ed. 5, St. Louis, 1971, The C. V. Mosby Co.
6. Biddle, B. J., and Rossi, P. H.: Educational media, education and society. In Rossi, P. H., and Biddle, B. J., editors: The new media and education; their impact on society, Chicago, 1966, Aldine Publishing Co., pp. 2-45.
7. Brown, E. L.: The social sciences and improvement of patient care, Am. J. Nurs. **56:**1148-1150, Sept. 1956.
8. Brown, E. L.: Nursing reconsidered: a study of change. Part I: The professional role in institutional nursing, Philadelphia, 1970, J. B. Lippincott Co.
9. Burling, T., Lentz, E. M., and Wilson, R. N.: The give and take in hospitals; a study of human organization in hospitals, New York, 1956, G. P. Putnam's Sons.
10. Chapman, J. S.: Effects of different nursing approaches upon psychological and physiological responses of patients, research report, Cleveland, 1969, Case Western Reserve University.
11. Christman, L.: Assisting the patient to learn the "patient role," J. Nurs. Educ. **6:**17-21, April 1967.
12. Condon, M., and Peters, C.: Family participation unit, Am. J. Nurs. **68:**504-507, March 1968.
13. Cowen, E. L., Gardner, E. A., and Zax, M.: Emergent approaches to mental health problems, New York, 1967, Appleton-Century-Crofts.
14. Curtis, E. B.: Medication errors made by patients, Nurs. Outlook **9:**290-291, May 1961.
15. Darbonne, A.: Crisis; a review of theory, practice and research, Int. J. Psychiatry **6:**371-379, 1968.
16. Davis, F.: Uncertainty in medical prognosis, clinical and functional, Am. J. Sociol. **66:**41-47, 1960.
17. Davis, J. A.: Education for positive mental health; a review of existing research and recommendations for future studies, Chicago, 1965, Aldine Publishing Co.
18. Duff, R. S., and Hollingshead, A. B.: Sickness and society, New York, 1968, Harper & Row, Publishers.
19. Dumas, R. G., and Leonard, R. C.: The effect of nursing on the incidence of postoperative vomiting, Nurs. Res. **12:**12-15, 1963.
20. Egbert, L. D., and others: The value of the preoperative visit by an anesthetist, J.A.M.A. **185:**553-555, 1963.
21. Egbert, L. D., and others: Reduction of postoperative pain by encouragement and instruction of patients, N. Engl. J. Med. **270:**825-827, 1964.
22. Felton, G., and others: Preoperative nursing intervention with the patient for surgery; outcomes of three alternative approaches, Int. J. Nurs. Stud. **13:**83-96, 1976.
23. Fink, D., and others: Effective patient care in the pediatric ambulatory setting; a study of the acute care clinic, Pediatrics **43:**927-935, 1969.
24. Fink, D., and others: The management specialist in

effective pediatric ambulatory care, Am. J. Public Health **59:**527-533, 1969.

25. Fortin, F., and Kirouac, S.: A randomized controlled trial of preoperative patient education, Int. J. Nurs. Stud. **13:**11-24, 1976.

26. Freidson, E.: Patients' views of medical practice, New York, 1961, Russell Sage Foundation.

27. Freidson, E.: Dominant professions, bureaucracy, and client services. In Rosengren, W. R., and Lefton, M., editors: Organizations and clients; essays in the sociology of service, Columbus, Ohio, 1970, Charles E. Merrill Publishing Co.

28. Gibson, W. B.: But who teaches the patient? Arch. Dermatol. **88:**935-936, 1963.

29. Glaser, B. G., and Strauss, A. L.: Time for dying, Chicago, 1968, Aldine Publishing Co.

30. Glasser, W.: Reality therapy; a new approach to psychiatry, New York, 1965, Harper & Row, Publishers.

31. Gregg, D. E.: Reassurance, Am. J. Nurs. **55:**171-174, Feb. 1955.

32. Gregg, D. E.: The therapeutic roles of the nurse, Perspect. Psychiatr. Care **1:**19-24, 1963.

33. Hall, L. E.: Nursing—what is it? Can. Nurse **60:**150-154, 1964.

34. Henderson, V.: The nature of nursing, Am. J. Nurs. **64:**62-68, Aug. 1964.

35. Hospitals must adapt patients' bill of rights or courts will tell them what it means, lawyer warns, Mod. Hosp. **120:**33, June 1973.

36. If you ask me: what encourages general duty nurses to teach patients? Am. J. Nurs. **60:**1236, Sept. 1960.

37. Janis, I. L.: Psychological stress; psychoanalytic and behavioral studies of surgical patients, New York, 1958, John Wiley & Sons, Inc.

38. Jenkin, S. A.: An investigation of how registered nurses felt regarding their responsibility for patient health teaching. Unpublished master's thesis, Seattle, 1961, The University of Washington.

39. Johnson, J. E.: The influence of purposeful nurse-patient interaction on the patient's postoperative course. In American Nurses' Association: Exploring progress in medical surgical nursing practice, New York, 1965, The Association, pp. 16-21.

40. Johnson, J. E., Dobbs, J. M., Jr., and Leventhal, H.: Psychosocial factors in the welfare of surgical patients, Nurs. Res. **19:**18-29, 1970.

41. Jowers, L. V.: Medicolegal aspects of diabetes, J. Legal Med. **3:**25-28, Feb. 1975.

42. Kauffman, E. L.: A study concerning patients' perception of stress within a university hospital setting and patients' perception of the nurse's role in reducing stress. Unpublished master's thesis, Seattle, 1965, The University of Washington.

43. Kinlein, M. L.: Independent nursing practice with clients, Philadelphia, 1977, J. B. Lippincott Co.

44. Kinlein, M. L.: The self-care concept, Am. J. Nurs. **77:**598-601, 1977.

45. Kinney, M. R.: Effects of preoperative teaching upon patients with differing modes of response to threatening stimuli, Int. J. Nurs. Stud. **14:**49-59, 1977.

46. Knapp, T. A., and Huff, R. L.: Emerging trends in the physician's duty to disclose; an update of Canterbury vs. Spence, J. Legal Med. **3:**41-45, Jan. 1975.

47. Knowles, J. H.: Responsibility for health, Science **198:**1413, 1977.

48. Kreuter, F. R.: What is good nursing care? Nurs. Outlook **5:**302-304, 1957.

49. Kutner, B.: Surgeons and their patients; a study in social perception. In Jaco, E. G., editor: Patients, physicians and illness, New York, 1958, The Free Press, pp. 384-397.

50. Lambertsen, E. C.: Nursing definition and philosophy precede nursing goal development, Mod. Hosp. **103:**136, Sept. 1964.

51. Lee, J. A.: The role of the occupational health nurse in the management of the pregnant employee, Am. Assoc. Industr. Nurses J. **14:**7-12, July 1966.

52. Levin, L. S.: Self-care; an emerging component of the health care system, Hosp. and Health Serv. Adm. **23:**17-25, 1978.

53. Levine, M. E.: The intransigent patient, Am. J. Nurs. **70:**2106-2111, 1970.

54. Lowe, M. L.: Effectiveness of teaching as measured by compliance with medical recommendations, Nurs. Res. **19:**59-63, 1970.

55. MacArthur, C.: We teach—do our patients learn? Can. Nurse **55:**205-210, 1959.

56. McBride, M. A. B.: Nursing approach, pain, and relief; an exploratory experiment, Nurs. Res. **16:**337-341, 1967.

57. McCaffery, M. S.: An approach to parent education, Nurs. Forum **6**(1):77-93, 1967.

58. McClure, M. J., and Ryburn, A. C.: Care-by-parent unit, Am. J. Nurs. **69:**2148-2152, Oct. 1969.

59. Mahaffy, P. R., Jr.: The effects of hospitalization on children admitted for tonsillectomy and adenoidectomy, Nurs. Res. **14:**12-19, 1965.

60. Malone, M., Berkowitz, N. H., and Klein, M. W.: Interpersonal conflict in the outpatient department, Am. J. Nurs. **62:**108-112, March 1962.

61. Matheny, A. P., Jr., and Vernick, J.: Parents of the mentally retarded child; emotionally overwhelmed or informationally deprived? J. Pediatr. **74:**953-959, 1969.

62. Mechanic, D.: Public expectations in health care, New York, 1972, John Wiley & Sons, Inc.

63. Mohammed, M. F. B.: Patients' understanding of written health information, Nurs. Res. **13:**100-108, 1964.

64. Monteiro, L. A.: Notes on patient teaching—a neglected area, Nurs. Forum **3**(1):26-33, 1964.
65. Moore, W. E., and Tumin, M. M.: Some social functions of ignorance, Am. Sociol. Rev. **14**:787-795, 1949.
66. National League of Nursing Education: Standard curriculum for schools of nursing, Baltimore, 1918, The Waverly Press.
67. National League of Nursing Education: A curriculum guide for schools of nursing, New York, 1937, The League.
68. National League of Nursing Education: Nursing organization curriculum conference, Glen Gardner, N.J., 1950, Libertarian Press.
69. Nedbor, P., and Averette, H. E.: Hospital institutes program for self-perineal care, Hosp. Top. **46**:81-82, May 1968.
70. Nite, G., and Willis, F. N., Jr.: The coronary patient; hospital care and rehabilitation, New York, 1964, The Macmillan Co.
71. Olivia, Sister M.: Aims of nursing administration, 1947, The Catholic University of America Press. Cited by Brown, E. L.: Nursing for the future, New York, 1948, Russell Sage Foundation.
72. Packard, R. B., and Van Ess, H.: A comparison of informal and role-delineated patient-teaching situations, Nurs. Res. **18**:443-446, 1969.
73. Patients' bill of rights could expose hospitals to liability, expert warns at AWH meeting, Mod. Hosp. **120**:26, May 1973.
74. Patterson, E. G., and Rowland, B. T.: Toward a theory of mental retardation nursing; an educational model, Am. J. Nurs. **70**:531-535, March 1970.
75. Peplau, H. E.: Interpersonal relations in nursing, New York, 1952, G. P. Putnam's Sons.
76. Peplau, H. E.: The changing view of nursing, Int. Nurs. Rev. **24**(2):43-45, 1977.
77. Pohl, M. L.: Teaching activities of the nursing practitioner, Nurs. Res. **14**:4-11, 1965.
78. Pratt, L., Seligmann, A., and Reader, G.: Physicians' views on the level of medical information among patients, Am. J. Public Health **47**:1277-1283, 1957.
79. Purdue University: Proceedings of the Purdue Farm cardiac seminar, Sept. 10-11, 1958, The University, Agricultural Experimental Station, Lafayette, Ind. Cited in Nite, G., and Willis, F. N., Jr.: The coronary patient; hospital care and rehabilitation, New York, 1964, The Macmillan Co.
80. Putt, A. M.: One experiment in nursing adults with peptic ulcers, Nurs. Res. **19**:484-494, 1970.
81. Reiter, F.: The nurse-clinician, Am. J. Nurs. **66**:274-280, Feb. 1966.
82. Roberts, B.: Research in educational aspects of health programmes, Int. J. Health Educ. **13**: No. 1 (Supplement), Jan.-March 1970.
83. Rogers, C. R.: Significant learning; in therapy and in education. In Hyman, R. T., editor: Teaching; vantage points for study, Philadelphia, 1968, J. B. Lippincott Co., pp. 152-165.
84. Rosengren, W. R., and Lefton, M.: Hospitals and patients, New York, 1969, Atherton Press, Inc.
85. Roth, J. A.: Some contingencies of the moral evaluation and control of clientele; the case of hospital emergency service, Am. J. Sociol. **77**:839-856, 1972.
86. Rubino, E.: Maternal and child nursing content for the associate degree nursing program, J. Nurs. Educ. **9**:5-41, Aug. 1970.
87. Safford, B. J., and Schlotfeldt, R. M.: Nursing service staffing and quality of nursing care, Nurs. Res. **9**:149-154, 1960.
88. Sarosi, G. M.: A critical theory; the nurse as a fully human person, Nurs. Forum **7**(4):349-364, 1968.
89. Schmahl, J. A.: Ritualism in nursing practice, Nurs. Forum **3**(4):74-84, 1964.
90. Schwartz, D.: Medication errors made by aged patients, Am. J. Nurs. **62**:51-53, Aug. 1962.
91. Simonds, S. K.: Health education and medical care; focus on the patient, Health Educ. Monogr. **16**:32-40, 1963.
92. Simonds, S. K.: "The educational care" of patients with congestive heart failure, Health Educ. J. **25**:131-141, Sept. 1967.
93. Skipper, J. K., Jr.: Communication and the hospitalized patient. In Skipper, J. K., Jr., and Leonard, R. C., editors: Social interaction and patient care, Philadelphia, 1965, J. B. Lippincott Co.
94. Skipper, J. K., Jr., and Leonard, R. C.: Children, stress, and hospitalization; a field experiment, J. Health Soc. Behav. **9**:275-287, 1968.
95. Skipper, J. K., Jr., and others: Child hospitalization and social interaction, Med. Care **6**:496-506, 1968.
96. Spearman, J. G.: A study of nutritional teaching done by a selected group of public health nurses on their home visits (unpublished master's thesis, Seattle, 1961, The University of Washington).
97. Steuart, G. W.: The specialist in health education; training for the future, Int. J. Health Educ. **9**:165-169, Oct.-Dec. 1966.
98. Streeter, V.: The nurse's responsibility for teaching patients, Am. J. Nurs. **53**:818-820, July 1953.
99. Strupp, H. H.: On the basic ingredients of psychotherapy, J. Consult. Clin. Psychol. **41**:1-8, 1973.
100. Travelbee, J.: Interpersonal aspects of nursing, ed. 2, Philadelphia, 1971, F. A. Davis Co.
101. Tryon, P. A., and Leonard, R. C.: The effect of the patient's participation on the outcome of a nursing procedure, Nurs. Forum **3**(2):78-89, 1964.
102. Ujhely, G.: Determinants of the nurse-patient rela-

tionship, New York, 1968, Springer Publishing Co., Inc.

103. Veenker, C. H.: A critical review of research in health education, Int. J. Health Educ. **8:**179-187, Oct.-Dec. 1965.

104. Vistainer, M. A., and Wolfer, J. A.: Psychological preparation for surgical pediatric patients; the effect on children's and parents' stress responses and adjustment, Pediatrics **56:**187-202, 1975.

105. Von Schilling, K. C.: The birth of a defective child, Nurs. Forum **7**(4):424-439, 1968.

106. Williams, T. F., and others: The clinical picture of diabetic control, studied in four settings, Am. J. Public Health **57:**441-451, 1967.

107. Woolridge, P. J., Skipper, J. K., Jr., and Leonard, R. C.: Behavioral science, social practice and the nursing profession, Cleveland, 1968, The Press of Case Western Reserve University.

108. Zola, I. K.: Medicine as an institution of social control, Sociol. Rev. **20:**487-503, 1972.

CHAPTER 2

Overview of the teaching-learning process

■ Teaching is an interactive process between a teacher and one or more learners. The role of the teacher centers on activities to promote learning and to assess learning that should take place or has taken place. The learner's role is to participate in or initiate activities that lead toward the desired behavior change. All students of nursing are aware of the learner's role because of their experiences in school. However, if the students are to function well in patient teaching, they must enlarge their perceptions to include a notion of how to function as teachers of health with individuals who are well and ill.

The purpose of this chapter is to describe the interrelationships between the various parts of the teaching-learning process. These parts will be separated for more thorough examination in succeeding chapters.

IDENTIFYING NEED FOR TEACHING

The process of teaching-learning often begins when an individual identifies a need for knowing or gaining an ability to do something. This person may be a community member or an inpatient, an outpatient, or a family member of someone under care. He or she may request information about promoting health and preventing disease, about a health facility, or about the disease or treatment. At other times, the

physician or other members of the health team recognize that patients need to learn even though they are not aware of their own needs.

How does the need to learn become known to the nurse? A patient may ask a direct question such as, "Why does my baby clench his fist that way?" "What will happen to me when they do the x-ray?" or "How do I use these crutches?" A member of the family may ask, "Why does my father cry when I come to visit him?" The women's club may wish to become informed about home nursing and may request that a public health nurse address the group. The physician may write an order for the nurse to teach a diabetic patient how to self-administer insulin. A group of obstetricians may agree on a postpartum teaching program to be given to all their patients after delivery. Or a community may suffer from high infant mortality, thus indicating there may be need for teaching as well as for other services that can prevent this problem.

It is easy to identify the opportunity for teaching when the request is direct. More difficult is inferring the need from observing physical condition and behavior and anticipating it from the treatment plan. For example, as nurses caring for diabetic patients notice that the skin on the feet is dry and cracking, it is their responsibility to question these patients to find out how much they know about foot care. Nurses have a responsibility to do this teaching, checking with the physician when necessary. They might also anticipate that a patient who has been put on a regimen of digitoxin will likely be receiving it for a while and might initiate teaching about the medication. Early in a hospitalization the physician should make plans for posthospitalization clear so that learning, which takes time, can begin.

The patient's failure to ask questions should not be construed as understanding. Indeed, nurses must become proficient at helping patients to identify their needs. Sometimes requests for concrete items of physical assistance such as a bedpan or glass of water are disguises for deeper emotional needs. [2]

WHAT CAN BE LEARNED

Since learning requires motivation, a realistic goal cannot be set without considering the learner's desires. Individuals who are not convinced that they need to learn will resist efforts to teach them. They will not be receptive. Nurses often try to help them become convinced that they need to learn. Sometimes lack of motivation is the result of difficulty in adapting to an illness, and sometimes it is the result of differences of value systems and concepts of health and illness between the professional health worker and the client. The nurse may be convinced that an individual needs to learn about immunizations and why they are important; however, the person's values may be fatalistic—"I will get the disease if I am meant to"—so that immunization is viewed as useless. Value systems vary by cultural group and socioeconomic class. Bridging these discrepancies is a major concern of public health, which is by and large a middle-class effort directed toward lower-class groups. [4]

The learner's abilities and the demands of the situation also determine learning goals. Given the prevalence of chronic disease today and the fact that the patient often functions with minimal medical supervision for long periods of time, a certain degree of independence is necessary. It is desirable for a mother to be able to care for her new baby, including recognizing common signs of illness. Other patients and their families are asked to assume considerably more responsibility, as in home hemodialysis. However, individuals vary in their readiness for health learning because of their general educational backgrounds, intellectual abilities, and attitudes toward acceptance of responsibility. Therefore, some patients and families would not be capable of understanding the purpose of hemodialysis or how to perform the procedure, or they would not be emotionally stable enough to live with this responsibility. Therefore, goals or objectives of health learning must vary a great deal even for individuals with the same disease. In addition, the special concerns brought by illness or suspicion of illness will alter the individual's usual emotional stability and interest in learning.

What a person is to learn is stated in the form of an objective, such as "To give an injection to himself." To further delineate behaviors to be learned, subobjectives are stated: "To use sterile technique in giving an injection"; "to measure dosage of medication accurately within 0.1 ml."; "to identify sites for injection"; "to redirect the needle if blood is aspirated." All these behaviors and others are necessary for acquisition of the main objective, to give an injection to oneself. If nurse-teachers force themselves to identify in precise terms the behavior to be attained, they will have a clearer notion of the content, the sequence of content, and the teaching methods that are most likely to be successful. In nursing, the scheduling of work time makes it necessary for many members of the staff to interact with the patient and do teaching. Therefore, communication of teaching goals must be absolutely clear.

STIMULATION OF LEARNING

Goals of learning have been classified into three domains: cognitive (understandings), affective (attitudes), and psychomotor (motor skills).[1] Nurses commonly teach material pertaining to all three domains. Patients learn to understand (cognitive domain) how diabetes affects their body, how insulin controls diabetes, and many other intellectual skills that are necessary for them to live healthfully with diabetes. Most important to this goal is an attitude of acceptance (affective domain) of their disease and of responsibility in caring for themselves. They must also learn motor skills (psychomotor domain), such as giving an injection.

Each of these domains responds best to particular methods of teaching. Facts and concepts are basic to intellectual learning and are taught by written materials, audiovisual aids representing the concepts, lectures, and discussion. Learning of attitudes does not automatically follow from a knowledge of facts; for example, accepting responsibility for following a medical regimen in diabetes does not necessarily result from an understanding of how diabetes affects the body. Attitudes can perhaps best be taught by discussing with patients, providing insight into their feelings and gaining acceptance of a new attitude, by providing a model to imitate, and by helping them to take actions. Motor skills are best learned through a demonstration of the skills, with subsequent practice until they are perfected.

Group learning can save a great deal of teacher time and can provide an opportunity for people to profit from each other's experiences. Commonly, there are groups to be taught in such situations as prenatal, postnatal, diabetes, or allergy care units.

The teacher plans to use both real and vicarious (substitute) experiences to produce learning. The combination used depends on the goals, available experiences, and ability to profit from vicarious experiences. Many people have limited skill in reading, following directions from written sources, interpreting diagrams, or performing skills viewed in a movie.

EVALUATION OF LEARNING

Teaching consists of assessing what the patient, family, or community member needs to learn, planning the lesson, and actually doing the teaching. It also includes ascertaining whether the desired behavioral change has occurred. This is accomplished by observation of the behavior and by oral and written questioning. Both the teacher and the learner should be constantly assessing the extent to which they are progressing toward the goals. In this way, their efforts can be redirected if necessary. Evaluation is also done at the end of a lesson or series of lessons and at later times to determine what learning has been retained over a period of time.

During a phase of health care when teaching is done, it is most important that there be a written record carefully communicating the plan and an evaluation of what was learned. This is particularly true when a major form of therapy has been teaching-learning, such as the initial orientation and regulation of a diabetic patient. Accumulation of health information, skills, and attitudes occurs throughout an individual's life. Records describing this development in a clinic, hospital, or public health situation can be most helpful in furthering development.

HOW THE PROCESS IS SYNTHESIZED IN PRACTICE

The process of teaching can be summarized as follows:

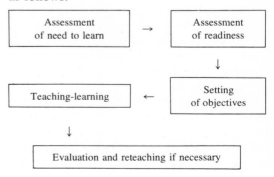

A few words must be said about the use of processes in practice and about how the teaching process fits with the nursing process. It is impossible not to use a process in professional practice. The amount of data that must be synthesized in order to do purposeful intervention requires a categorizing system, because people cannot keep any more than seven items at most in their short-term memories. Very little is known about how process is actually used by practitioners, but what seems clearest is that it does not flow in an orderly, sequential fashion, as shown in the diagram on p. 25. Data about physician decision making may be instructive.

One study showed that most of the clinical workup was used by physicians to test specific hypotheses they formed very early in their contact with the patient. The number of hypotheses at any one time seemed to be four, plus or minus one, and they were ranked according to probability, seriousness, treatability, and novelty, as well as by other criteria. Adhering to a strict routine of problem solving can help to compensate for the characteristic in human thinking of becoming wedded to a hypothesis even though it is incorrect.[3] The implications for use of the teaching process may be: (1) One starts at the beginning of the process but subsequently skips from step to step; and (2) the elements do serve as check points for safety to ensure that the relevant variables that affect the teaching-learning activity have been considered. Although teaching does not have commonly used diagnostic categories, the objectives can serve such a purpose. Pioneering work on nursing diagnosis does include learning needs. Indeed, in medicine, diagnosis may never be known, and it is not unheard of to have started and completed the treatment plan without a named diagnosis.

The teaching process can be seen as parallel to the nursing process in that each has an assessment, diagnosis, and intervention phase. Since the necessity for learning about health is one state pertinent to nursing practice, some general screening questions as to what patients know and how they see their present problems should be part of the general nursing assessment. If at any time during care the ongoing assessment indicates a learning problem for which teaching is relevant, a more refined assessment of need and readiness is then made, and that problem is dealt with through the teaching process.

Of course, the most cogent question of all concerns the quality of use of either the nursing process or the teaching process and whether, at

Table 1. Relationship of teaching process to nursing process

Assessment	Diagnosis	Goals	Intervention	Evaluation
Nursing process				
General screening questions to detect patient's need to learn. If positive, use teaching process.	One of the problem statements may be a need to learn.	Learning goals are a subset of the goals.	Teaching intervention may be delivered with other intervention.	
Teaching process				
Refined assessment of need to learn and readiness.		Setting of learning goals.	Doing teaching.	Evaluating learning.

least in the psychosocial realm, fine points in use of the process make any difference in patient outcome. I believe that there are gross errors in the practice of patient education that do make a difference. Errors in practice are probably made in this order: (1) omissions of assessment of need to learn and thus no activity in patient education even if needed, and (2) omissions of any given step—such as assessment of readiness, setting of goals, or systematic evaluation—but not of the actual intervention. Of course, it is impossible not to have at least implicit goals when one teaches, but the goals may not be related to a particular patient's readiness, and the instruction may not be constructed to meet those goals.

With adequate practice one becomes very efficient in thinking through the required steps of the teaching process. The nurse-teacher becomes very sensitive to expressions of readiness that may be part of an ordinary conversation with the patient and learns to organize care to elicit measurements of readiness. The teaching that many patients require can be done in the same amount of time that the nursing process is already taking if done at the proper level of proficiency.

SUMMARY

Health teaching requires that nurses be able to make judgments about what patients need to know, what they are capable of learning, how they can best be taught, and what they have learned. Since knowledge of human behavior is at best tentative, particularly with regard to motivation and learning processes, teachers must be aware of the extent of evidence about the teaching-learning process. This will be the topic of succeeding chapters.

STUDY QUESTIONS

Read Marilyn E. Schima's article, "Starting Sex Instruction for Sixth-Grade Boys" (Am. J. Nurs. **62**:75-76, Sept. 1962). Identify these parts of the teaching-learning process:
1. Assessing readiness for learning
2. Determining learning goals (objectives)
3. Preparing a plan for teaching, and also preparing teaching materials
4. Carrying out the teaching
5. Evaluating in terms of desired learning

REFERENCES

1. Bloom, B. S., editor: Taxonomy of educational objectives: the classification of educational goals. Handbook I: Cognitive domain, New York, 1956, David McKay Co., Inc.
2. Elder, R. G.: What is the patient saying? Nurs. Forum **2**(1):25-37, 1963.
3. Elstein, A. S., and others: Methods and theory in the study of medical inquiry, J. Med. Educ. **47**:85-92, 1972.
4. Simmons, O.: Implications of social class for public health. In Jaco, E. G., editor: Patients, physicians and illness, New York, 1958, The Free Press.

CHAPTER 3

Readiness for health education

■ There are two facets of readiness to learn. One is emotional readiness, or motivation, which determines the individual's willingness to put forth the effort necessary to learn. A second facet is experiential readiness, the individual's background of experiences, skills, and attitudes and his or her ability to learn that which is considered desirable. These two facets are closely interrelated. Inability to understand an idea such as immunization (lack of experiential readiness) contributes to a lack of motivation to learn. Probably more commonly, a feeling that the material is unimportant to the individual (lack of motivation) contributes to the lack of knowledge about immunization. Major factors that help to explain this relationship for health education are the influence of beliefs about health, often culturally defined, and the impact of a health crisis.

The focus on this chapter is on describing the multiple factors that affect readiness to make a health behavior change. Knowledge of these and ability to identify them in potential learners will help the nurse to predict the degree of a person's readiness to change particular health behaviors.

THEORY ABOUT MOTIVATION IN HEALTH

Notions about motivation in health are still somewhat disorganized, although this situation is improving. Detailing of trends in theories on psychologic adjustment to physical disability is instructive in showing the larger frame in which theories of motivation have been seen to fit. Over the years, ideas about the causes of psychologic maladjustment to physical illness and disability have developed considerably, moving away from emphasis on the mental traits of patients or the somatic properties of disabilities and toward physical and social environments as critical factors that shape patients' psychologic reactions to their conditions. Serious study of the psychologic aspects of physical disability began in the late 1940's, and it became clear that removal or circumvention of disability alone was not always enough to ensure success in rehabilitation. An early explanation for such failures was that certain individuals lack the necessary energy or drive to take advantage of the opportunities provided them—they are "unmotivated." Later interpretations were that few patients truly lacked motivation but that there was a blocking or misdirection of it; this explained why the patient's motives failed to correspond with those of the treatment staff. Subsequently, lack of motivation became transformed into a problem of mental health, with explanations from psychoanalytic theory. The sociologic view that disability and illness are social judgments based on normative standards of health, disease, and handicap was followed by behaviorism, which early focused almost entirely on the environment as the cause of behavior. It is suggested that several of these theories are useful for particular problems in rehabilitation but that none is adequate as a comprehensive theory.[107]

Generally, within the health field, the cognitive component of motivation is being seen more clearly; the Health Belief Model (explained later in this chapter) is derived from expectancy theory, which has a high component of cognition. The cognitive model of motivation sees a motive as a cognitive representation of a desired future state that the organism has the potential to achieve and that is more satisfying than its current state. The energy for behavior comes from the awareness of the potential satisfaction. Emotions can serve to organize either approach or avoidance behaviors; they serve as motives to energize, direct, and sustain behavior and as one input of information in formation of the goal.[31] In addition to the cognitive focus, static hierarchies of drives are giving way to notions of associative networks of motives with a hierarchy of strength or importance to an individual; these hierarchies can be shifted.[107]

A pattern of response receiving considerable attention is the theory of learned helplessness. The expectation that an outcome is independent of responding: (1) reduces the motivation to control the outcome; (2) interferes with learning that responding controls the outcome; and, if the outcome is traumatic, (3) produces fear for as long as the subject is uncertain of the uncontrollability of the outcome, and then produces depression.[106]

This notion of the perception of the individual about whether he can affect his environment is prominent today as evidenced in the work on locus of control and internal motivation. Optimal arousal, optimal incongruity, and competence and self-determination are seen as explanatory of intrinsic motivation; direction is often provided by developmental tasks. An internal locus of control is an expectancy seen as a necessary condition for internal motivation; the

individual believes he can affect his environment and is generally proficient in information acquisition and utilization. A person with high external locus of control does not perceive that he can affect his environment—things just happen to him. There is a suggestion that negative encounters with the environment tend to weaken intrinsic motives. Indeed, lack of control is a situation variable as well as a personality variable; a high average level of internality in an individual does not mean that he necessarily has a high level in every situation. We know very little about how to induce changes in locus of control beliefs and indeed very little about their origin.[87]

Clinical studies are being done with locus of control, since different intervention methods may well be required to deal with these very different notions about causality of events. One done with individuals undergoing dental surgery showed that patients with high internal locus of control adjusted poorly in surgery when given general, marginally relevant information about the impending operation; however, they showed good adjustment if they viewed a tape that imparted specific information about procedures and sensations they might expect. The reverse was true of patients with high external locus of control.[5] A study of individuals with diabetes showed surprising outcomes. "Internals" did have more diabetic information but seemed to incur more problems with disease than did "externals" as the disease progressed. It is suggested that since the major features of diabetes and its treatment are still too poorly understood to permit adequate therapeutic recommendations for many patients, the person with internal locus of control may find himself in a situation in which the environment cannot be completely controlled. He may give up some of the control he originally exercised. For the person with external locus of control, the mode of coping is compliance with authority (physician), which may be the more adaptive set of responses in this situation.[64]

HEALTH BELIEFS AND BEHAVIOR— FACTORS AFFECTING CHANGE

Health beliefs and behavior are the targets of teaching, and at the same time they affect the probability that change will occur. There are many instances in which the nurse's goal is to maintain existing beliefs and behavior since they are adequate. In other circumstances, change is desirable.

The Health Belief Model

The Health Belief Model, although only partially developed, is probably the most complete theory regarding readiness to take health action. Its original form, developed in the early 1950's, says that people are not likely to take a health action unless (1) they believe they are susceptible to the disease in question; (2) they believe that the disease would have serious effects on their lives if they should contract it; (3) they are aware of certain actions that can be taken and believe that these actions may reduce their likelihood of contracting the disease or reduce the severity of it; (4) they believe that the threat to them of taking the action is not as great as the threat of the disease itself.[95] The model is an example of the value-expectancy approach to predicting behavior. The first two elements constitute a readiness.

A major addition to the model has been the concept of motivation; a factor that serves as a cue or trigger to action appeared to be necessary. This element of the model has not been subjected to careful study; the required intensity of the cue presumably varies with differences in the level of perceived susceptibility and severity.[98] Examples of triggers that are believed to affect timing include interpersonal crisis, interference of the symptoms with a valued social activity, and the nature and quality of the symptoms. Samples of the modified model for preventive health behavior and for explaining sick-role behavior may be seen in Figs. 1 and 2. A few studies show that it is possible to modify the perceived threat of disease (that is, the combination of perceived susceptibility and severity) as well as the perceived efficacy of professional intervention and that such modifications lead to predictable changes in health behavior.[10,97]

Some limitations of the model, important for those who would use it in health education, should be explained. There needs to be a balance between vulnerability, severity, and the psychologic benefit/cost ratio; perceived severity can reach such high levels as to be dysfunctional. There is some evidence of a threshold level, but neither theory nor research has disclosed what the optimal levels of readiness are. Little is known about the stability of the beliefs.[9] Perceived severity is the most doubtful of the elements, although it seems to be more useful in illness than in preventive behavior. The causal roles of the beliefs have not been studied. The beliefs are more prevalent in whites than in other racial groups, in high socioeconomic status than in low, in women than in men, and in the relatively young than in the old, but we do not know why.[98] The relationship among the elements—that is, whether they are additive, multiplicative, or interactive—is not clear. Some evidence shows them to be relatively independent.[51] A critical body of evidence regarding the Health Belief Model for understanding chronic illness behavior[51] or preventive dental behavior[44] has not yet been accumulated. Significant elements missing from the model are: the social environment, including lay referral and social support, the physician-patient interaction, and perception of symptoms and lay construction of illness and the sick role.[51]

The model does not imply or prescribe strategies for changing health behavior. Whereas an obvious strategy is direct persuasion to modify the beliefs, perhaps more useful is modification of the health care delivery system,[99] which could then alter the beliefs.

Present knowledge about some health problems is sufficient to allow identification of major gaps in health motivation according to the Health Belief Model. For example, it is known that only about 15% to 20% of the population in the United States follow practices likely to lead to better dental health. Research suggests that this lack of care for so many people is related in part to a belief that the disease does not have serious effects on life.[54] Perhaps health educators might emphasize the potential seriousness of dental problems (step 2 of the model) as well as the benefits of prophylaxis by professionals (step 3 of the model).

Another example of a motivation gap was identified in a study of individuals' beliefs about their chances of avoiding serious diseases, particularly cancer. The study encompassed 1,500 adults in the United States, representing a typical cross section of the adult population living in private households. Only 3.5% took cancer tests on a purely voluntary basis,

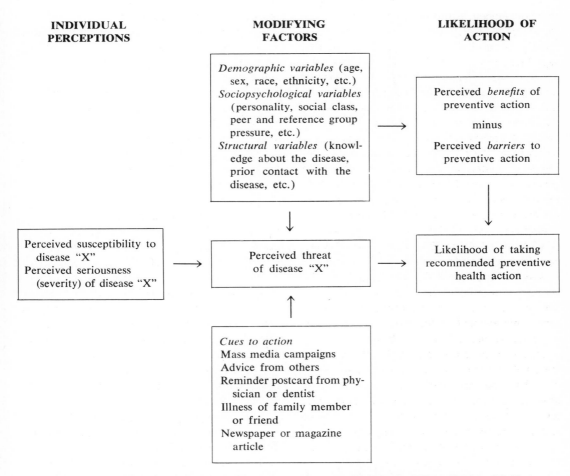

Fig. 1. The Health Belief Model as predictor of preventive health behavior. (From Becker, M. H., and others: A new approach to explaining sick-role behavior in low-income populations, Am. J. Public Health **64:**205-216, 1974.)

READINESS TO UNDERTAKE RECOMMENDED SICK-ROLE BEHAVIOR	MODIFYING AND ENABLING FACTORS	SICK-ROLE BEHAVIORS

Motivations
Concern about (salience of) health matters in general
Willingness to seek and accept medical direction
Intention to comply
Positive health activities

Value of illness threat reduction
Subjective estimates of:
Susceptibility or resusceptibility (including belief in diagnosis)
Vulnerability to illness in general
Extent of possible bodily harm*
Extent of possible interference with social roles*
Presence of (or past experience with) symptoms

Demographic (very young or old)
Structural (cost, duration, complexity, side effects, accessibility of regimen; need for new patterns of behavior)
Attitudes (satisfaction with visit, physician, other staff, clinic procedures and facilities)
Interaction (length, depth, continuity, mutuality of expectation, quality, and type of doctor-patient relationship; physician agreement with patient; feedback to patient)
Enabling (prior experience with action, illness or regimen; source of advice and referral)

Likelihood of
Compliance with prescribed regimens (e.g., drugs, diet, exercise, personal and work habits, follow-up tests, referrals and follow-up appointments, entering or continuing a treatment program)

Probability that compliant behavior will reduce the threat
Subjective estimates of:
The proposed regimen's safety
The proposed regimen's efficacy (including "faith in doctors and medical care" and "chance of recovery")

*At motivating, but not inhibiting, levels.

Fig. 2. Summary Health Belief Model for predicting and explaining sick-role behaviors. (From Becker, M. H.: The health belief model and sick-role behavior, Health Educ. Monogr. **2**:409-419, 1974. Copyright 1974 by the Society for Public Health Education, Inc., 655 Sutter Street, San Francisco, Calif. 94102.)

and 70% had had no cancer tests within the past 10 years. It is suggested that it may be intolerable for these people to believe that diseases such as cancer or tuberculosis are terribly serious, that one can contract them, and that they can progress to an incurable stage, so that people chose not to believe they were susceptible. The recommendation of the authors of this study is that health educators place less emphasis on the seriousness of these diseases and more emphasis on science's ability to detect them before symptoms appear.[120] In other words, their recommendation is to strengthen knowledge of the third factor in the model previously described.

More recent work with the model has shown that for a group of mothers of obese children, it predicted quite well dietary compliance and appointment keeping.[12] Study of its usefulness with asthmatics, who are an example of those with a regimen not consistently effective, shows that the model works as well as for diseases with consistently effective treatment.[13] Also, in the area of participation in genetic screening for Tay-Sachs disease, some interesting results have been obtained. It may be that low knowledge of the disorder yields low perceptions of susceptibility.[68] Another study found high susceptibility and low severity to be optimal; the perception that being a carrier would be highly disruptive of future family planning seems to have an inhibiting effect on participation.[11]

Changing beliefs

Both the desirability of changing health beliefs and the ability to do so require scrutiny. The well-being of an individual or group may be poorly served if health beliefs are altered so that they do not conform to the cultural norm or if a denial that is helping to maintain an individual's stability is destroyed. An example of such an effect occurred in the study of Prairie Town, where investigators' efforts to liberalize the town's views of mental illness incurred great hostility. The townspeople were resisting change in a definition around which they had built a system for handling the mentally ill and that they believed resulted in stability in their community. Since this belief was central to the moral code of the community, the resistance was great.[25]

Even if one is convinced that a health belief ought to be changed, reaching this goal can be very difficult because of the complexity of little-understood factors that contribute to a health belief or a health action. Since many studies of health attitudes are performed on a one-time basis, there is limited knowledge about whether the beliefs that underlie such expressions persist or are present only at the particular time the data are gathered and about the association between attitudes and beliefs and behavior.[55] Literally hundreds of evaluation studies in the field of health education have documented the fact that knowledge is rarely a sufficient basis for actions.[117] However, there is still a considerable gap in our understanding of the extent to which knowledge affects attitudes and the ways in which both can be used to predict behavior. There are almost no data that help define how and what a message should be in order to persuade specific populations to take health actions.[55]

A study of poisoning in children under 6 years of age suggests a multiplicity of factors involved in health behavior and a limitation of an educational program. For many years, attention has been directed toward improved storage of medicines and toxic chemicals and toward education of the public to the potential toxicity of these agents. In the study a group of families whose children had been treated for poisoning were compared with families randomly selected from neighbors of the poisoned children and not differing in a number of variables such as race and family size. There were no statistically significant differences in mothers' knowledge of toxicity of medicines and household products or in the number and storage pattern of potentially toxic substances accessible to children. A positive relationship was found between pica and daredeviltry in children and poisoning accidents. This study suggests that parental ignorance of toxicity and carelessness are mainly secondary environmental factors, which may be manipulated to decrease the ease and frequency with which the accident occurs. Perhaps national attempts to control poisoning among children should focus on high-risk groups and the more susceptible child and family life periods, for which there are clues.[6]

In American culture there are several general factors that affect the probability of changing beliefs. One factor affecting the possibility of change is that health competes for attention with other values of life. There is evidence to suggest that health motives as a whole are perhaps less potent or salient for most people than are other motives, such as those concerning social approval[95] or economic pressures, and that other motives often win out. It has been suggested that raising health values to predominance is a hopeless task and that health workers should utilize social motives, such as a desire to conform, as a means for motivating health actions. For example, sometimes a mother may be persuaded to take her child to a pediatrician, not because she is concerned with its importance for the child's health, but because all the other mothers do it.

The relationship of the public to health practitioners has presented barriers. The large difference in values and beliefs that seems to exist between much of the population and upper-middle-class physicians yields a series of difficulties for the health teacher. The status gap between these two groups becomes as serious as the financial gap, making it emotionally expensive for a lower-class person to seek help from an upper-class physician.

Health practitioners have considered much of the population to be apathetic and nonreceptive to health teaching. However, there is today widening recognition of the fact that these people are not devoid of health motives and that they do have a system of health beliefs consistent with their whole cultural system of beliefs. The lower-class individual may use the pharmacist or chiropractor as health practitioners because they have less prestige. In addition, the chiropractor bridges the cognitive gap between patient and health practitioner by explaining disease and treatment in terms of a mechanistic theory that most patients are able to grasp. The concept of a chance event and the coincidence of several factors that come together to allow disease to occur is psychologically difficult for many people who want to think in terms of cause and effect.[59,88] This finding should be relevant to the activities of the nurse in teaching lower-class patients.

Knowledge of how to introduce change into a cultural system is still very limited, as is knowledge of how to channel existing cultural beliefs toward positive health goals. Indeed, the task set for introducing change in health beliefs and practices seems to go beyond that accomplished by any other concern in our society. Although motivation research for advertising is useful, pertinent differences make the task of health motivation much more difficult. For public health programs to be effective, as much as 70% (smallpox) to 100% (polio) of the audience must be motivated, in contrast to the much smaller percentages that most commercial products hope to capture. Also, consumers are asked to perform the fairly simple act of buying, whereas in health programs people are being asked to submit to procedures often painful, inconvenient, expensive, and difficult to perform.[95]

Much is unknown about the motivating effects of general approaches to health education. An early tactic was production of fear, but fear was found to incapacitate some persons. Then an emphasis referred to as "sweetness and light" became popular, with health viewed as both an end and a means to a wonderful, joyous life. Later came a reliance on facts, with the assumption that people would act if they knew.[103] Today there is considerable evidence that health teaching involves changing of attitudes and values and willingness to take actions and that these are not altered by mere teaching of facts.[113] Indeed, there is much need for research relating the personalities of learners to the motivating approaches for particular subject matter.

Research workers are now concerned with describing systems of health belief of various cultures and socioeconomic groups and with relating these beliefs to health actions taken. This effort is based on the belief that all behavior is motivated and that it can be predicted and guided only to the extent that motivations are understood. Indeed, the facts and principles that make up the core of behavioral science fall to a large extent in the area of determinants of behavior.[95] Eventually, theories of behavior regarding health will be derived.

The next section of this chapter will present descriptions of health beliefs in further detail, with subsequent sections focusing on how these beliefs relate to the behaviors of seeking medical care and following health advice.

Systems of health belief and behavior

There are many accounts of the health beliefs of cultures throughout the world. A comprehensive bibliography of these descriptions can be found in an article by Polgar.[88] What an individual or group will learn regarding health depends at least in part on the orientation of its culture to such questions as whether man's nature is good or evil; how independent of nature man can be; whether the basic orientation is present, past, or future; whether an individual's cultural role is primarily active or passive; and how the individual is bound to other individuals.[58] For example, in most technologically underdeveloped areas, the limited-future time orientation makes education for disease prevention difficult. Therefore, preventive programs are combined with those that meet immediate needs. Bloom describes an Italian patient in America who did not seem to respond to her physician's directions. On investigation, it was found that her cultural values—the great importance of family, present-time orientation, fatalism, and passivity—were conflicting with her physician's individualism, belief in the importance of sacrificing for the future, optimism regarding illness, and belief in an active role in becoming well.[20] Nationality groups have also been found to differ in the way members reacted to pain and in their relationship with their physicians.[121]

Perhaps the most insightful comparative studies of groups of population in the United States have focused on socioeconomic status. Although the studies have been of limited populations, their potential for explaining health behavior is great, for socioeconomic status seems to be one of the major variables in health behavior.[50] Such a statement seems reasonable, since these classes vary in educational level, economic level, family structure, and other variables that affect health beliefs. Other factors thought to be important in explaining health behavior, such as sex and age, have been studied in relation to socioeconomic status.

Probably the most information is available regarding the lower class, since it is seen as being most deviant from the views of professional health workers. As a group, these people are reported to be indifferent to their symptoms and to view health as important only as it becomes poor health and interferes with daily maintenance of independence.[35,59] Their view of life has been described as characterized by powerlessness, meaninglessness, and isolation.[47]

Lower-class people are less likely than persons in higher social strata to recognize the signs of major illnesses, to understand body functioning, and to use preventive health services but are more likely to hold irrational ideas about illness, rely on folk medicine and fringe practitioners, and delay seeking medical treatment.[73] The lower class is often quite isolated from the middle class, including middle-class sources of information about health. For example, black patients in a Southern rural hospital, many of whom were of lower socioeconomic status, were found to have vague concepts of the body and its organ systems. They described their symptoms in folk terms. Pain was called "the miseries" or "something got in there," particularly head pain. Some patients suggested that diseases were associated with witchcraft.[65] Pregnant adolescents of low socioeconomic status seemed to one author to be trapped in a maze of almost bizarre and frightening fantasies about what was happening to them and to lack resources to get correct information. They often misinterpreted the prepping procedures being done to them, such as shaving and enemas, as being strongly punitive.[27] The challenges and problems of everyday living are much more real to these people than are the postponed rewards of preventive medicine, which are valued by the middle class. For example, parents of low socioeconomic status were less likely to allow their children to get Salk vaccine and knew less about the vaccine and about poliomyelitis than did parents in other classes.[30]

A study of prenatal care in one urban setting revealed that once the need for care was defined, the lower socioeconomic class had the least wherewithal to meet the needs and the longest duration of care once it was received but the least overall care in spite of great need.[94] They have been described as having difficulty in working with health workers who may wrongly assume that patients can describe symptoms, understand diagnoses, carry out treatments, keep appointments, and follow up referrals.[114] In contrast, upper-class persons more often defined themselves as being ill and were more likely to seek treatment when afflicted.[59]

In spite of these descriptions of deficiencies, the validity of middle-class standards of health behavior is not to be assumed. Adherence to an "ideal" maternal activity pattern prenatally was not found in one investigation to be essential in its entirety to normal birth. This suggests that this ideal is a dominant cultural pattern and not a physiologically based requirement and, therefore, ought not to be imposed.[76]

Perhaps the greatest body of evidence regarding health behavior by classes exists for mental illness. A study in one community found that the person with high socioeconomic status was more aware of psychologic problems than the person from the lower class, who was more apt to tolerate abnormal behavior without any awareness that it was pathologic. This person would attribute his troubles to unhappiness, tough luck, laziness, meanness, or physical illness rather than to psychogenic factors. The classes shared generally negative attitudes toward psychiatrists and psychiatric agencies, a fact that resulted in persons' turning in many directions for help before they sought psychiatric help—usually only after a serious breakdown in social relationships. The view of persons from the lowest class that suffering is a result of ill fate rather than something amenable to remedial action further hampered motivation to seek help.[45] The same effect for a different reason is suggested in a study of upper-class persons who tried too long to cope with psychosocial illness before seeking help, probably out of a powerful sense of personal responsibility toward health maintenance characteristic of this class. This prolonged attempt to cope did not occur with physical illness.[17]

A study of patients under psychiatric care in a New England community showed that the higher the socioeconomic status, the more likely an individual was to be accepted for psychiatric treatment and to be treated by highly trained personnel. Upper-class patients went to private physicians for individual psychotherapy, whereas lower-class patients received directive therapies and custodial care in institutions, partly because they were rejected by their families and communities. These lower-class people rarely entered therapy voluntarily. They were viewed by psychiatrists as being unable to participate in therapy. They were described as being passive; expecting to be given advice, pills, needles, and sympathy; often leaving therapy; and being unable to grasp the notion that they could be helped by obtaining insight into their own problems. Many were described as viewing mental illness as a somatic disease caused by "bad blood" or "too much booze." A group of psychiatrists reported that they were frustrated, repelled, and irritated by the lower-class patient's inability to think in their terms. The psychiatrists found the upper-class patient able to think in symbolic terms and desiring to reach his potential effectiveness.[45]

Health beliefs and actions vary by religious belief, ethnic group, and family group, all of which are related to socioeconomic class. Encompassing these variations, Suchman has described two major constellations of health belief: parochial life style, related to popular health orientation, and cosmopolitan style of life, related to scientific health orientation. The parochial orientation includes close relationships with one's ethnic group and friends and a family pattern of tradition and authority. This finds expression in the health area in lack of factual knowledge about disease, suspicion of outside professional medical care, and reliance on members of one's own group for help and support during illness. People with the cosmopolitan style of life have less close relationships with the groups indicated; their scientific orientation toward health includes considerable knowledge regarding disease, with more acceptance of professional medical help than reliance on members of their own close social group.

Suchman found the lower class much more likely to be parochial, with a popular health orientation, whereas the upper class was more often cosmopolitan, with scientific health orientation. However, class did not always explain

the beliefs of the subjects studied. Women tended to be more parochial in their ideas than men but actually showed a lower commitment to a popular health orientation. Women were likely to be better informed about disease than were men and less skeptical of medical care. It may be that health care is more important to women, who as mothers are responsible for the health of their families and who for this reason learn more about disease and place more faith in physicians. The more one is exposed to illness and medical care, the more likely one is to have a scientific health orientation.[115]

The significance of these differences in health beliefs is that as modern medicine becomes increasingly scientific, formal, specialized, complex, impersonal, objective, and oriented toward the disease rather than toward the patient, it comes into increasing conflict with the parochial types of social groups (traditional, dependent, closed, and local). As a result, the more parochial the individual and the more popular his health orientation, the more likely he is to seek lay diagnosis and help, to delay treatment, to stress folk remedies and self-medication, to be more concerned with immediate symptom relief than long-term cure of disease, to use marginal or lay practitioners, to find it difficult to adjust to hospital routines, and in general to be poorly informed about health or medical services. Thus parochialism and anti-scientific health orientation are major sources of resistance to modern health care. Some professionals feel that there is a need to interpret scientific progress to such people in terms that make it seem less foreign to them[115] and that health programs should be more available to them. Methods of implementing these suggestions are not clear; also, the notion that these people are irresponsible and therefore not deserving of help holds strong in middle-class values.

Some of the beliefs found in the folk medical system of a group of low income black Americans in Tucson are of interest. A recurring theme in their belief in witchcraft is that animals are introduced into the body by magical means. The mere fact that an illness has not been cured may signal to believers that it is unnatural in origin. Maternal impression was found to be nearly universal. Very few informants believed in contagion; more commonly slime and impurities in the body were believed to be the cause of respiratory tract infections, fever, and rashes. Since they believe that all one has to do to change the state of the blood is to wait for different weather conditions or to make minor dietary changes, an explanation about a condition that will last a lifetime makes little sense. The informants recognize high blood (too much blood) as a syndrome and terminologically confuse it with high blood pressure. They believe strokes are caused by excess blood backing up into the brain. Low blood is conceptually allied with anemia and terminologically confused with low blood pressure. According to their beliefs, low blood (too little blood) is a condition that makes it difficult for the heart to pump the blood through the body, and it can be brought up to normal by eating something red or by eating yeast. Moreover, blood moves faster when environmental conditions are unsettled. "Bad blood" means venereal disease. Blood viscosity is affected by outside temperatures. Prescription medicine is believed to be quite strong; therefore, if taken, it should produce practically instantaneous results.[110] There are many other such beliefs described for this group. There are many folk beliefs about pregnancy (Table 2), producing considerable difference between women holding these beliefs and their caregivers in regard to risk factors and priorities.

A study of child rearing among Appalachian families in eastern Kentucky found that the infancy of the children was strongly emphasized, there was a marked lack of emphasis on developing verbal skills, and that sexual functioning was a virtually taboo topic. Many of these poor families lacked the psychologic mobility to seek specialized care outside their local communities

Table 2. Folk beliefs concerning effect of maternal behavior on fetus*

Maternal behavior	Believed outcome
Pregnant woman worked too hard or breathed paint fumes	Miscarriage
Pregnant woman lifted arms over head	Fetus strangled by cord
Pregnant woman slept too much and baby stuck to uterus	Difficult delivery
Pregnant woman cursed by enemy or punished for sin	Neonatal death
Pregnant woman craved food and touched self	Birthmark
Pregnant woman pitied or mocked retarded person; had unfulfilled desire	Retarded infant
Pregnant woman saw something frightening	Malformed infant
Pregnant woman went out during lunar eclipse without protection	Cleft palate or body part missing
Pregnant woman saw someone suffer seizure and pitied or mocked them	Infant suffers seizures

*From Snow, L. F., and others: The behavioral implications of some old wives' tales, Obstet. Gynecol. **51**:727-732, 1978.

and cooperated better if the public health nurse aided with child training.[62]

One study of intergenerational families found the senior generation appallingly lacking in knowledge and ability to perform such rudimentary home care techniques as taking a temperature orally (39% did not know how) or rectally (70% did not know how), giving an enema (37% did not know how), taking a pulse (74% unable), using a rectal suppository (43% unable), stopping bleeding (65% did not know how), or providing artificial respiration (84% could not).[61]

This description of beliefs is meant to help the nurse anticipate health behavior individuals may display. There are certain stages in the health-illness cycle when these beliefs and behavior become crucial. One of these times is when the individual seeks care, either preventive or diagnostic.

Seeking care

The behavior persons display when they seek care has been studied because it is viewed by the medical community as important for a satisfactory medical outcome. Many diseases can be treated best with early diagnosis. People with chronic illness may, because they fail to seek treatment, function inefficiently for long periods of time; such a pattern creates economic and social loss for the family as well as the possibility of communicating illness to the family, as is believed may occur with schizophrenia.[16] Community surveys have repeatedly noted large numbers of individuals, both aware and unaware of their disorders, who were not under medical care.[112] One such report came from Britain where, despite the fact that health service is free, 37% of the families, as reported by the mothers, had a member suffering pain or discomfort without being treated.[88]

Although there is information available describing patterns of utilization of health care, very little is known about the reasons for differences in these patterns.[3] Studies of delay in seeking treatment have been done about disease entities, particularly cancer, but there are diseases, such as psychoneurosis, about which almost no inquiry has been made. In addition, many of these studies are retrospective; that is, they require the patient to recall feelings and actions. The fact that feelings are changed by intervening events reduces the reliability of recall as a means of gathering these data.[16] One should also be careful in interpreting the findings of such studies, so that the professed belief in the desirability of health actions is not confused with actual taking of action. Indeed, one study shows that, although more than 80% of a sample of the adult population in this country believed that annual physical examinations are a good thing, less than 30% had had such ex-

aminations in the year preceding the study, and then usually to fulfill insurance or job requirements. The same kind of pattern was found for annual visits to the dentist.[3,41]

There are data regarding differences by sex in preventive health behavior. In our culture, men engage in more risk-taking behavior and take preventive measures less frequently than do women, whereas women avoid risks and take more preventive action, particularly those actions associated with medical intervention. These behavioral differences are consistent with certain aspects of the socialization and adult role patterns deemed appropriate for each sex in our society. Ironically, it is women's positive orientation toward medical care that may be responsible for the one class of risk-taking behavior in which women clearly predominate: women are more frequent users than men of psychotropic medications, the most common substances obtained by entry into the medical system.[80]

Available evidence indicates that seeking medical care is influenced by many factors and by the interplay among them. A single factor, such as ignorance, is often not solely responsible for delay or promptness in seeking medical care.[92] The previous discussion of health behavior by socioeconomic class revealed that economic ability to pay for care is bound up with health beliefs and with values about the priority of health among many motivations. The individual's, the family's, and the culture's answers to the following questions help to determine whether or not care will be sought: What is the meaning attached to the body site of the symptom? How are hospitals, medical personnel, surgery, and the body itself viewed? Does the family support the health action psychologically and financially? How is a person's responsibility for his own health viewed? How important is the person himself? What kinds of care facilities are acceptable for use? All these factors influence the way in which people select, perceive, and interpret information and services available to them.

Certainly the development of anxiety helps to determine action in seeking health care. It is known that mild anxiety is useful in that it yields a tendency to act; however, greater degrees of anxiety interfere with adaptive action.[96] It has been suggested that the educational campaign regarding the seven danger signals of cancer may produce too much fear and too little support for seeking care.[92] In other words, there is more to seeking medical care than mere factual knowledge regarding the disease. Fear of negative reactions from high-status medical personnel may inhibit individuals from going to the physician with an "insignificant" symptom. Since 1946, when the method for breast self-examination was introduced, there has been a decrease in delay in seeking care for breast cancer. It is believed that part of this change may have occurred because women now have a concrete "confirmation tool" that is viewed by the physician as valid and something on which to act. It is as if the physician were conferring on the patient permission to ask for an examination. Rejection by health personnel can become a barrier to the use of any knowledge the individual may have.[16] One of the functions of health education should be to provide sufficient knowledge of health and of care systems to sanction seeking help when dysfunction is suspected.

For many people, inadequate knowledge of symptoms, particularly early ones, produces delay in seeking medical care. Patients with the nephrotic syndrome were found to define "edema" as "illness"; edema was the symptom for which the patient sought advice regardless of other symptoms of his renal disease.[33] For many patients with bronchitis and emphysema the so-called cigarette cough is normal and is not viewed as a reason to consult the physician.[63] Such patients may see the physician only when they have dyspnea and, even then, only when the symptom interferes with the performance of their usual tasks. In general, the individual has no clear idea of his disorder

and must rely on critical symptoms that he considers worthy of medical attention and treatment. These may include cough, fever, pain, bleeding, nervousness, or the location and frequency of symptoms.[112] Many chronically ill patients are old, and some of them tolerate functional impairments unnecessarily because they erroneously associate their symptom with aging rather than with illness and fail to adhere to their medical regimen.[2,52]

A study regarding well-child supervision in a clinic serving lower-class patients serves to exemplify the multiple factors relating to failure to obtain care. Although there are many such factors, they are related and can be predicted to some extent. Those mothers whose children received less preventive care were less educated, were married to men in the lowest occupational stratum, were of higher parity, lived farther from the clinic, were less likely to have a car and had more difficulty in getting to the clinic, were less impressed with the purpose and potentialities of well-child care, and felt powerless and socially isolated. Maternal-child health care seeking was found to form a consistent pattern for individual mothers. If the mothers received prenatal care early, it was more probable that their children would receive postnatal care than if the mothers had neglected prenatal care.[78]

Evidence now available questions the assumption that individuals at most times during their lives are really asymptomatic. There is little medically to distinguish many minor disorders brought to the doctor from those that are ignored, tolerated, or self-medicated.[122] Much of this "illness" is never brought to physicians. Illness, defined as the presence of clinically serious symptoms, is the statistical norm. On the average, we may have a new "illness" episode every 6 days. Usually we ask what makes people delay in getting medical aid; it might be more fruitful to ask, what on earth makes people consult?[93] One study finds the crux of the decision to seek medical aid based on a break in the accommodation to the symptoms, not usually at the physically sickest time. Triggers to seek aid include the occurrence of interpersonal crises, perceived interference with vocational or physical activity and with social or personal relationships, and sanctioning. Where the physician paid little attention to the specific trigger, the patient was most likely to break off treatment.[122] A very common response to symptoms is taking medications, both prescription and over-the-counter medications. A British study found that although 91% of the adults reported they had symptoms during the 2 weeks before the interview, only 16% had consulted a doctor during that time. Fifty-five percent of the adults said they had taken or used some medicine during the 24 hours before the interview.[38]

A social psychologic model of the process of seeking help has been described by Mechanic. There are seven groups of variables that appear to be particularly important[74]:

1. Number and persistence of symptoms.
2. The individual's ability to recognize symptoms.
3. Perceived seriousness of symptoms.
4. The extent of social and physical disability resulting from the symptoms.
5. The cultural background of the defining person, group, or agency in terms of emphasis on qualities such as tolerance or stoicism.
6. Available information and medical knowledge.
7. Availability of sources of help and their social and physical accessibility.

Note that a number of the variables are the same as those in the Health Belief Model or have been suggested to be included in it.

Follow-through behavior

The health worker is also interested in patterns of behavior regarding cooperation with treatment or follow-up behavior. The patient controls this facet, which is vital to the cure process.

The literature regarding compliance is immense. Marston, who has written a summary article, finds published reports of compliance behavior to show wide variations—4% to 100% default. Generally, about 30% to 35% of patients fail to follow their physicians' medical recommendations. Little or no correlation has been found between compliance behavior and sex, age, race, marital status, socioeconomic status, or education. Use of personality tests to predict compliance has been disappointing. It is unclear whether actual severity of illness is related to compliance, although severity as perceived by the patient probably results in increased compliance. Noncompliance increases with the complexity of the regimen. In general, no clear picture of the determinants of compliance emerged from the author's review of the literature.[69]

The requirements of carrying out the physician's orders can be more or less difficult for the patient. Patients with difficult illnesses (involving infectiousness, complications, chronicity, interference with life, costly treatment, need for ancillary services, and a number of medical visits per year) were found in one study to do more poorly in following restrictions and taking medications and treatments than those with less difficult illnesses. Also, follow-through is not a unitary phenomenon but consists of a series of behaviors, such as taking medicines, having treatments, returning to see the physician when requested, and following through on referrals. Even after performing one behavior, the patient may or may not carry out another.[15] A study has been done of follow-through behavior of farmers with cardiac disease, many of whom had to comply with changes in diet, work restrictions, and personal habits such as smoking. Most commonly, these individuals reported that they complied with two out of three regimens, with the activity restrictions and personal habits being the most difficult to control. A higher proportion of educated persons than of those with less formal education stopped complying.[29]

In Schwartz and co-workers' study of follow-through behavior, a group of 178 ambulatory chronically ill elderly patients showed considerable difficulty. Forty percent of the patients said that they had difficulties arising from the prescribed medical regimen, most frequently in adhering to a diet. They were eating too much, were hungry, disregarded the diet, or did not like the diet food. Fifty-nine percent of the patients interviewed were found to be making medication errors. An error was defined as (1) taking a medicine not ordered by the physician, (2) not taking a medicine ordered by the physician, or (3) taking a medicine ordered by the physician but in incorrect dosage, at the wrong time, or with a total lack of understanding of its purpose.[105] An additional study of elderly patients attending a private clinic in Seattle supported these general findings.[81]

Forty percent of the error makers in the study done by Schwartz and co-workers were confused or wrong about the general purpose of at least one of the medications they were taking. About one fifth of those who made errors had inaccurate knowledge about their medications that could have had dangerous repercussions. Most of the patients' mistaken notions about the purpose of their medications appeared to stem from having begun to take two or more different medications simultaneously without ever having a clear idea of which was in which bottle. It appeared that patients identified the most impressive-looking tablet with the symptom or organ causing them the greatest concern, referring to it, for example, as "my heart medicine." Others simply never separated which instruction belong to which medication, apparently because instructions were given before the prescriptions were filled, and the patients did not know which was which. This suggests that medications should be more carefully labeled and that medical personnel should give slower and more thoughtful instructions, with the medications used as visual aids.

The nurse interviewing the patient should not expect to get a satisfactory answer to, "Are you having any trouble with your medications?" or "Are you doing exactly what the physician told you?"[105] Rather, the nurse might ask questions regarding what medications are being taken, how much, when, and why and might query the patient regarding those symptoms that represent desired action and side effects. Among ambulatory chronically ill elderly patients like those studied, the nurse may anticipate more errors by those who are over 75 years of age, those living alone, those with a large number of illnesses, and those with less formal education.[105]

There is considerable evidence that patients often do not take medications prescribed for them. In interpreting these investigations, it must be borne in mind that interview and pill count can be unreliable; much more reliable is analysis of a body fluid, such as urine, for the substance. Again, multiple factors seem to determine whether or not the health action will be taken. A study of families whose children were to take penicillin orally for 10 days for rheumatic fever prophylaxis found that 80% of the families understood the diagnosis, 90% knew the medicine was penicillin, and 95% knew the proper directions for giving the medication. Yet, by the third day of the 10-day regimen, only 44% were taking the penicillin; by the sixth day, only 29%; and by the ninth day, only 18%. Particularly the younger children were not receiving the medication, possibly because of the difficulty of getting them to take any pill. The interview data suggested that parents stopped giving the medicines when they were no longer concerned about the child—that is, when symptoms ceased. Perhaps a better method of meeting the objective would be to give long-acting penicillin by injection.[14]

Considerable difficulty can occur when long-term chemotherapy is a major method of treatment but patients do not reliably take medications. For example, tuberculosis is now treated with drugs, with periods of isolation and hospitalization being shorter than those used previously. The course of treatment often runs at least 18 months. The approach of the nurse must be to assess the ability of the patient to learn independence in taking the course of treatment. For those for whom this objective is not possible, supervision of drug taking is suggested, partly because the daily costs of hospitalization are at least three to four times as much as a nurse's home visit.[79]

Some research with regard to the patient reliability in taking medicines has identified some very interesting reasons for failure to follow through. Interviews with patients with peptic ulcers have indicated that failure to follow the diet and medicine regimen is common. Reasons that the patients gave for not taking antacids include cost and inconvenience during work. A study showed, however, that patients took less than one-half the prescribed dose of antacids even when their symptoms were not severe and when they were in a hospital under close supervision.[100] A subsequent study of patients' and their families' understanding of ulcer diagnosis and treatment showed a particular lack of knowledge regarding acid, its significance, and the relation of medications to it. Few of these individuals understood that acid is secreted from the stomach; rather, they believed it came from foods. It is doubtful that these people understood that between-meal or nighttime doses of antacid were prescribed to decrease acidity. Rather, patients seemed to conceive of the medication as having only a direct and curative effect on the "ulcer sores"—as coating them physically, protecting and soothing them. Such ideas do not seem conducive to an understanding of the preventive rationale of long-term therapy with the goal of maintenance of gastric pH at prophylactic levels. Since such a concept is abstract and difficult for many to understand, it is tempting for health workers to explain it in physical terms that patients are likely to understand. In this instance, patients seemed to construct their ideas about the healing process by analogy to what they knew regarding healing of visible sores on the skin. Many of them therefore believed that an ulcer is a sore that heals through a process of scab formation. They saw the healing process as doubtful because the sore was constantly wet and irritated by rough foods and chemical irritants such as alcohol. Conceivably, the patient who thinks of the medicine as having a coating action may view the action of this medication as superfluous from the time he believes the ulcer is healed or "covered over."[102]

From a companion study of the dietary regimen for patients with ulcers it was found that patients believed that they had to follow a diet, such as the modified Sippy, for a long time or forever. They showed little understanding of the abstract concept that foods that stimulate acid secretion should be restricted; rather, patients excluded food they thought to cause a direct physical irritation of the stomach, such as bananas because of the black seeds or foods that contained acid. Patients were avoiding fats because of the common knowledge that they are hard to digest, when in reality fats are recommended because they diminish gastric motility and secretion. Some data from this study suggested that patients were ignoring the literal rules of the diet and were employing a simple test of whether or not symptoms were relieved. In this way patients may actually be obtaining the major benefits of the diet, since its value in relieving symptoms has been demonstrated whereas its value in healing has not.[101]

Interviews with 60 parents of children attending a rheumatic fever clinic evidenced that the parents' all-pervading anxiety about heart disease and death led them to impose or continue restrictions contrary to medical advice, even on children with normal hearts.[56] These kinds of investigations are most pertinent to patient teaching, for they point up misconceptions that medical personnel might not anticipate and contribute to an understanding of why patients may not follow the prescribed regimen.

As might be expected, persons of lower socioeconomic status seem to have added barriers to follow-through. Even if the very poor seek prenatal care, they may be unable to follow advice regarding diet and rest unless some supplementation of income can be arranged. If the family's attitude toward care differs significantly from patient's attitude, the patient may be so burdened by anxiety that she is unable to follow medical instructions. For example, relatives whose childbearing was aided only by a midwife may be scornful of the idea that any special care is necessary during pregnancy.[28] There is some evidence that if barriers like these are removed, patients respond. A small study concerned with encouraging low-income blacks with poor health levels to use modern health facilities showed that those who were helped with their social problems were more likely to follow through on medical referrals. Removal of barriers such as long waiting periods for appointments and complex procedures involving many trips to obtain necessary documents yielded more follow-through. It was also found that these persons needed to have health goals and values interpreted to them so that they could accept health information.[42]

The studies cited sample only specific categories of patients and kinds of follow-through behavior. Perhaps the emphasis on taking medicines exists because this is a widely used therapy and because behavior required is relatively clear-cut. At any rate, the nurse should be aware that follow-through behavior does not occur automatically; it needs to be directed in various ways, one of which is patient teaching.

EXPERIENTIAL READINESS

Examples of experiential readiness have already been introduced in the discussion of health beliefs and behavior. Experiential readiness merely refers to whether or not the individual has had experiences that make him able to learn what is desired. Thus it may be said that certain people show lack of experiential readiness to utilize modern medical care. They may not have enough knowledge of anatomy and physiology of the human body to follow an explanation of their disease or sufficient understanding of cleanliness and sterility to adequately carry out sterile dressing changes by themselves. An individual from any social class who has been irresponsible all her life may not begin to understand and value the concept of responsibility in motherhood, even according to the expectations of her own socioeconomic class. Indeed, many behaviors necessary for optimal functioning in relation to health require quite a background of knowledge, physical skills, and attitudes. If this background on which to build is not available, either individuals must learn much more before they are ready to function, or someone else, such as a family member, neighbor, or health worker, will have to help them function.

Experiential readiness is closely tied to emotional readiness, because individuals tend to be motivated to do those things that are familiar and interesting to them and to resist those that are foreign.

Maturation, which occurs throughout life, greatly influences experiential readiness. Within a culture, individuals usually have developed certain physical skills, intellectual skills, and attitudes by a particular age. Knowledge of normal growth and development helps the nurse to determine what health education goals may be possible for the learner. Although this must be supplemented with information about a particular individual's readiness, it guides the assessment.

Knowledge of what is commonly known by groups of people is also useful so that the probable level of understanding can be anticipated. For example, from a 1964 study in one city it was found that more than 33% of the respondents thought tuberculosis was inheritable, and nearly 30% did not know whether it was or not.[118] Middle-class persons may have little knowledge of the various medical specialties.[88]

Knowledge of possible misunderstandings is very useful in helping the nurse anticipate confusion or errors. For example, some patients believe that the cardiac monitor paces their heart. Some pregnant adolescents of low socioeconomic status believed that there was danger of the cord strangling the fetus if they lifted their arms to hang the family wash.[27] Faced with similar situations, people often reason out similar answers, which may be untrue. A nurse who visited parents after loss of a child by sudden death syndrome found that the parents had formulated certain concepts about the death and what caused it, such as smothering or suffocation; choking on mucus or regurgitated food, especially if the baby was left with a propped bottle; unsuspected illness; virus affecting the brain; or crying himself to death. All these reasons are false, but each is an interpretation of the signs that are present. The nurse brings information to the families and a chance for resolution of confusion and concern.[90]

Health workers can possess quite inaccurate concepts of the learner's level of knowledge about a subject. One kind of inaccuracy was illustrated in a study of the amount of knowledge 214 clinic patients had about cause, symptoms, and treatment of ten common diseases. Physicians thought patients would be able to answer correctly 82% of the test items, whereas patients could actually answer only 55%.[91] A second kind of error, which I have noted to be common among nursing students, is the assumption that individuals who have had an illness or have been in a hospital understand the illness and the hospital and do not need further teaching. One wonders whether these errors are really caused by an inability to determine what patients know or by a lack of concern about what they ought to know and imprecision in defining it. Certain ideas common in the medical subculture can lead to unwarranted assumptions. The literature typically describes parents of the mentally retarded child as having neurotic mechanisms that tend to prevent or distort

changes toward realistic expectations for their child, the implication being that staff should help provide amelioration of these reactions through short-term psychotherapeutic approaches. Another point of view is that what the parents require most is specific, clearly transmitted, honest information about the child, implications for his future, and knowledge of what concrete steps they can take to deal with the problems. Perhaps parents' lack of acceptance of limitations on their child's life might result from lack of knowledge about retarded children and inability to translate the child's present abilities into future capabilities.[71] The point is that one should not accept one explanation for behavior without exploring others.

Before teaching, nurses must analyze what behaviors are prerequisite, so that they can determine whether the learner possesses them. For example, the following abilities are considered necessary before hemiplegics can learn to transfer themselves from bed to wheelchair:

1. Ability to balance in sitting position
2. Ability to turn over and push up in bed
3. Ability to follow simple directions about movement of the unaffected side
4. Ability to bear a goodly portion of the body weight on the arm
5. Ability to pay attention to a series of actions and commands for the span of a few minutes[46]

Unless the patient has the necessary skills, trying to reach the objective of self-transfer is unrealistic.

It is obvious that learning requires an adequately functioning nervous system and that some patients with whom the nurse is working will have more or less obvious disruptions. There are a legion of examples. With kidney failure, rising levels of waste products in the system first affect attention and concentration, and then, with these involved, the higher intellectual functions of abstraction, generalization, and language skills cannot be effectively executed. There is some support for the notion that every dialysis candidate is experiencing at least mild organic brain dysfunction, which affects learning.[26] One of the reasons that preoperative teaching is important is that postoperatively the patient's attention span is shortened because of the effect of medications and pain. Fatigue also decreases the quality of thinking. As a result of brain injury, the hemiplegic patient may be a poor observer of his environment, may fluctuate in mental ability, may have a short attention span, and may be highly suggestible.[21] Obviously, teaching will be most effective if timed to coincide with periods of maximum cognitive functioning, such as may occur after rest or dialysis or relative to the effects of a particular medication.

A state called hypovigilance, described as a disturbance in awareness affecting receptivity and reactivity, encompasses but is different from both withdrawal and lowered level of consciousness. The patient's decreased ability to sustain attention may cause him to be unable to accurately perceive his enviornment and thus may result in confusion and disorientation. He may appear to be indifferent to everything and may have a reduction in activity, initiative, and interests. An influencing factor with some patients may be powerlessness—an expectancy that their behavior cannot influence the outcomes they seek.[75] Although powerlessness is thought to be a more or less permanent personality trait and therefore difficult to alter,[49] helping the patient to increase his control by providing information and helping him to solve problems may have merit. Another hypothesized cause of hypovigilance is restriction of sensory input or perceptual monotony. Nursing intervention includes introduction of orienting stimuli, such as a clock, calendar, television, colors, flowers, different foods, or conversation. It also includes a pattern of questioning patients to see if they understand what is happening; if they do not, it includes a pattern of providing information, then requestioning, and so forth, in the form of a drill.[75]

MOTIVATING FACTORS IN ROLE OF PATIENT

A person's beliefs regarding health and a background of physical and mental skills and attitudes are with him as he undergoes a health crisis. The situation places special stresses on him and his family and affects their motivation to learn. Models of the psychosocial adaptation to illness suggest some variations in readiness during this process. The hospital, which is the setting in which the patient often finds himself, supports him during the adaptation but at the same time creates stresses of its own.

Implications of psychosocial adaptation to illness

The threat of illness and the later confirmation of it precipitate a series of redefinitions of the self, a process that allows a person to adapt to being sick. The degree of adaptation that occurs will vary with the self-concept before illness, the severity of the illness and change in living pattern it necessitates, and the meaning that the altered function has to the person and those close to him. Effective nursing supports and guides the patient and family as they move through the stages of adaptation.[24] Teaching, properly timed, is a nursing skill that can facilitate adaptation.

Several authors have described the process of psychosocial adaptation to illness. They agree on its general characteristics but focus on slightly different behavioral aspects and divide the process into different numbers of stages. Table 3 presents the descriptions of selected authors.

Variations in receptivity to teaching are suggested by these models. During the first stage, denial may be present to interfere with the patient's learning about his diagnosis and restrictions and with his orientation to the hospital. The nurse must expect to reinterpret this information for him. Studies of persons with tuberculosis suggest that, if the diagnosis is not clear-cut or is slow to be made, it seems less credible that illness exists.[34] Features of denial include suppression and distortion of information that has been presented to the patient in unambiguous terms, a grandiose approach to his situation, and withdrawal from the demands of his role. An example could be given of a patient on a dialysis program for several months who, although having had considerable instruction, says he did not know he could not use salt in his diet,[26] or a patient who, avoiding speaking about his heart attack, rationalizes another cause ("It must be gas pains") or outwardly denies its occurrence ("This couldn't happen to me"). It is believed that if during this stage of disbelief the nurse tries to force the patient to look at how sick he is, the patient may be angered and draw away from the nurse.[16] Presentation of "the facts" may cause patient resistance,[77] but it also has been viewed as a technique by which to move the patient toward reality.[26]

In later stages of adaptation, the person becomes better able to consider himself as sick, to hear facts about his illness, and to participate in his own care.[24] For example, one would expect that during the stages of assumption of sick role and medical care contact, the patient would be more receptive than he previously was to teaching regarding diagnosis, treatment, and course of the illness. A study of information that a group of patients wanted to have regarding their diagnostic tests reflects the heightened self-concern characteristic of early stages of adaptation. The information they desired was why the test was being done, how the equipment would concern them (including the part of the body the test would affect), what they could do to help with the test, what the results meant, and whether more tests would be necessary.[36] During the period of accepted illness, patients might be quite ready to learn about body functions, although one would question their ability to develop complex learning because of the usual preoccupation with self.

Convalescence has been described as involving three tasks: life reassessment, dealing with threat to self-image, and dealing with dependence. A patient may have morbid and ridiculous thoughts with haunting vignettes from the past and fantasies of the future. Because he realizes these are partly irrational, he may not talk much about them. Patients do talk about the emptiness of their lives, the neglect of family and friends, and their profound loneliness, which can be frightening or embarrassing to the nurse. Short hospital stays put the patient back into the home when much of this work must still be accomplished. He may have rapid mood swings, pain, restlessness, sleeplessness, and other behavior for which family members are ill prepared and in which the roles of both patient and family members are not clearly defined.[83]

Different disease processes might be expected to produce slightly different patterns of adaptation. Table 3 contains an example of the process found in patients with multiple sclerosis.[72] These patients may regress from an advanced stage of adaptation to an earlier one when exacerbation occurs, or they may remain forever in one stage if the disease does not progress. Integration not only was found to take a relatively long time to achieve but also had to be reestablished with each exacerbation, because each new "attack" reminded the patient of his true vulnerability. This may account for the finding that as the disease (disability and symptoms) worsens, the self-concept gets better—in many cases, markedly better.[72] This model is different from the Suchman and Lederer models, which assume convalescence, recovery, or rehabilitation. The illnesses that are known to bring death within a forseeable time seem to be associated with a different pattern of adjustment, described by the well-known Kübler-Ross model.

Adaptation of the family is crucial to the tasks of reorganization and rehabilitation. During the stages concerned with convalescence and rehabilitation, the patient's apparent inability to learn self-care may result from the fam-

Table 3. Stages of psychosocial adaptation to illness

CRATE*

Disbelief	Development of awareness	Reorganization	Resolution and identity change
This begins when person learns by diagnosis or change in function (symptoms) that he has a particular condition. He may express denial by "I don't have it," a claim to have something else, avoidance by forgetting or refusing to do things required of him, attempts to control treatment, or diverting attention to other issues.	Patient becomes less able to maintain denial, more aware of what has happened to him and the implications of it. Dependence on others causes conflict yielding anger, at first diffuse and later more specifically focused on being sick. Anger may be expressed openly, projected, or directed toward oneself in depression.	Patient accepts increased dependence. There is reorganization of feelings between family members.	Patient resolves his loss; he begins to acknowledge changes in how he sees himself. He begins to identify with others who have same problem.
Nurse should allow patient to deny but does not join him in the denial.	Nurse should avoid joining patient in his anger. Nurse assumes responsibility for care so that patient is free to deny.	Nurse is safety valve when family cannot accept patient.	Nurse encourages patient to express his views of himself. Goal of this process is for patient to be better able to live with his illness, rather than repressing it. If he has chronic illness, he is likely to undergo this process again and again.

LEDERER†

Transition from health to illness	Accepted illness	Convalescence
Apprehension and anxiety are present. Many patients ignore symptoms and use denial to allay anxieties, reinforced by plunge into health. Denial may be expressed by minimizing importance of symptoms by identifying them with common, benign, or trivial indispositions. Some patients meet anxiety aggressively and are irascible and ill-humored. Others allay anxiety by passivity and are compliant. Patient is driven by his symptoms to seek diagnosis and therapy but is anxious and so displays vacillating behavior, reflecting indecision. Urgent requests for diagnostic examinations are rapidly alternated with failure to appear for examination.	Patient has accepted diagnosis and initial therapeutic procedures. He views himself as ill and abandons pretenses of health. He is preoccupied with symptoms and illness, is greatly concerned with functioning of his body, and is dependent. He assumes that physician and nurse share these preoccupations and is highly subjective in judging things. In people who have elaborate defenses against regression and expression of dependency, there is little or no phase of "accepted illness." These people continue to deny and do not follow medical advice; rather, they challenge it. This phase ends gradually after pathologic process has been reversed or arrested.	There is return of physical strength and reintegration of personality. This stage may be prolonged if previous life pattern was not satisfying or if person believes he cannot return to a life that was satisfying. Some patients wrench themselves quickly from dependency and overdo. This stage has been likened to adolescence. Nurse must not encourage dependency with protection.

SUCHMAN‡

Symptom experience	Assumption of sick role	Medical care contact	Dependent patient role	Recovery or rehabilitation
Decision that something is wrong is made in these ways: 1. Physical experience (pain, discomfort, change of appearance) 2. Cognitive aspect (interpretation of physical experience) 3. Emotional response of fear or anxiety There is often denial of illness or "flight to health."	Person decides that he is sick and needs professional care. He seeks symptom alleviation, information and advice, and temporary acceptance of his condition by family and friends. How they react has much to do with his ability to enter sick role. Patient wants confirmation of his feelings and permission to suspend normal obligations.	Patient seeks professional medical diagnosis and course of treatment. He seeks authoritative sanction to become "legitimately" ill or return to normal activities. If he refuses to accept diagnosis or treatment, this stage is prolonged as he searches for another diagnosis. Patients, who perceive their symptoms as less serious use self-treatment rather than going to the physician.	There is decison to transfer control to physician and to accept and follow prescribed treatment—to be a "patient"; 74% of people studied felt this task to be difficult for them.	Person relinquishes patient role. For many with chronic illnesses or physical impairments, this is a long and demanding stage with with recurring episodes of illness. Person reestablishes relationships changed by illness.

MATSON AND BROOKS§

Stage I: Denial	Stage II: Resistance	Stage III: Affirmation	Stage IV: Integration
"It's not true; it can't be happening to me." Concealing symptoms. Seeking an authority who will deny the diagnosis. Refusing help. Holding to past life and values.	"It won't get me down!" Searching for a cure or treatment. Active in programs seeking other patients. Reluctant to accept help. Initial recognition of change in life-orientation.	"I guess I have to face it." Grieving for loss of former self. Publicly explaining about M.S. Learning to accept help. Subjectively rearranging priorities in life.	"I know it's there, but I don't think much about it." Living with it. Spending time and energy on other matters. Accepting help when necessary. Integration of life style with new values.

*Crate. M. A.: Am. J. Nurs. 65:72-76, Oct. 1965.

†Lederer, H. D.: J. Soc. Issues 8(4):4-15, 1952.

‡Suchman, E. A.: J. Health Hum. Behav. 6:114-128, 1965. This description is based on a study of the 137 persons who had been ill at some time during the two months before the study was conducted, out of a population of 5,340 persons in New York City representing an area probability sample.

§Reprinted with permission from Matson, R. R., and Brooks, N. A.: Adjusting to multiple sclerosis; an exploratory study, Soc. Sci. Med. 11, copyright 1977, Pergamon Press, Ltd.

ily's difficulty in making this adaptation. Indeed, an individual may experience difficulty or be unable to move through any of the phases, with the result that assistance from special therapy is needed for adjustment.

The literature regarding psychosocial adaptation to illness and the implications regarding teaching represent a suggested theoretic framework rather than an adequately proved set of recommendations. There have, however, been observations of patient learning that lend credibility to the framework. In a study of patients with myocardial infarction, it was noted that during the first 2 weeks after the attack patients often were resentful of limits placed on their activity and repeatedly expressed hostility. These behaviors are characteristic of the stages of disbelief or transition to illness. Patients apologized for having services of a personal nature performed for them (developing awareness stage). In the third and fourth weeks of hospitalization, they began to evidence interest in their surroundings and in increasing their activities. Patients asked many questions such as, "How bad was my attack?" and "Will I get sick again?" suggestive of the stages of accepted illness or dependent patient role. Much of the information given to the patients during this time was not retained. During the fifth and sixth weeks the patients felt good; their activities were increasing. They repeated many questions previously asked, but the questions were more specific, dealing with the future.[84] This behavior follows that described in the stage of recovery or rehabilitation, convalescence, or resolution of identity change. For many disorders, the stages of adaptation seem to have a characteristic length and characteristic behavior pattern, probably because the effects of the illness and the treatment are similar.

Adaptation to motherhood is a process with some of the same psychosocial components as the models described above—disbelief followed by acceptance and later a desire to return to the usual state. During the first trimester, women are often ambivalent about their pregnancy. At this time they are most concerned about their own health and about how to get medical care. The second trimester involves an increasing awareness of the child rather than just the pregnancy, accompanied by interest in learning what a baby is like and what is involved in being a mother. After the seventh month, the pregnancy may become a burden; the mother wants to separate from the baby. At this time, she seeks other women with an intimate knowledge of pregnancy for support. She is most receptive to learning how to relieve pressure and congestion in order to promote comfort, how to look attractive, how to control weight, how to prepare her breasts for lactation, and how to know the signs of labor and what to do at that time. Thus the natural course of the pregnancy progressively precipitates these needs for learning.[28,119]

The notion of what an individual is ready to learn about health is also suggested by analyzing systems of human needs and human development. Maslow's hierarchy is one such system. It describes physiologic needs as most basic, with safety, love and belonging, esteem, and self-actualization needs as steps up the hierarchy. Needs at the lower end of the hierarchy must be satisfied before the person can attend to those at the upper end.[70] Thus it may be inferred that a person suffering with pain (physiologic need) is not likely to be receptive to teaching about how to adjust to his illness (love and belonging or esteem needs). Nor is the individual who is concerned about acceptance of his altered self by his family (love and belonging) likely to be efficient at learning about creating something new in his profession. Similarly, Erikson's theory of stages of ego development is a system of hypotheses about readiness, in that attainment of each stage is regarded as necessary for progression toward a later stage. For example, a person can lose himself in a relationship of genuine intimacy only after his identity has been stabilized.[40]

If nurses have an understanding of the processes of adaptation and an ability to identify them in their patients, they should, when possible, time their teaching to take advantage of natural readiness. They will also find instances in which lack of attention to the patient's progress in the adaptation process has contributed to teaching failure.

Receptivity during hospitalization

Patients may be in the hospital as they are progressing through the stages of adaptation just described. The hospital is an institution that has as its purpose helping sick people; however, there is evidence that this goal is a difficult one to meet in its entirety. A factor significant to patients' well-being is communication of information and attitudes that they need to have. Since the hospital is considerably unlike other social systems persons encounter, it seems safe to assume that most people enter it with a great deal of role ambiguity. They are uncertain as to their expectations for themselves as well as for others, and many appear to be searching for the means of clarifying mutual expectations to decrease the uncertainty.[22]

Orientation to the hospital has long been considered a teaching action within the province of the nurse. Its purpose has been to enable patients to function within this new setting so that they can attend to coping with the illness.

From one study of 40- to 60-year-old patients with cardiovascular and gastrointestinal illnesses, it was found that patients wanted answers to the following questions: "What do the physicians and nurses really expect of patients?" "Which of the hospital regulations may be stretched a bit?" "To whom can I turn for help with personal problems?" "How soon will the nurse answer my call?" "How can I identify the head nurse?" These patients were often preoccupied with safety factors in the hospital, and many were fearful of being neglected or being made the subject of gross mistakes. They desired to secure information about

what was supposed to be happening to them so that they could exercise more control over the situation and be able to protect themselves against errors. Even though all patients in the group studied had had previous hospital experience, they still lacked knowledge about technical medical procedures and found it difficult to foresee forthcoming events; at times anxiety and fear resulted from their lack of psychologic preparation.[109]

Two studies in university hospitals showed that many of the patients (all 30 in Kauffman's study and more than one half in Newman's study) desired more information about such things as hospital routines and their illness.[53,82] The lack of knowledge was identified as generally stress producing by patients[53]; at least some expressed this as worry about future security in their jobs and families.[82] These concerns no doubt represent to some extent the heightened self-concern present during illness. The desire of patients for personal contact with staff and the loneliness that they express represent similar kinds of feelings.

Although these studies are based on small samples, they support the view that more than a cursory explanation of the physical environment and schedule is required for hospital orientation. Attention must be given to continued adjustment throughout the hospitalization, not just as the patient enters. Actions of personnel speak far louder than do words; the staff that professes to answer patients' call lights immediately but does not do so in practice confuses and angers patients. By their own social systems, patients do much to orient each other to "how things really are." This system is generally helpful, but the demise of large wards seems to have reduced its effect. Observation of the "grapevine" in operation can do much to inform the nurse of the adequacy of communication with the staff.

Other studies, composed of interviews of patients in individual hospitals midway through their hospitalization and at discharge, showed that these patients felt that they needed information about the diagnosis, the cause of their condition, the effect on their short- and long-term futures, activity restrictions, and symptoms they wished explained.[1,37] These represent topics that it has been the physician's prerogative to initiate but that the nurse can reinforce and interpret.

Reactions of children to illness and hospitalization affect their readiness to learn. The major question that should reveal learning needs is: In what respects does the child's illness or handicap interfere with the learning that normally takes place and with the reception of gratifications necessary for optimal growth at his particular age level? Nurses need knowledge of normal growth and development in order not only to support it but also to predict the disruptions with which they must deal. For example, it is important for nurses, when working with a child less than 3 years old, to know that those of his age are predominantly afraid of separation from the mother, of disapproval, of physical pain, of punishment, and of their own aggressiveness. It is known that children aged 7 months to 7 years are susceptible to damange by hospitalization. There has been much less study of effects on those of school age and on adolescents. However, many of these older children have not acquired the capacity of thinking into the future and waiting for health; meanwhile, they have to cope with immobilization in the hospital and loss of normal ways of expressing themselves.[18,19]

A concern of the nurse is how to ascertain patients' needs for information and for other services. One study of 41 patients on a semiprivate surgical unit revealed that they often did not express their needs clearly to the nurse in their initial behavior. Some first requested concrete physical assistance, such as a bedpan, glass of water, or change in height of the bed; only as these needs were satisfactorily met did others emerge, frequently categorized as emotional. Other patients reversed this pattern; only

when they felt relief from pent-up tensions were they able to be aware of specific areas of bodily discomfort. In 30 of the 60 nurse-patient contacts, the patients' behavior was nonverbal only. The investigator also found initial behavior not to be a reliable basis for assessing the degree of discomfort.[39] These persons may therefore need considerable help in identifying and expressing their needs, and the nurse must be skilled at anticipating needs, interpreting behavior, and encouraging expression of feelings.

Compare these recommendations for determining learning needs with the behavior described in a postoperative study of 52 adult patients. These patients generally viewed nursing personnel as too busy, as disapproving, and as persons who they hated to bother. Although 76% of patients' requests were answered after the initial request, 52% of the nurse responses to those regarding medicines were delayed from 15 minutes to 2 hours and 30 minutes. Twenty-three percent of the requests were repeated by patients. Interviews with patients revealed that the number of unstated requests they had was very high.[43] This kind of environment is not conducive to helping patients become skilled at identifying and expressing their needs, both of which are educational goals for them.

It seems that hospitalization can be a time of many stresses, some of which might be relieved by teaching. Knowledge of common patient concerns and means of expressing them can help the nurse to be alert to these needs.

UTILIZING GENERAL PRINCIPLES OF MOTIVATION

There do exist basic principles of motivation that are applicable to learning in any situation.

The environment can be used to focus the patient's attention on what he is to learn. A businesslike yet warm and accepting atmosphere created by the teacher has been shown to promote continued effort and favorable attitude toward learning in children.[57] It would seem also to be successful with adults. Having in the department visual aids such as booklets for new mothers to read, posters of postpartum exercises, or equipment for practicing how to draw fluid into a syringe motivates learners by capturing their attention and curiosity.

Incentives motivate learning. These include privileges such as leaving the ward, having special treats of food, and receiving praise from a medical person or a family member. The teacher tries to determine an incentive that is likely to motivate an individual at a particular time. For some individuals and families, being able to care for their own health needs is incentive enough; they are eager to learn. For many patients, still startled that they have an illness, there is much need for the nurse-teacher to guide learning and reward appropriate behavior until they have a clearer view of their situation and become more self-motivating. In the areas of prevention of disease and promotion of health without the threat of illness, there may be very little self-motivation without rewards. It is desirable for persons to find satisfaction in learning based on their belief that the goals are useful to them or, less commonly, based on pure enjoyment of exploring new things. *This internal motivation is longer lasting and more self-directive than is external motivation, which must be repeatedly reinforced by praise or concrete rewards.* Some individuals—particularly children of certain ages but also some adults—have little capacity for internal motivation and must be guided and reinforced constantly. The use of incentives is based on the principle that learning occurs more effectively in situations from which the individual derives feelings of satisfaction.[104]

Learning is most effective when an individual is ready to learn, that is, when he feels a need to know something. The purpose of this entire chapter is to describe factors that affect readiness to learn about health so that the nurse can utilize the state when it exists or analyze why it may not be present. Sometimes readiness comes with time, and the nurse's role is to encourage its development. Depending on how urgent the desired change in behavior is, the nurse may need to use direct supervision to see that the desired behavior occurs. An example is the patient with a recent myocardial infarction who has been instructed to limit physical activity but refuses to listen because he is not intellectually convinced that he has a myocardial infarction or has not emotionally accepted it. In this instance, the nurse must expect that the patient may not be reliable in following instructions, that he must be supervised and instructions repeated again and again.

Motivation is enhanced by the way in which the material to be learned is organized. In general, the best organization is that which makes the information meaningful to the individual. One method of organization consists of relating new tasks to those already known. For example, if patients know that care for a surgical wound utilizes many of the same principles they have been using in dressing superficial wounds with Band-Aids, they are oriented to what needs to be learned. Other ways of stimulating meaning include determining whether the persons to be taught understand the final outcome desired and instructing them to compare and contrast ideas.[57]

None of the aforementioned techniques will produce sustained motivation unless the goals are realistic for the learner. The basic learning principle involved is that *success is more predictably motivating than is failure.* Ordinarily, people will choose activities of intermediate uncertainty rather than those that are very difficult (little likelihood of success) or very easy (very high probability of success); for goals of high value there is even less tendency to choose more difficult conditions.[66] Having learners assist in defining goals increases the probability that they will understand them and want to reach them. However, patients and families sometimes have very unrealistic notions of what they can accomplish. This may occur either because they do not understand the precision with which a skill must be carried out or the depth of knowledge necessary to provide adequate care—such as in the administration of insulin—or the amount of skill, strength, and determination necessary to care adequately for an invalid relative. Nurses do have this perspective and are responsible for assessing the abilities of the learners to meet the goals. The nurse may suggest that the family utilize the services of a home health aide to provide them with some of the skill and physical energy necessary for caring for the invalid. Patients with diabetes may be helped to learn routines of general hygiene and insulin administration by having a person with medical background available to assess the effectiveness of their self-care. These limited goals may be intermediate to more advanced goals, or they may be all that the individual can accomplish. In order to identify realistic goals, nurse-teachers must be skilled in assessing readiness and progress toward goals.

Sometimes the accepted goals of a health education program are beyond the readiness of a whole group of individuals who need to learn. This seemed to be the case in one study of medically indigent blacks with diabetes. This study resulted in the suggestion that the traditional teaching and therapeutic programs for the management of diabetes have been planned for the middle or upper-class patient. The diets called for a generous amount of the more expensive protein foods and a three-meal pattern. The administration of insulin requires a concept of asepsis and purchase of equipment and medicine. Keeping written records and understanding signs and symptoms necessitate abstract thinking. Many of these behaviors are unrealistic goals for the medically indigent, uneducated individual.[4]

Because it requires change in beliefs and behavior, learning normally produces a mild level of anxiety, which is useful in motivating the individual; however, severe anxiety is incapacitating.[57] A high degree of stress is inherent in some of the situations nurses encounter. During an emergency, teaching-learning is at a mini-

mum, because other goals are more important and anxiety is very high. Individuals with less severe health crises may also react with intense anxiety because they are threatened by what has occured. As anxiety becomes severe, the individuals' perception of what is going on around them becomes limited; they are oriented more toward gaining relief than toward attending to learning, and they show advancing physical signs and symptoms of anxiety.[85] For this reason, mothers who are highly distressed because of their children's illness may be quite unable to learn skills with which to care for them. Nurses must be able to identify such anxiety and realize its effect on learning. They also have an obligation to avoid needlessly inducing severe anxiety by such behavior as setting ambiguous or unrealistically high goals.

These general principles of motivation are interrelated. A single teaching action can utilize many of them simultaneously. For example, having a display of teaching pamphlets available in the patient lounge of a maternity floor may focus the patients' attention on things to be learned, utilizing their natural curiosity about such subjects as breast feeding or postpartum exercises. The content in these pamphlets is aimed at helping patients set and attain realistic goals and often is organized to relate new material to that which most women know. Such a display can also communicate to the patients the staff's interest in their learning and encourage questions.

Finally, let it be said that an enormous gap exists between knowing that health behavior is motivated and identifying the specific motivational components of any particular act. The nurse-teacher's focus has to be on learning patterns of motivation for an individual or group, with the realization that errors will not be uncommon.

ASSESSING READINESS

Nurse-teachers must possess certain knowledge and skills in order to assess readiness. They must understand the subject matter to be learned, for this allows them to compare the difficulty of the skill with what the patient already knows or is able to do. For example, they cannot assess whether a patient can learn to care for a colostomy if they know little or nothing about a colostomy and its care. Nurses should also know the desired degree of independence for patients with a particular condition. For the person with a colostomy, the goal is daily care of it, knowledge of factors that affect it (such as diet), and ability to recognize complications that require medical attention. The question facing nurses is: Is the person capable of learning these behaviors?

These decisions are based on information about an individual's knowledge and beliefs gathered by interview and study of available records. Then, the patient behaviors essential to effective treatment are written out, and educational experiences are planned. The same approach is used when the family, a neighborhood, or a community is the learner.

General information collected when a patient is admitted to a health agency is useful in assessing need for and acceptance of teaching. Knowledge of socioeconomic class, which can be judged by occupation and amount of education, suggests certain kinds of health beliefs and behavior. Age indicates the developmental tasks with which the individual probably is concerned and allows speculation as to willingness to accept certain restrictions or to experience growth. Knowledge of the basic composition of the family helps the nurse to anticipate the patient's responsibilities and sources of influence on his or her health beliefs and actions. Knowledge of the diagnosis brings to mind the patient behaviors essential to successful treatment. Information recorded by the physician on history, physical examination, and progress provides some information as to what the physical and mental capabilities of the patient may be. Goals of medical care are recorded, and what the patient needs to know to reach these goals may be surmised. The medical history, although rarely concerned with the person's knowledge and

health beliefs, does indicate what medical experiences the patient has had and how he has acted in relation to seeking and following medical care. Having old charts available increases the amount and detail of available information. From data such as these, contained in hospital and medical records, nurses can gather some beginning notions about the individual's readiness. They must then validate and extend these notions through their communication with the patient.

One of the techniques for validation is the interview. Such a means is often used to obtain information for a nursing history, which is then used in planning nursing care. Since patient learning is part of the general plan of nursing care, the history should be structured to include items useful for accomplishment of teaching-learning as well as other goals. Both the history and the plan of care that an agency or an individual nurse uses reflect the philosophy of nursing. A philosophy that values the meaning of illness and hospitalization to the patient and his family might include obtaining the following kinds of information about an ill patient:

1. Patient's perceptions and expectations. Why he sought care, what he thinks caused him to get sick, and how his illness has affected his usual way of life tend to reveal his understanding of his condition and how it has affected him. What hospitalization means to him is learned by asking what he expcts will happen to him, what it is like to be in the hospital, and how long he expects to stay. How he expects to manage after hospitalization and his view of the effects of his illness and hospitalization on his family or on other significant persons are also important.

2. Patient's ability to meet his basic needs, such as rest, elimination, nutrition, comfort, safety, personal hygiene, and, from that description, nursing intervention on which he and the nurse agree.[67]

For children, part or all of this information may be obtained from the adult responsible for their care; questions may be included about how they communicate verbally and nonverbally. An approach used with children 4½ to 7 years of age includes asking simple questions about why they came to the hospital, what bothers them, and what their parents have told them. This may disclose fantasies that might be missed if the nurse merely begins to tell them what is going to happen. Not infrequently, children deny any knowledge, which can be merely an expression of their hope that if they deny the event, it will not take place.[86]

Besides the interview, observations of children at play reveal mastery of experiences, levels of intellectual functioning, relationships with other children, and perceptions of illness and treatment.

There are several purposes for obtaining this kind of information. One is to use it to provide conditions that will help patients function in a strange environment, such as a hospital, and to allow them to follow, as much as possible, patterns of living that are satisfying to them at home. Second, the staff then knows more about the person's health behavior, and this aids in determining what an individual might need to learn. Although nurses gather this kind of information from conversing with patients while they are giving care, the advantage of writing down the results of the interview is that they can be found as part of the record and therefore are consistently available for all patients and are more easily utilized.

There is no substitute for informal nurse-client interaction to gain rapport and assess the client's basic concerns, some of which can be alleviated by teaching. Under these conditions, the patient may ask such questions as how to follow the physician's instructions or what a particular symptom means. A patient may also present cues, as is true of the lady with congestive heart failure who says, "My feet look swollen today"; the 20-year-old girl who says she does not brush her teeth because her gums bleed; or the patient who tells the nurse that she

wants to save the menu from her tray so that she can follow her special diet at home. A patient who is newly paraplegic is commonly not ready to participate in a bladder training program and during the first few months may tend to ignore the bladder disability and refuse to take part in the necessary procedures. A cue of readiness is presented when the patient shows interest in what the nurse is doing and/or asks to participate.[32]

These responses require further probing to determine how much the patient does know, since patients may ask questions for many reasons other than lack of understanding, such as wanting the nurse to stay with them or wanting someone in the role of parent-surrogate. Sometimes the cues are not verbal but present themselves as the nurse observes the patient's body and behavior. The mother who is obviously inept in handling her baby but who does not ask for instruction needs to be questioned further to assess her readiness.

Although much can be learned about readiness by providing a milieu in which natural behavior will occur, there are also times when a specially structured situation will provide the most accurate information. An example is asking a mother and father separately what they have been told by physicians and others about their mentally retarded child and what is their own estimation of the child's condition and mental age.[77]

There are many kinds of disorders with which nurses work that require special knowledge of common learning deficits and skill in assessing the extent and quality of the deficit. Although such special instruction is beyond the scope of this book, which deals with the process common to all teaching-learning in nursing, it is readily available elsewhere. Nursing of patients with aphasia is an especially pertinent example, since nurses do use techniques of speech reeducation in their dealings with such patients. Valuable resources for nurses working with aphasic patients may be found in an article by

Miller[77] and in filmstrip-tape format.[23] Similarly, nurses who work with retarded children learn skill in evaluating growth and development that deviates from normal and in determining readiness for further learning. For teaching complex motor skills like walking, they must determine whether component parts are present, such as head control and truncal support while sitting, equilibrium responses while sitting or kneeling, or parachute responses. A nurse working with a child who did not possess these skills in sufficient amount to begin walking set up a program of exercises specific for helping to develop the prior walking behaviors the child did not have, such as swaying and learning to catch himself in the sitting posture. After equilibrium responses were evident in this posture, the nurse followed the same schedule for the kneeling posture.[7]

There are currently only a few written instruments available for assessment of readiness for health teaching. One such instrument is a Semantic Differential Test that measures beliefs about particular diseases. The significance of measuring these beliefs is that what the public thinks and feels about any disease can be a strong determinant of its response to preventive case finding and therapeutic programs, and many of these beliefs are not easily verbalized. Various diseases arouse feelings of different qualities and intensities that may contribute to differences in motivation for seeking health care. Some scales of this Semantic Differential Test are intended to measure beliefs about susceptibility to disease (how many people get it, at what age, the chance *you* have of getting it), the severity of a disease (amount of pain caused, how frequently it causes death, how fast-moving it is), and its prominence in public thought and discussion (how often it is talked about, how often you think about it).[48] The Semantic Differential Test provides information about two of the four beliefs thought important in taking health action—susceptibility and effect on life. It does not consider preventive actions or the threat of taking these actions weighed against the threat of the disease. Besides being useful in assessing current beliefs in preparation for an educational program, the instrument can also be used to evaluate belief change as a result of an educational program.[48]

Through these techniques, assessment is made of what individuals want and need to learn and what their levels of understanding, skill, and motivation are. Every member of the nursing team ought to be able, to some degree, to identify readiness for learning. Those workers with the least formal education are often with patients a great deal and may be quite perceptive regarding the meaning of their behaviors. In addition, some patients may relate to these individuals better than they would to a registered nurse or physician. Of the nursing team, it is professional nurses who study in greatest depth the meaning of behavior and the teaching-learning process. They are likely to be best prepared to know what information should be gathered and how it can be obtained and used to formulate realistic learning goals. It would seem useful to gather material regarding learning readiness in one section of the patient's chart, perhaps on a teaching record. A form is suggested in a later chapter.

SUMMARY

This chapter deals with assessing readiness, which is composed of motivation, experiential background, and ability to learn. Knowledge of patterns of health beliefs, behavior, and the psychosocial impact of illness helps the nurse to anticipate certain levels of readiness. General principles of motivation, valid in any learning situation, should be utilized to attain efficient learning. Assessing readiness requires of the nurse an understanding of the aims of health teaching and skill in gathering and validating information, by means of interview, informal conversation, observation, available tools, and health records.

STUDY QUESTIONS

1. Design a nursing interview, to be used at hospital admission, that you believe contains the major items needed to assess learning readiness.
2. What questions would you ask to assess readiness to learn in each of the following nursing situations?
   a. You are going to catheterize a patient after delivery.
   b. As a public health nurse you visit the home of a sick 3-year-old child and must help the mother carry out the physician's orders to force fluids.
   c. As a nurse working in a gynecology clinic, you are to teach breast self-examination to groups of women in the waiting room.
   d. As a public health nurse you are to teach a 10-year-old boy who is mentally retarded, blind, and suffering from cerebral palsy how to feed himself.
3. For each description of patient behavior that follows, indicate possible explanations in terms of the psychosocial adaptation to illness model.

   The importance of proper timing and sensitivity to the patient's feelings was made evident in the case of Mike S., a 21-year-old college student who sustained a T10 fracture in a skiing accident. His first admission lasted three months; during this time he was apathetic and easily discouraged. He preferred to stay in bed as much as possible, covering himself from head to toe with a sheet. A common statement heard in reference to Mike was, "He certainly has potential but just won't use it. . . ."

   A trial of voiding was attempted even though Mike indicated he didn't care if it worked or not. Needless to say, the trial was unsuccessful. . . .

   It was true that Mike did have potential for rehabilitation, but he was unable to mobilize this potential because he did not yet have the necessary strength to accept his disabled body. Not only was his bladder in shock, but also his mind and spirit. Mike was discharged to his home to return in three months. He left as an angry, depressed young man, unable to see much future in his life as a paraplegic. . . .

   On readmission, there was a noticeable change in Mike's attitude toward himself. He had obviously used his three-month vacation from the hospital in a constructive way. He had developed many plans and ideas to improve his self-care. He was also interested in getting rid of the catheter. . . .*

4. Do you agree or disagree with the following statement: The better nurses understand the patient, the more success they should have in getting him to follow their advice in matters related to his health? Explain why you agree or disagree.
5. The following statement is from Conte and others:

   Some of our patients revealed that when they were first advised to take anti-hypertensive medications, they had doubts as to the accuracy of the diagnosis. Some said they had taken their hypertension seriously only after an unusual or frightening event had occurred as a result of their hypertension or after they learned of its dangers. This suggests that early patient education regarding hypertension could prevent many unnecessary complications.*

   Do you agree?

REFERENCES

1. Alt, R. E.: Patient education program answers many unanswered questions, Hospitals **40:**76-78, 166, Nov. 16, 1966.
2. Anderson, H. C.: Newton's geriatric nursing, ed. 5, St. Louis, 1971, The C. V. Mosby Co.
3. Anderson, O. W.: The utilization of health services. In Freeman, H. E., Levine, S., and Reeder, L.G., editors: Handbook of medical sociology, Englewood Cliffs, N.J., 1963, Prentice-Hall, Inc.
4. Anderson, R. S., Gunter, L. M., and Kennedy, E. J.: Evaluation of clinical, cultural and psychosomatic influences in the teaching and management of diabetic patients; a study of medically indigent Negro patients, Am. J. Med. Sci. **245:**682-690, 1963.
5. Auerbach, S. M., and others: Anxiety, locus of control, type of preparatory information and adjustment to dental surgery, J. Consult. Clin. Psychol. **44:**809-818, 1976.
6. Baltimore, C. L., and Meyer, R. J.: A study of storage, child behavioral traits, and mother's knowledge of toxicology in 52 poisoned families and 52 comparison families, Pediatrics **42:**312-317, 1968.
7. Barnard, K.: Teaching the retarded child is a family affair, Am. J. Nurs. **68:**305-311, Feb. 1968.
8. Becker, M. H.: The health belief model and sick role behavior, Health Educ. Monogr. **2:**409-419, 1974.
9. Becker, M. H., and Maiman, L. A.: Sociobehavioral determinants of compliance with health and medical care recommendations, Med. Care **13:**10-24, 1975.
10. Becker, M. H., and others: A new approach to explaining sick-role behavior in low-income populations, Am. J. Public Health **64:**205-216, 1974.
11. Becker, M. H., and others: Some influences on public

*Delehanty, L., and Stravino, V.: Achieving bladder control, Am. J. Nurs. **70:**312-316, Feb. 1970.

*Conte, A., and others: Group work with hypertensive patients, Am. J. Nurs. **74:**910-912, 1974.

participation in a genetic screening program, J. Community Health **1:**3-14, 1975.

12. Becker, M. H., and others: The health belief model and prediction of dietary compliance; a field experiment, J. Health Soc. Behav. **18:**348-366, 1977.

13. Becker, M. H., and others: Compliance with a medical regimen for asthma; a test of the health belief model, Public Health Rep. **93:**268-277, 1978.

14. Bergman, A. B., and Werner, R. J.: Failure of children to receive penicillin by mouth, New Engl. J. Med. **268:**1334-1338, 1963.

15. Berkowitz, N. H., Malone, M. F., and Klein, M. W.: Patient care as a criterion problem, J. Health Hum. Behav. **3:**171-176, 1962.

16. Blackwell, B.: The literature of delay in seeking medical care for chronic illnesses, Health Educ. Monogr. **16:**3-31, 1963.

17. Blackwell, B.: Anticipated pre-medical care activities of upper middle-class adults and their implications for health education practice, Health Educ. Monogr. **17:**17-36, 1964.

18. Blake, F. G.: Immobilized youth; a rationale for supportive nursing intervention, Am. J. Nurs. **69:**2364-2369, Nov. 1969.

19. Blake, F. G., Wright, F. H., and Waechter, E. H.: Nursing care of children, ed. 8, Philadelphia, 1970, J. B. Lippincott Co.

20. Bloom, S. W.: The doctor and his patient; a sociological interpretation, New York, 1963, Russell Sage Foundation.

21. Burt, M. M.: Perceptual deficits in hemiplegia, Am. J. Nurs. **70:**1026-1029, May 1970.

22. Christman, L.: Assisting the patient to learn the "patient role," J. Nurs. Educ. **61:**17-21, April 1967.

23. Concept Media: The stroke patient (filmstrips and records), Costa Mesa, Calif.

24. Crate, M. A.: Nursing functions in adaptation to chronic illness, Am. J. Nurs. **65:**72-76, Oct.1965.

25. Cumming, J., and Cumming, E.: Mental health education in a Canadian community. In Paul, B. D., editor: Health, culture, and community, New York, 1955, Russell Sage Foundation.

26. Cummings, J. W.: Hemodialysis—feelings, facts, fantasies; the pressures and how patients respond, Am. J. Nurs. **70:**70-75, Jan. 1970.

27. Daniels, A. M.: Reaching unwed adolescent mothers, Am. J. Nurs. **69:**332-335, Feb. 1969.

28. Davis, M. E., and Rubin, R.: DeLee's obstetrics for nurses, ed. 18, Philadelphia, 1966, W. B. Saunders Co.

29. Davis, M. S., and Eichorn, R. L.: Compliance with medical regimens; a panel study, J. Health Hum. Behav. **4:**240-249, 1963.

30. Deasy, L. C.: Socio-economic status and participation in the poliomyelitis vaccine trial. In Apple, D., editor: Sociological studies of health and sickness, New York, 1960, McGraw-Hill Book Co.

31. Deci, E. L.: Intrinsic motivation, New York, 1975, Plenum Press.

32. Delehanty, L., and Stravino, V.: Achieving bladder control, Am. J. Nurs. **70:**312-316, Feb. 1970.

33. Derow, H. A.: The nephrotic syndrome (concluded), N. Engl. J. Med. **258:**124-129, 1958.

34. Deuschle, K., and Hochstrasser, D.: Doctors and patients; some human factors in tuberculosis control, Bull. Int. Union Tuberc. **36:**74-82, 1965.

35. DiCicco, L., and Apple, D.: Health needs and opinions of older adults. In Apple, D., editor: Sociological studies of health and sickness, New York, 1960, McGraw-Hill Book Co.

36. Dlouhy, A., and others: What patients want to know about their diagnostic tests, Nurs. Outlook **11:**265-267, 1963.

37. Dodge, J. S.: Factors related to patients' perceptions of their cognitive needs, Nurs. Res. **18:**502-513, 1969.

38. Dunnell, K., and Cartwright, A.: Medicine takers, prescribers and hoarders, London, 1972, Routledge & Kegan Paul.

39. Elder, R. G.: What is the patient saying? Nurs. Forum **2**(1):24-37, 1963.

40. Erikson, E. H.: Identity; youth and crisis, New York, 1968, W. W. Norton & Co., Inc.

41. Freidson, E., and Feldman, J. J.: The public looks at dental care. Research series No. 6, New York, 1958, Health Information Foundation. Cited in Anderson, O. W.: The utilization of health services. In Freeman, H. E., Levine, S., and Reeder, L. G., editors: Handbook of medical sociology, Englewood Cliffs, N.J., 1963, Prentice-Hall, Inc.

42. Getting people to accept modern medical service, Public Health Rep. **3:**229-230, 1966.

43. Gowan, N. M., and Morris, M.: Nurses' responses to expressed patient needs, Nurs. Res. **13:**68-71, 1964.

44. Haefner, D. P.: The health belief model and preventive dental behavior, Health Educ. Monogr. **2:**433-454, 1974.

45. Hollingshead, A. B., and Redlich, F. C.: Social class and mental illness; a community study, New York, 1958, John Wiley & Sons, Inc.

46. Hurd, G. G.: Teaching the hemiplegic self-care, Am. J. Nurs. **62:**64-68, Sept. 1962.

47. Irelan, L. M., editor: Low-income life styles, Washington, D.C., U.S. Government Printing Office.

48. Jenkins, C. D.: The semantic differential for health; a technique for measuring beliefs about diseases, Public Health Rep. **81:**549-558, 1966.

49. Johnson, D. E.: Powerlessness; a significant deter-

minant in patient behavior? J. Nurs. Educ. **6:**39-44, April 1967.

50. Kariel, P. E.: The dynamics of behavior in relation to health, Nurs. Outlook **10:**402-405, June 1962.

51. Kasl, S. V.: The health belief model and behavior related to chronic illness, Health Educ. Monogr. **2:**433-454, 1974.

52. Kassebaum, G. G., and Baumann, B. O.: Dimensions of the sick role in chronic illness, J. Health Hum. Behav. **6:**16-27, 1965.

53. Kauffman, E. L.: A study concerning patients' perception of stress within a university hospital setting and patients' perception of the nurse's role in reducing stress (unpublished master's thesis, Seattle, 1965, The University of Washington).

54. Kegeles, S. S.: Why people seek dental care; a review of present knowledge, Am. J. Public Health **51:**1306-1311, 1961.

55. Kegeles, S. S.: Attitudes and behavior of the public regarding cervical cytology; current findings and new directions for research, J. Chronic Dis. **20:**911-922, 1967.

56. Kennell, J. H., and others: What parents of rheumatic fever patients don't understand about the disease and its prophylactic management, Pediatrics **43:**160-167, 1969.

57. Klausmeier, H. J., and Ripple, R.: Learning and human abilities; educational psychology, ed. 4, New York, 1975, Harper & Row, Publishers.

58. Kluckhohn, F. R., and Strodtbeck, F. L.: Variations in value orientations, Evanston, Ill., 1961, Row, Peterson & Co.

59. Koos, E. L.: The health of Regionville, New York, 1954, Columbia University Press.

60. Lederer, H. D.: How the sick view their world, J. Soc. Issues **8**(4):4-15, 1952.

61. Litman, T. J.: Health care and the family; a three-generational analysis, Med. Care **9:**67-81, 1971.

62. Looff, D. H.: Appalachia's children, Lexington, 1971, University of Kentucky Press.

63. Lowell, F.: Personal communication. Cited in Stoeckle, J. D., Zola, I. K., and Davidson, G. E.: On going to see the doctor, the contributions of the patient to the decision to seek medical aid, J. Chronic Dis. **16:**975-989, 1963.

64. Lowery, B. J., and DuCette, J. P.: Disease-related learning and disease control in diabetics as a function of locus of control, Nurs. Res. **25:**358-362, 1976.

65. McCabe, G. S.: Cultural influences on patient behavior, Am. J. Nurs. **60:**1101-1104, Aug. 1960.

66. McDaniel, J. W.: Physical disability and human behavior, New York, 1969, Pergamon Press.

67. McPhetridge, L. M.: Nursing history; one means to personalize care, Am. J. Nurs. **68:**68-75, Jan. 1968.

68. McQueen, D. V.: Social aspects of genetic screening for Tay-Sachs disease; the pilot community screening program in Baltimore and Washington, Soc. Biol. **22:**125-133, 1975.

69. Marston, M. V.: Compliance with medical regimens; a review of the literature, Nurs. Res. **19:**312-323, 1970.

70. Maslow, A. H.: A theory of human motivation, Psychol. Rev. **50:**370-396, 1943.

71. Matheny, A. P., Jr., and Vernick, J.: Parents of the mentally retarded child; emotionally overwhelmed or informationally deprived? J. Pediatr. **74:**953-959, 1969.

72. Matson, R. R., and Brooks, N. A.: Adjusting to multiple sclerosis; an exploratory study, Soc. Sci. Med. **11:**245-250, 1977.

73. Mechanic, D.: Illness and cure. In Kosa, J., Antonovsky, A., and Zola, I. K.: Poverty and health; a sociological analysis, Cambridge, Mass., 1969, Harvard University Press.

74. Mechanic, D.: Public expectations and health care, New York, 1972, John Wiley & Sons, Inc.

75. Meinhart, N. T., and Aspinall, M. J.: Nursing interventions in hypovigilance, Am. J. Nurs. **69:**994-998, May 1969.

76. Milio, N.: Values, social class, and community health services, Nurs. Res. **16:**26-30, 1967.

77. Miller, L. G.: Toward a greater understanding of the parents of the mentally retarded child, J. Pediatr. **73:**699-705, 1968.

78. Morris, N., Hatch, M. H., and Chipman, S. S.: Deterrents to well-child supervision, Am. J. Public Health **56:**1232-1241, 1966.

79. Moulding, T.: New responsibilities for health departments and public health nurses in tuberculosis—keeping the outpatient on therapy, Am. J. Public Health **56:**416-427, 1966.

80. Nathanson, G. A.: Sex roles as variables in preventive health behavior, J. Community Health **3:**142-155, 1977.

81. Neely, E., and Patrick, M. L.: Problems of aged persons taking medications at home, Nurs. Res. **17:**52-55, 1968.

82. Newman, M. A.: Identifying and meeting patients' needs in short-span nurse-patient relationships, Nurs. Forum **5**(1):76-86, 1966.

83. Norris, C. M.: The work of getting well, Am. J. Nurs. **69:**2118-2121, Oct. 1969.

84. Nite, G., and Willis, F. N., Jr.: The coronary patient; hospital care and rehabilitation, New York, 1964, The Macmillan Co.

85. Peplau, H. E.: A working definition of anxiety. In Burd, S. F., and Marshall, M. A., editors: Some clinical approaches to psychiatric nursing, New York, 1963, The Macmillan Co.

86. Petrillo, M.: Preventing hospital trauma in pediatric patients, Am. J. Nurs. **68:**1469-1473, July 1968.

87. Phares, E. J.: The locus of control in personality, Morristown, N.J., 1976, General Learning Press.

88. Polgar, S.: Health and human behavior; areas of interest common to the social and medical sciences, Curr. Anthropol. **3:**159-179, 1962.

89. Political and economic planning: Family needs and the social services, London, 1961, George Allen & Unwin Ltd. Cited in Anderson, O. W.: The utilization of health services. In Freeman, H. E., Levine, S., and Reeder, L. G., editors: Handbook of medical sociology, Englewood Cliffs, N.J., 1963, Prentice-Hall, Inc.

90. Pomeroy, M. R.: Sudden death syndrome, Am. J. Nurs. **69:**1886-1890, Sept. 1969.

91. Pratt, L., Seligmann, A., and Reader, G.: Physicians' views on the level of medical information among patients. In Jaco, E. G., editor: Patients, physicians and illness, New York, 1958, The Free Press.

92. Roberts, B. J.: A framework for consideration of forces in achieving earliness of treatment, Health Educ. Monogr. **19,** 1965.

93. Robinson, D.: The process of becoming ill, London, 1971, Routledge & Kegan Paul.

94. Rosenfeld, L. S., and Donabedian, A.: Prenatal care in metropolitan Boston, Am. J. Public Health **48:**1115-1124, 1958.

95. Rosenstock, I. M.: What research in motivation suggests for public health, Am. J. Public Health **50:**295-302, 1960.

96. Rosenstock, I. M.: Public response to cancer screening and detection programs; determinants of health behavior, J. Chronic Dis. **16:**407-418, 1963.

97. Rosenstock, I. M.: The health belief model and preventive health behavior, Health Educ. Monogr. **2:**354-386, 1974.

98. Rosenstock, I. M.: Historical origins of the health belief model, Health Educ. Monogr. **2:**328-335, 1974.

99. Rosenstock, I. M., and Kirscht, J. P.: Practice implications, Health Educ. Monogr. **2:**470-473, 1974.

100. Roth, H. P., and Berger, D. G.: Studies on patient cooperation in ulcer treatment. I. Observation of actual as compared to prescribed antacid intake on a hospital ward, Gastroenterology **38:**630-633, 1960.

101. Roth, H. P., and Caron, H. S.: Patients' misconceptions about their peptic ulcer diets; potential obstacles to cooperation, J. Chronic Dis. **20:**5-11, 1967.

102. Roth, H. P., and others: Patients' beliefs about peptic ulcer and its treatment, Ann. Intern. Med. **56:**72-80, 1962.

103. Russell, R. D.: Motivational factors as related to health behavioral change. In Veenker, C. H., editor: Synthesis of research in selected areas of health instruction, Washington, D.C., 1963, The School Health Education Study.

104. Sand, O.: Curriculum study in basic nursing education, New York, 1955, G. P. Putnam's Sons.

105. Schwartz, D., Henley, B., and Zeitz, L.: The elderly ambulatory patient; nursing and psychosocial needs, New York, 1964, The Macmillan Co.

106. Seligman, M. E. P.: Helplessness, San Francisco, 1975, W. H. Freeman and Co.

107. Shontz, F. C.: Psychological adjustment to physical disability; trends in theories, Arch. Phys. Med. Rehabil. **59:**251-254, 1978.

108. Simonds, S. K.: Emerging challenges in health education, Int. J. Health Educ. **19**(Suppl. to No. 4), 1976.

109. Skipper, J. K., Jr.: Communication and the hospitalized patient. In Skipper, J. K., Jr., and Leonard, R. C., editors: Social interaction and patient care, Philadelphia, 1965, J. B. Lippincott Co.

110. Snow, L. F.: Folk medical beliefs and their implications for care of patients, Ann. Intern. Med. **81:**82-96, 1974.

111. Snow, L. F., and others: The behavioral implications of some old wives' tales, Obstet. Gynecol. **51:**727-732, 1978.

112. Stoeckle, J. D., Zola, I. K., and Davidson, G. E.: On going to see the doctor; the contributions of the patient to the decision to seek medical aid, J. Chronic Dis. **16:**975-989, 1963.

113. Suchman, E. A.: Sociology and the field of public health, New York, 1963, Russell Sage Foundation.

114. Suchman, E. A.: Social factors in medical deprivation, Am. J. Public Health **55:**1725-1733, 1965.

115. Suchman, E. A.: Social patterns of illness and medical care, J. Health Hum. Behav. **6:**2-16, 1965.

116. Suchman, E. A.: Stages of illness and medical care, J. Health Hum. Behav. **6:**114-128, 1965.

117. Suchman, E. A.: Evaluative research; principles and practice in public service and social action on programs, New York, 1967, Russell Sage Foundation.

118. Utah Tuberculosis and Heart Association: Downtown Salt Lake City socio-cultural study, Salt Lake City, 1964, The Association. Cited in Drenckhahn, V. V.: Educational role of the nurse in chronic disease control, Public Health Rep. **80:**1103-1106, 1965.

119. Wiedenbach, E.: Family-centered maternity nursing, ed. 2, New York, 1967, G. P. Putnam's Sons.

120. You can be too optimistic about your health, Public Health Rep. **80:**130-131, 1965.

121. Zborowski, M.: People in pain, San Francisco, 1969, Jossey-Bass, Inc., Publishers.

122. Zola, I. K.: Pathways to the doctor—from person to patient, Soc. Sci. Med. **7:**677-689, 1973.

CHAPTER 4

Objectives of health teaching in nursing

■ The objectives, or goals, of health teaching are the behaviors desired as a result of the learning process. They are determined by the health team and are based on what the individual's state of health and social situation require and what he is capable of learning. Objectives guide teaching and learning activities, and the major purpose of evaluation is to determine whether or not objectives have been met, that is, whether the individual can perform the desired behavior. Knowledgeable decisions as to what the goals should be and precise, complete statement of them provide clear direction in teaching the client. Poorly determined goals or poor statement of them produces confusion throughout the entire teaching-learning process. This chapter is concerned with determination of goals, with rules for statement to make them functional, and with the usefulness of a system of classifying behaviors to be attained.

BEHAVIORAL OBJECTIVES AS EDUCATIONAL TOOLS

With present knowledge of teaching and learning, it is not possible to predict all the goals that should or will be met during a particular teaching episode. Because of this inadequacy, some individuals take the position that specification of objectives before instruction is restrictive. This position challenges the teacher's ability to predetermine what the learner needs and also charges that the narrow focus of predetermined objectives restricts instruction that does not serve to meet those goals but that might be of considerable value. Although the degree of validity of this argument is not really known, the weight of present opinion does support the use of objectives, with the caution to avoid letting them become overprescriptive and with constant alertness to the fact that unintended objectives do occur.

At this time, behavioral objectives form the only well-worked-out system of planning in education. Since the lack of an adequate model of learning is one of the particular weaknesses of the systematic approach that requires prespecification of objectives, other useful schemes, such as disjointed incrementalism and correction of determination of objectives through feedback, are adopted. Many people combine all three of these approaches and use them when appropriate. Disjointed incrementalism involves moving toward short-term goals, without a clear notion of what long-range goals are, or specifying objectives in terms of moving away from what everyone agrees is a bad situation. In the feedback model, one may have either a general or fairly specific notion of the learning goals, but these goals are at least seen as fallible tools and at most made clear by outcomes of teaching-learning. Constraints of time, especially when one is entering a new area of learning, are best suited to nonspecified approaches. Teachers, however, should not allow themselves to construct excuses for avoiding the hard work of determining what needs to be learned.

Other weaknesses of behavioral objectives are: (1) They do not show the complex manner in which ideas are related and therefore have no higher-level structure; (2) other than hunch or intuition, there exist no procedures for justifying the exclusion or inclusion of a given objective, unless it relates to an obviously unnecessary task; (3) there is no consistent view of the origin of objectives; (4) they conflict with exploratory learning; and (5) they often communicate intent ambiguously.[27]

Work on nursing diagnoses provides other classification systems that serve to integrate nursing activity, including learning and teaching. A diagnostic category such as "lack of understanding" is primarily focused on teaching-learning[18]; for other categories, such as "inadequate mobility-device management," inadequate information and skill can form one possible cause.[8] Other diagnostic categories, such as "anxiety" or "confusion," provide information about readiness. The category systems also provide a goal by naming a patient state believed to be desirable or undesirable.

RELATIONSHIP OF A PHILOSOPHY TO OBJECTIVES

A philosophy is a statement of beliefs regarding the conduct of human affairs. Nurses face several questions of philosophy with regard to patient teaching. One such issue concerns how much and what information should be shared with clients and how much independence should be allowed clients or should be required of them while participating in health care. Beliefs regarding this matter may be altered when researchers are able to describe more fully the effects of giving information to or withholding it from patients and the effects of teaching them independence or dependence. Following are

questions relating to this issue, which nurses will encounter: Is it the patient's right to know about results of the diagnostic process and about prognosis? Should a patient's denial of his own imminent death be allowed or broken? How much care is it desirable for parents to be taught to give to their hospitalized child? Should prospective parents be prepared to make choices with regard to the care that their children receive or be taught to accept one method of care? One children's hospital has organized its patient-teaching program around the philosophy of helping parents to be partners in furthering the recovery of their child, since the ultimate care of that child rests with the parent.[1]

A related question is who should determine what the patient is to be taught. A moderate and generally accepted position is that the health team respects the physician's general philosophy of management unless they feel that it is having a deleterious effect on the client. From this position there are variations. At one extreme are those who believe that the physician's judgment regarding patient teaching should not be challenged; at the opposite extreme are those who support the position that members of the health team have areas of special competence in which their judgment regarding teaching should be paramount. The usefulness of agreement between the members of the health team cannot be denied, since it prevents presenting the patient with conflicting directions that may immobilize learning.

Another facet regarding how much the patient should know has to do with the roles of the patient and family as members of the health team in determining what they are to learn. Patients are in the unique position of being able to control what is finally learned, but they should participate in a much more positive way. The line between trying to motivate patients and invading their privacy can be very thin and depends on the nurse's philosophy about the patients' ability and right to determine their own course. Increasingly, groups of health care consumers, in neighborhood clinics and elsewhere, are demanding the right to determine their own courses, and philosophies of many professionals are being challenged and altered or are being reaffirmed. Teaching seems to be more effective when the patient's and nurse's goals are similar; however, even if goals are divergent, intervention is possible. In this instance, professional responsibility may be seen by some as promotion of readiness in the patient.

In order to promote a unity of purpose on the part of staff and patients, the nursing services of many health agencies have developed statements of philosophy and goals by which they function. Although the term "teaching" is not always used, one finds goals stated that imply teaching, such as the goal to assist the patient in his acceptance of and adjustment to his condition and the goal that:

As coordinator of the patient's care the nurse supports his right to make decisions regarding his care. Nursing also has the responsibility to interpret daily hospital experiences and to provide emotional, physical, and spiritual support for the patient as well as to help him to maintain his family and community roles.[40]

It is recommended that nurses compare an agency's statement of philosophy and goals with their own beliefs and, if they find conflict, question whether or not they can function satisfactorily in that agency. An agreement in philosophies would mean, for example, that nurses who strongly believe that patients must be helped to see the religious significance of their illnesses would best function in an agency with the same philosophy. In contrast, nurses who do not have this orientation or do not possess training in religious doctrine cannot fulfill the expected role in such an institution. The same comparison might be made regarding the commitment to and expected degree of proficiency in the teaching function on the part of the nurse and on the part of the agency.

At times, nurses, patients, families, or members of a health agency staff challenge an agency's stated philosophy or point out violations of it by members of the agency, hoping to force a resolution of the discrepancy. Indeed, all staff members must be alert to such discrepancies and be aware that they can undermine the purpose of the institution, but that at times they represent a redefinition of purpose that is essential to progress.

In the ways just discussed, then, philosophies regarding the role of patient education in health care and the roles of members of the health team in meeting the goals of patient education affect what the nurse might teach the patient.

DETERMINATION OF LEARNING OBJECTIVES

In determining the objectives for a particular client, nurses need to consider not only the philosophic setting in which they are working but also the goals that can be accomplished by teaching and the readiness of the person to learn.

Objectives for patients in general

The general goal of health teaching is to assist individuals in developing their optimal health potential. For example, an objective of nursing maternity patients is to strengthen the parents' inner resources so that they may be better able to participate in the childbearing experience and gain satisfaction from it.[42] Part of this objective is achieved through teaching. General goals for all patients might be as follows: to make rational decisions about health, to participate effectively in care and cure, to adjust to realities of the health situation, to feel satisfaction in working toward health.[31]

Besides having an orientation to general goals in health teaching, nurses need to know the feasibility of meeting particular goals by means of teaching. For example, it is doubtful that nurses could expect to be successful in teaching unwed mothers not to become involved in any more out-of-wedlock pregnancies. A more realistic goal might be to develop added awareness of reality, which may influence the mother's behavior in the future.[3] Some patients with hypertension apparently cannot be persuaded of the dangers of the disorder until a frightening event has occurred as a result of it.[11] On the other hand, preoperative instruction of patients about to undergo surgery is apt to be successful. The series of studies about preoperative instruction, reviewed in Chapters 1 and 10, provide confidence that teaching-counseling techniques can be used by nurses to aid in successful postoperative recovery.

There are a number of examples of objectives that have been considered important for persons in certain situations. Analysis of skills required and influencing factors can help to provide a perspective regarding the teachers' and learners' tasks.

Family member caring for sick person

Skills required. The family member must report to the home-care team and carry out their instructions concerning administration of medications and measuring of sugar and other elements in urine; regulation of diet, fluid, and exertion; supervision of active exercises including proper use of braces, crutches, prostheses, or wheelchair; use of special equipment for treatments, as in oxygen administration, intermittent positive pressure breathing, catheter and tube care, wound care, and heat therapy; bathing and dressing; physical assistance in moving, such as help with transfers, use of patient lift, and passive exercises; toilet care and incontinence care; full-time supervision of feeding and other activities; courage and determination.

Influencing factors. Sicker and more fragile patients can be maintained at home more easily now than previously. Often one person, either spouse, son, or daughter, is caring for the patient. This person may have special attributes of motivation and emotional commitment that no professional would have.[19]

Parent education

General goals. These are prevention of future difficulties as parents, early case finding of the beginnings of problem behavior, and growth in self-knowledge and individual competence for parenthood.[2]

Skills required. The parents need to learn to handle child rearing in the manner they choose or toward which they tend—there are many types of good parents.[28] They need to understand the dynamics of behavior and how people react to and feel about each other. Independent problem solving regarding parenting can be used as a tool.

Influencing factors. There is a lack of tradition in parenting, and there are conflicting recommendations available through the mass media, which may be in opposition to one's values and may intensify feelings of uncertainty.[28]

Education of parents of exceptional children

Skills required. The parents must be able to initiate growth-producing activities when the child shows signs of readiness, even when the rate of social, physical, intellectual, and emotional development is very uneven and in the absence of usual bases for assessment such as mental, chronologic, or social age.

Influencing factors. There are few models available in the family's everyday life or from the mass media that interpret the altered readiness behavior of these children. For retarded children, the paucity of response in their development results in limited feedback from their environment, so that inactivity and lack of development add to each other.[4] The mentally retarded may find it difficult to verbalize their feelings and ideas.[34]

At ages 6 to 12 years, when normal children are utilizing church, school, and other social institutions, retarded children find these experiences unavailable or frustrating, thus adding to the parents' burden.

Training of patients with cord bladders

Skills required. The patients must have adequate bladder emptying with low amounts of residual urine and a predictable socially accepted voiding pattern.

Upper motor neuron bladder. When patients are voiding in good amounts on a regular basis, they learn to schedule 300 to 400 milliliters of intake spaced over waking hours and attempt to void every 4 hours. They learn to stimulate "trigger areas," which initiates the voiding reflex.

Lower motor neuron bladder. The patients learn to use Credé's method, straining or contracting abdominal muscles to assist in bladder emptying.

Influencing factors. Readiness is assessed by a trial of voiding procedure.[13]

Training of patients after head and neck surgery

Skills required. Patients who will have a feeding tube for a long period of time will need to feed themselves through it and change the tube when necessary. Some patients may have a tracheostomy and will need to care for it. Patients who have had oral surgery will need to irrigate their mouths with salt and soda solutions.[32]

Training of patients with chronic obstructive lung disease

Skills required. The patients will need to perform abdominal breathing exercises, pursed lip breathing, daily bronchial hygiene. They will need to take adequate amounts of warm fluids to thin and moisten secretions. Patients discharged from the hospital with tracheostomies will need to change and clean the tubes. They will also need to note any changes in secretions that sig-

nal infection and to note symptoms of carbon dioxide narcosis, which may include headache, increased drowsiness, and confusion.

Teaching of family health tasks

Skills required. The family must be able to recognize interruptions of health development, such as illness or a child's failure to thrive; to make decisions about seeking health care; to deal effectively with health and nonhealth crises that have an effect on health; to provide nursing care to sick, disabled, or dependent members of the family; to maintain a home environment conducive to health maintenance and personal development; to maintain reciprocal relationship with the community and its health institutions.[17]

All these examples indicate that it is desirable for patients to have a considerable amount of independence and an attitude of sufficient emotional acceptance to function adequately and to be able to interpret the meaning of a variety of behaviors. Most of these tasks require physical skills. It is extraordinary that, although such skills are required, they are supported by a very haphazard system of patient education. Nurses, as well as patients and families, are constantly caught in the confusion of this system. Consider patients with diabetes, for whom ordinary indiscretions and forgetfulness can be serious. These people also have to cope with confusion created by many different types of equipment and techniques available as well as by differing professionals' interpretations of a prescribed regimen. They are faced not only with unpleasant alterations in their daily living, usually for the rest of their lives, but also with having to decide how to process the conflicting data.

Health workers are constantly frustrated by dealing with learning needs that could be met but not within the time restrictions that exist. To some extent, this situation is the result of a segmented health care delivery system, but, in addition, it reflects lack of value by society, and thus the resources necessary, for adequate health education. Those with learning difficulties, including limited potential, who require slow, repetitious teaching or lack well-developed basic thought skills, often do not get much help. Persons who live with chronic diseases should learn problem-solving skills so that they can alter their regimen within safe limits. For example, Mr. K., hospitalized for hemiplegia and congestive heart failure, tested with his nurses three ways to get in and out of a bathtub before deciding on the best plan. On the basis of this and other experiences with problem solving, he was prepared to work through several tedious trials of tub bathing at home.[10] Consider all the other parts of his daily life for which the same preparation was necessary and all the other persons in Mr. K.'s situation who are not able to solve problems even with help.

Health situations often offer the possibility for considerable growth of persons, families, or communities, which can be realized if the resources are available. Nurses learning to be leaders in work with unwed pregnant black girls of low socioeconomic status were shown how to open for these girls the possibility of suitable behavioral choices, a greater understanding of their own potentials as persons, a widening sense of responsibility toward bringing new life into the world, and increasing sense of self-worth. This can be done in a variety of ways— by listening to their concerns, by helping them think about the role of mother, by opening up for them the possibility of further education and a job suited to their capabilities.[12]

Besides needing these openly stated goals commonly accepted by professionals, nurses need skills in identifying missing and hidden objectives and in resolving goal conflicts. Cogswell believes that the social skill necessary for paraplegics to relate successfully with nondisabled people has been a missing goal. The results of her study suggest that the patients received help with the physical skills necessary for independent mobility, with acceptance of the reality of their disability, and with occupa-tional choices, training, and placement but that they were left without knowledge of steps necessary for social reintegration.[9] A hidden objective is one that is assumed or inherent in the approach used; it is seldom examined and has the potential for being detrimental. Such an objective may exist in health care delivery systems that indicate to people that they have to change their life style in order to get the care they are seeking. Conflict in goals is not uncommon. Often, teaching is involved in the resolution of the goal. The public health nurse may see the need for an elderly disabled woman to become more independent even though this will cost much effort or pain. The family may believe the goal should be to do everything humanly possible for a beloved parent, relieving her of effort or pain whenever possible. The goal acceptable to both nurse and family may be to prevent damage, and from this consensus, agreeable subgoals may be defined.[17]

Objectives for specific learners

Against this background knowledge of the philosophy and general goals of health teaching, nurses assess the teaching needs and readiness of particular clients, the philosophy of their physicians when appropriate, and the treatment plan being instituted. Of considerable importance is what clients want to learn—what their objectives are. Taking these factors into account, nurses are able to develop a set of objectives that is likely to be attainable.

For common teaching tasks, such as orientation to the hospital or participation in tests and procedures, there are basic objectives that may need to be altered only slightly for particular patients. A plan stating such basic objectives may be found as part of the written procedure for a health agency. In some instances a single physician or a group of physicians may have agreed to standing orders regarding patient teaching, such as the orders for teaching prenatal or infant care, for well-child guidance, or for diabetic and colostomy care. These orders or guidelines worked out between the physicians and the nurses are preferably written and describe behavior that the patient should learn. Written orders regarding the teaching of patients are most usual for those health conditions that are common or those in which the need for patient teaching is well accepted. For some subjects, such as health teaching for patients with diabetes, there seems to be substantial agreement among professionals on the general content to be taught and consensus that, unless the teaching is effective, the patient is poorly equipped to handle his health problems.[37] Other people have very individualized teaching requirements because they have uncommon health needs, because their physicians wish them to follow a regimen not used by other physicians, or because they have particular problems in learning. In these instances, the nurses who teach must be more skilled in identifying the behaviors to be learned than they have to be when the pertinent behaviors are already identified for them. In addition, they have to be able to judge the probability that particular behaviors can be attained. A nurse in the Mississippi delta wondered how to teach a woman with hypertension, who could not read or write and who had always eaten salt pork, to follow a low-sodium diet. Her compromise was to show the woman how to trim the fat off the pork and how to lift the greens up out of the fat instead of dishing them out swimming in fat. She also recognized that it was local practice to eat fresh green vegetables, which contain less sodium than do canned ones.[25]

Readiness is a crucial element in defining learning objectives and health programs for communities, as well as for individuals and small groups. Vital statistics provide clues to health needs, part of which are learning needs. For example, it may be apparent that a particular community will not respond well at a particular time to a crash program for tuberculosis control. Supportive evidence for this hypothesized state of readiness might be that many community members accept the disease as inevitable, that prevalent folk medicine beliefs and practices are a powerful deterrent, and that relationships between the organized health unit and indigenous practitioners are characterized by a lack of understanding and trust. The first thrust might, therefore, be toward caring for individuals and postponing mass action, the former being used as a means of developing readiness in community members.[17]

The fact that patients ask many questions does not necessarily indicate the need for a special teaching plan. Some of these questions fall under objectives that have already been defined, such as orientation to the hospital; others represent a fleeting need for information. When patients' questions reveal a serious lack of knowledge or when they form a pattern indicating their concern, objectives should be defined in preparation for teaching. Indeed, with clearly defined objectives, the learners are provided the means to evaluate their own progress during instruction, and they are often able to learn by themselves—from observation of others or from reading materials.[29]

When developing a teaching plan, nurses need to express objectives in written form so that they can be communicated to the learner and to other health workers. Writing the objectives also helps the teacher envision how they might be taught.

Objectives over a period of time

Many things that patients need to learn require days, weeks, or months of instruction, during which the individual may be in more than one setting. Examples of such objectives include the development of skills and knowledge and an attitude of confidence in giving infant care, which may be begun by the hospital staff and continued perhaps by a public health nurse or by a clinic nurse as the mother receives postpartum health supervision. A patient who has suffered paralysis from a cerebrovascular accident may begin work toward the objectives

---

EXAMPLE OF GOALS FOR LEARNING EXTENDED OVER TIME

Main objective: To follow a restricted sodium diet

Week 1	Week 2	Week 3
To name all foods common to the usual eating pattern that have high sodium content	To plan from memory nutritious menus that are within the sodium allotment	To accommodate the new eating pattern to situations such as social functions and being away from home
To agree that a restricted sodium diet may have some merit	To verbalize willingness to follow a restricted sodium diet	To follow the restricted sodium diet without fail
	To prepare foods without using salt	

---

of understanding what a stroke means and learning to reuse muscles while in the hospital and subsequently continue rehabilitation in a nursing home. Since health care is organized so that an individual uses many agencies, continuity must be assured in patient teaching as in other phases of nursing care. Precise statements of behavior to be developed (objectives), with description of progress that the patient has already made toward these goals, are significant aids in attaining this continuity. The hospital nurse may indicate that a mother can hold her baby in several positions and change his diapers but that she is not yet adept at controlling his motions for bathing and breast feeding and lacks confidence in doing these activities. With this statement, public health or clinic nurses know where they must take up the teaching in order to help the learner meet the objective of handling her baby confidently.

If the behavior to be learned will require several weeks or months to attain, statements of intermediate objectives, as indicated in the box above, are helpful. These goals may be individualized, that is, some persons learning this same material may do so in 1 week or in 4 weeks, with appropriate weekly goals, or some individuals may already be able to function at the level of the second week's goals when teaching begins.

Consideration must also be given to the sequential arrangement of the behavior to be learned. In general, individuals master behaviors that are simple to them before they attempt those that are complex and that build on the simple. Thus individuals must learn to stand on crutches before they can manipulate them well enough to walk. An illustration of sequential arrangement may be seen in the box above.

Another consideration is priority, that is, learning first that which is necessary for safe and adequate functioning. The nurse-teacher is concerned that a new mother knows how to handle her baby safely and how to recognize signs and symptoms of common illness before leaving the hospital and, hopefully, that she is committed to seeking regular medical care. Anticipatory guidance regarding the baby's development in the next several months or an understanding of the baby's system of reflexes has lower priority in learning.

STATEMENT OF OBJECTIVES

As has been shown to this point, objectives reflect decisions regarding philosophy, the use of research results, learner readiness, continuity in learning, sequential arrangement of the behavior to be learned, and priority of learning. However, even if a teacher is quite capable of making such decisions, they are of limited use unless they can be adequately communicated to the learner and to other workers. Objectives must express the manner in which learners are to change their thinking, feelings, and actions by the educative process.

Each objective must point out a behavior and a content. Statements such as "Develop critical thinking" lack of content. Develop critical thinking about what? "Read a chapter of the textbook." What should the student read? Behavior is not defined in the statements "Display a positive attitude," "Babies need protection," "Smoking is a hazard," and "Antibiotics fight infection." What is the learner to do with these generalizations or topics—memorize them, apply them, believe in them? With either content or behavior missing, the objective cannot guide teaching and learning. As shown below, the objectives from the box on p. 69 specify both behavior and content, behavior being indicated by italics and content by regular type.

To name all foods common to the usual eating pattern that have high sodium content
To agree that a restricted sodium diet may have some merit
To plan from memory nutritious menus that are within the sodium allotment
To verbalize willingness to follow a restricted sodium diet
To prepare foods without using salt
To accommodate the new eating pattern to situations such as social functions and being away from home
To follow the restricted sodium diet without fail

It should also be noted that each of the objectives presented contains a single behavior and a single content. Examples of multiple behaviors and areas of content are as follows:

To plan and serve nutritious menus that are within the sodium allotment (Two behaviors)

To verbalize willingness to follow a restricted sodium diet and activity limitations (Two behaviors and two content areas)

This error in objective writing—specifying multiple behaviors or areas of content in one objective—is not as serious as is failure to define the objectives precisely. If the multiple behaviors vary in level of accomplishment, area of content, or both, they may be taught at quite different periods of time, with resulting awkwardness in using the objectives for particular lessons.

An objective may be made precise in its meaning by describing the important conditions under which the behavior is expected to occur and by specifying the criteria of acceptable performance. These techniques are not useful with all objectives but may greatly clarify some.[29] In an objective previously stated, the learner is required to accommodate his sodium allotment to the conditions of social functions and being away from home. Another objective requires planning of menus under the conditions of recalling from memory. An acceptable level of functioning is indicated in several of the objectives. The learner is expected to name *all* the foods common to his usual eating pattern that have high sodium content, rather than to name five, or ten, or some. The goal is for him to follow the restricted sodium diet without fail, rather than sometimes or usually. The minimum acceptable performance may sometimes be defined by a time limit, such as when a mother must learn to avoid chilling her baby by not prolonging his bath, or it may be defined by an acceptable deviation, such as taking a particular medication within a half hour of the designated time or measuring a dosage of medicine for injection within two minims of the correct dosage. Defining the social and physical settings in which and the level of stress at which a patient should be able to function also is a means of communicating learning goals precisely. As nurses become proficient in formulating objectives, they will no doubt find themselves using other means of obtaining specificity. For further discussion of these methods in an excellent self-learning presentation, I suggest that the student read *Preparing Instructional Objectives* by Robert Mager.[29]

Objectives are more accurately stated in terms of what the student is to learn rather than what the teacher is to teach, since learning is the ultimate goal and does not always follow from teaching. The objectives in learning to follow a restricted sodium diet were correctly stated in terms of the learner. Another possible wording of these objectives may make more explicit the description of learner behavior:

The student names all foods common to his diet that have high sodium content.

The student plans from memory nutritious menus that are within the sodium allotment.

The infinitive form used previously to state the objectives merely eliminates repetitious words. Examples of objectives stated in terms of teacher behavior, which are not desirable, are the following:

To teach the patient to name all foods common to his diet that have high sodium content.

To teach the patient to plan from memory nutritious menus that are within the sodium allotment.

Depending on the words used, a description of behavior may be more or less precise. When behavior is described, it is best to use verbs that have fewer interpretations. In addition, there are verbs that denote an internal state such as thinking, believing, feeling. These verbs should be avoided since such states cannot be evaluated except as they are manifested in observable behavior. The following two lists give examples of verbs that have relatively broad and relatively specific interpretations, respectively:

Terms with many interpretations

To know (recall, relate, understand, identify?)
To understand (know, relate, identify?)
To be familiar with (know, understand, recognize?)

To realize (discover, appreciate, comprehend?)
To appreciate (realize, know, understand?)
To believe (realize, have faith in?)
To have faith in (believe, hope, trust?)
To be interested in (be aware of, to like?)
To enjoy (relish, love, be pleased with?)
To value (appreciate, hold in high esteem?)
To feel (receive an impression, be impressed with, respond?)
To think critically (evaluate, apply, synthesize?)
To think (understand, conceive, imagine, reflect, infer, judge?)
To really understand[29]
To fully appreciate[29]

Terms with few interpretations

To identify
To list
To compare and contrast
To predict
To interpret
To recall
To translate
To apply
To recognize
To state
To classify
To differentiate[29]
To construct
To order
To describe
To demonstrate

It is not possible to list all behavioral terms that may be used in objectives. Rather, the nurse should think about the broadness or specificity of meaning that the term has and choose that which is specific and denotes observable action. Lists of verbs classed by domain and level of learning within that domain are available.[33]

It is entirely acceptable to state in general terms a main objective describing the overall goal of teaching, as long as components of this main objective are expressed more specifically in subobjectives. Two such examples are shown on p. 72. Of course, the group of subobjectives should represent all components necessary for accomplishment of the main objective. The

RELATIONSHIP BETWEEN MAIN OBJECTIVES AND SUBOBJECTIVES

Situation 1: The patient is a person with a newly diagnosed case of diabetes.
Main objective: To administer insulin to oneself without assistance (Psychomotor; cognitive; affective)
Subobjectives:
   A. To identify injection sites according to a system of rotation, avoiding tissue where absorption will not take place (Cognitive, comprehension)
   B. To use aseptic technique in caring for equipment and giving the injection (For classification, see text.)
   C. To draw a determined amount of solution into a syringe, using only U 40 insulin and syringe, accurate within two units of insulin (Psychomotor, mechanism)
   D. To inject the insulin into subcutaneous tissue, avoiding the bloodstream (Psychomotor, mechanism; cognitive, comprehension)
   E. To assume responsibility for insulin administration, without fail (Affective, valuing)
   F. To take appropriate therapy for complications—mild hypoglycemia, insulin reaction, or skin breakdown (Cognitive, comprehension or application, depending on how different the situation is from that which the patient has encountered before)

Situation 2: A public health nurse is teaching a wife and a daughter how to care for a bedfast elderly father and husband. The patient moves little but has not been incontinent. He has had no skin breakdown to the present but, according to the wife, has been allowed to lie in one position for 4 hours. The main objective is part of the more encompassing objective, to avoid harmful consequences of bed rest.
Main objective: To avoid decubitus ulcer formation (Psychomotor; cognitive; affective)
Subobjectives:
   A. To recognize any evidence of tissue breakdown by criteria of color, sensation, and response to massage (Cognitive, comprehension; psychomotor, perception)
   B. To reposition the patient at least every 2 hours, so that the body is resting on the same surface only every fourth time (Psychomotor, mechanism; cognitive, comprehension)
   C. To keep all linen wrinkle free (Psychomotor, mechanism; cognitive, knowledge)
   D. To massage vigorously, at every turning, the skin that has been receiving pressure from body weight (Psychomotor, mechanism)
   E. To report to the public health nurse or physician evidence of incontinence or skin breakdown, within 4 hours after it is observed (Cognitive, knowledge)

main objective may, in turn, be part of a larger overall goal, such as the goal in Situation 1 for a patient with diabetes to attain independence in daily living. The terms in parentheses will be explained in the next section of the chapter.

The terms in main objectives must be general in order to communicate the breadth of the goal and guide large segments of learning. However, teaching cannot be adequately carried out from main objectives alone. The specific content of a lesson derives from careful definition of specific behavior and content, at approximately the level of generalization of the subobjectives for the learning plans in the two situations just presented.

Readers should test their understanding by comparing these objectives with the criteria for precise statement: containment of a single behavior and content, definition of conditions for behavior and criteria of acceptable performance, statement in terms of learning rather than teaching, description of specific observable behavior, and comprehensiveness of the subobjectives in relation to the main objective.

In situations in which the teacher is inexperienced, the subject being taught is rapidly changing, or the abilities of the learners vary, objectives are continually being revised, giving the nurse an opportunity to practice devising a functional learning plan. Such a situation assumes, of course, a continuing program of instruction on a particular topic. For the once-only, often short-term teaching that nurses do, skill in stating objectives can still be gained by noting their effectiveness in guiding teaching, learning, and evaluation.

Since a meaningfully stated objective is one that succeeds in communicating to the reader the writer's instructional intent, a further test of its clarity is to have another nurse-teacher, a family member, or a patient indicate what behaviors should be expected to occur if the learner reaches the objective. Analysis of the evaluation instruments that the nurse intends to use or has used may show that the behavior desired is quite different from that which the objective states. This may be brought to the nurse's attention by the learner who complains about being expected to know something when it was not part of the instruction or is not useful to him. Such a situation requires an analysis of what behavior really is desired.

Nurses sometimes say they cannot put their objectives into words or that nursing cannot be measured—it is too intangible and personal.[38] These comments may indicate lack of skill with objectives.

Each nurse is not likely to attain a high level of skill in writing objectives. The same can be said of an elementary or secondary teacher; for just that reason, objectives exchanges have been developed. That is, educators can write to the exchange and obtain sets of objectives for a particular content area in a particular grade level. Obviously, the exchange does more than provide well-written objectives; the sets represent someone else's thinking about what goals ought to be and so are instructive to the teacher. Such an endeavor would be excellent for the field of patient education although probably not economically feasible because of the lack of stable financial bases for most patient education programs at this time. Perhaps areas in which instruction is common, such as diabetes education, could initially test the idea. It seems that nurses who can choose from a list of well-stated, potential objectives for a particular patient are more motivated to teach. The skills required for choosing objectives—recognizing a well-stated objective and matching the patient's situation to the right objectives—are simpler and less time consuming than those required for composing objectives—conceptualizing and expressing goals in precise language.

TAXONOMIES OF EDUCATIONAL OBJECTIVES
Development of the taxonomies

In the late 1940's a group of psychologists and educators became concerned about the need for defining levels of behavior according to complexity and about agreeing on terms to denote these levels. Such a step was vital not only to communication among all those concerned with learning but also to progress in research on the relationship between educating and evaluating. A committee approached the problem by developing taxonomies of behaviors found in objectives used in educational institutions and in the literature. The behaviors were divided into three domains: the cognitive, dealing with intellectual abilities; the affective, including expression of feelings in interests, attitudes, values, and appreciations; and the psychomotor, dealing with skills commonly known as motor skills. Each domain was to be ordered in taxonomic form of hierarchy: that is, those complex behaviors at the upper end of the taxonomy (numbered 5.0 or 6.0) included the simple behaviors at the lower end (numbered 1.0). Effort was made to incorporate results of personality and learning research into the structure. At the completion of the cognitive domain taxonomy, the authors believed that they had not succeeded in obtaining complete and sharp distinctions between behaviors.[7] When the taxonomy is used in patient teaching, this weakness is compounded by the fact that the taxonomy was developed from school objectives, which, particularly in the affective domain, seem to differ from some of the behaviors that health learners need to develop. Although the exact classification of behaviors may not always be clear-cut, general classification is sufficient for the nurse-teacher to reap the benefits of using the taxonomy.

An abbreviated adaptation of the completed parts of the taxonomy is given on pp. 75-78 and that of a tentative part on pp. 79 and 80. More complete descriptions of the behaviors may be found in the original sources. The reader should become familiar with the levels of behavior and be able to classify educational objectives at least into low, middle, and high levels of each domain. Further detail is provided here only to broaden the reader's concept of the major categories.

The cognitive and psychomotor domains are ordered on the concept of complexity of behavior, whereas the affective domain represents increasing internalization or commitment to a feeling, thus also requiring more complex behavior at higher levels. It can easily be seen that classification into domains represents emphases only, with objectives belonging only more or less clearly in one domain rather than another.[26] Classifications of the objectives in the box on p. 72 were indicated in parentheses following the statement of each objective, with multiple entries listed in order of decreasing emphasis. For example, the objective regarding identifying injection sites is primarily cognitive in that the basic essential behavior is knowledge of good sites for the purpose of injection. However, there is also a psychomotor element—the individual must find the sites through visual and tactile inspection—and a much lesser affective component—belief in the value of identifying sites correctly. The objective regarding drawing solution into the syringe is primarily psychomotor, but the individual must also possess an intellectual grasp of how to do this task and an understanding of and belief in the importance of accurate measurement.

The group formulating the cognitive and affective taxonomies found that there was much more concern in educational settings with cognitive than with affective matters. That is, attention to definition of terms and to methods of evaluation was considerably greater for cognitive objectives than for affective objectives. It was found that, because of inadequacy in the evaluation of affective objectives, they were used in school curricula only with hesitation. Perhaps a more compelling reason is that the individual's beliefs, attitudes, and values are viewed, in the democratic traditions of the Western world, as being private matters, with education and indoctrination sometimes very closely related.[26] These same difficulties with justifying objectives, defining behaviors, and knowing how to teach them pertain to patient teaching in the affective domain. For example, is it an invasion of privacy and an unrealistic goal to teach children to value cleanliness when they cannot be expected to maintain this value at home?

Besides establishing definitions that facilitate communication, the taxonomy of educational objectives also clarifies certain teaching decisions. There is considerable evidence that in the cognitive domain, learning at the lowest level—acquiring information—can be achieved by a great variety of learning experiences, including lectures, printed material, and pictures or illustrations. Attainment of the higher categories of the domain requires much

COGNITIVE DOMAIN*

1.00 Knowledge

Knowledge, as defined here, involves recall or remembering of information.

   1.10 *Knowledge of specifics*
      1.11 Knowledge of terminology
      1.12 Knowledge of specific facts

   1.20 *Knowledge of ways and means of dealing with specifics*
      1.21 Knowledge of conventions (characteristic ways of treating and presenting ideas and phenomena)
      1.22 Knowledge of trends and sequences
      1.23 Knowledge of classifications and categories
      1.24 Knowledge of criteria
      1.25 Knowledge of methodology

   1.30 *Knowledge of the universals and abstractions in a field*
      1.31 Knowledge of principles and generalizations
      1.32 Knowledge of theories and structures

2.00 Comprehension

This represents the lowest level of understanding. It refers to a type of understanding . . . such that the individual knows what is being communicated and can make use of the material or idea being communicated without necessarily relating it to other material or seeing its fullest implications.

   2.10 *Translation*
      Comprehension as evidenced by the care and accuracy with which the communication is paraphrased or rendered from one language or form of communication to another. Translation is judged on the basis of faithfulness and accuracy, that is, on the extent to which the material in the original communication is preserved although the form of the communication has been altered.

   2.10 *Interpretation*
      The explanation or summarization of a communication. Whereas translation involves an objective part-for-part rendering of a communication, interpretation involves a reordering, rearrangement, or new view of the material.

   2.30 *Extrapolation*
      The extension of trends or tendencies beyond the given data to determine implications, consequences, corollaries, effects, and so forth which are in accordance with the the conditions described in the original communication.

3.00 Application

The use of abstractions in particular and concrete situations. The abstractions may be in the form of general ideas, rules of procedures, or generalized methods. The abstractions may also be technical principles, ideas, and theories, which must be remembered and applied.

4.00 Analysis

The breakdown of a communication into its constituent elements or parts such that the relative hierarchy of ideas is made clear or the relations between the ideas expressed are made explicit,

*Adapted from Bloom, B. S., editor: Taxonomy of educational objectives; the classification of educational goals. Handbook I: Cognitive domain, New York, 1956, David McKay Co., Inc., pp. 201-207. (Used by permission of David McKay Co., Inc.)

Continued.

COGNITIVE DOMAIN—cont'd

or both. Such analyses are intended to clarify the communication, to indicate how the communication is organized and the way in which it manages to convey its effects, as well as to indicate its basis and arrangement.

4.10 *Analysis of elements*
Identification of the elements included in a communication.

4.20 *Analysis of relationships*
Identification of the connections and interactions between elements and parts of a communication.

4.30 *Analysis of organizational principles*
Identification of the organization, systematic arrangement, and structure which hold the communication together. This includes the "explicit" as well as "implicit" structure. It includes the bases, necessary arrangement, and mechanics which make the communication a unit.

5.00 Synthesis
The putting together of elements and parts to form a whole. This involves the process of working with pieces, parts, elements, and so forth and arranging and combining them in such a way so as to constitute a pattern or structure not clearly present before.

5.10 *Production of a unique communication*
The development of a communication in which the writer or speaker attempts to convey ideas, feelings, or experiences or all three to others.

5.20 *Production of a plan, or proposed set of operations*
The development of a plan of work or the proposal of a plan of operations. The plan should satisfy the requirements of a task that may be given to the student or that he may develop for himself.

5.30 *Derivation of a set of abstract relations*
The development of a set of abstract relations either to classify or explain particular data or phenomena, or the deduction of propositions and relations from a set of basic propositions or symbolic representations.

6.00 Evaluation
Judgments about the value of material and methods for given purposes: quantitative and qualitative judgments about the extent to which material and methods satisfy criteria; use of a standard of appraisal. The criteria may be determined by the student or given to him.

6.10 *Judgments in terms of internal evidence*
Evaluation of the accuracy of a communication from such evidence as logical accuracy, consistency, and other internal criteria.

6.20 *Judgments in terms of external criteria*
Evaluation of material with reference to selected or remembered criteria.

AFFECTIVE DOMAIN*

1.00 Receiving (attending)

1.10 *Awareness*
Awareness is almost a cognitive behavior. But unlike knowledge, the lowest level of the cognitive domain, awarenes is not so much concerned with a memory of or ability to recall an item or fact as with the phenomenon that, given an appropriate opportunity, the learner will merely be conscious of something—that he will take into account a situation, fact or event, object, or stage of affairs.

1.20 *Willingness to receive*
At a minimum level we are here describing the behavior of being willing to tolerate a given stimulus, not to avoid it.

1.30 *Controlled or selected attention*
There is an element of the learner's controlling the attention here, so that the favored stimulus is selected and attended to despite competing and distracting stimuli.

2.00 Responding

2.10 *Acquiescence in responding*
The student makes the response, but he has not fully accepted the necessity for doing so.

2.20 *Willingness to respond*
There is the implication that the learner is sufficiently committed to exhibiting a behavior so that he does so not just because of a fear of punishment, but "on his own" or voluntarily.

2.30 *Satisfaction in response*
Behavior is accompanied by a feeling of satisfaction, an emotional response, generally of pleasure, zest, or enjoyment.

3.00 Valuing

3.10 *Acceptance of a value*
The learner is sufficiently consistent that others can identify the value and sufficiently committed that he is willing to be so identified, but there is more of a readiness here to reevaluate his position than would be present at higher levels of valuing.

3.20 *Preference for a value*
Behavior at this level implies not just the acceptance of a value to the point of being willing to be identified with it, but more, a seeking it out and wanting it.

3.30 *Commitment*
Belief at this level involves a high degree of certainty. There is a real motivation to act out the behavior.

4.00 Organization

4.10 *Conceptualization of a value*

*Adapted from Krathwohl, D. R., Bloom, B. S., and Masia, B. B.: Taxonomy of educational objectives; the classification of educational goals. Handbook II: Affective domain, New York, 1964, David McKay Co., Inc., pp. 76-85. (Used by permission of David McKay Co., Inc.)

Continued.

AFFECTIVE DOMAIN—cont'd

At this level the quality of abstraction or conceptualization is added. It permits the individual to see how the value relates to those that he already holds or to new ones that he is coming to hold.

4.20 *Organization of a value system*
Objectives properly classified here as those that require the learner to bring together a complex of values, possibly disparate values, and to relate them in an ordered fashion with one another. Ideally, the ordered relationship will be one which is harmonious and internally consistent.

5.00 Characterization by a value or value complex

5.10 *Generalized set*
A generalized set is a basic orientation that enables the individual to reduce and order the complex world about him and to act consistently and effectively in it. The generalized set may be thought of as closely related to the idea of an attitude cluster.

5.20 *Characterization*
Here are found those objectives that concern the individual's view of the universe, his philosophy of life . . . a value system having as its object the whole of what is known or knowable.

more investment of time and energy on the part of the teacher and learner, with the learner actively working through problems and the teacher helping the learner to attain insight into the processes to be learned. It is believed that the same is probably true of the levels of the affective domain[26] and could reasonably be so for the psychomotor. Thus, along with evidence that the individual learner has the background to reach objectives at higher levels of the domain, there must be consideration of whether the learner and a teacher wish to commit sufficient time and energy to the venture.

A couple of other taxonomies of the psychomotor domain have become available; they mainly focus on skills for particular activities, such as athletics, and are very useful for researchers. One taxonomy that focuses on perception, which is basic to all psychomotor functioning, is most useful (see pp. 81-82).

Perception is the act of extracting information from the welter of stimuli impinging upon the sense organs. It can be distinguished from the cognitive domain, which refers to judgments made from memory and to mental operations performed in the absence of stimuli. The taxonomy of perceptual domain is said to be based on a summary of research. It is arranged in a hierarchy of increasing information extraction and is not limited to any single modality of sensory input. Moore notes that the difference between behavior termed "intuitive" and that not so termed may lie in the amount of information extracted from the stimulating situation and the degree of its association with previously extracted information.[30]

A word must be said about undeveloped taxonomies that would be most helpful in patient education. We have no taxonomies of situations; yet it is known that behavior varies con-

PSYCHOMOTOR DOMAIN: A TENTATIVE SYSTEM*

1.00 Perception
Process of becoming aware of objects, qualities, or relations by way of the sense organs.

1.10 *Sensory stimulation*
Impingement of a stimulus(i) on one or more of the sense organs.
1.11 Auditory
1.12 Visual
1.13 Tactile
1.14 Taste
1.15 Smell
1.16 Kinesthetic

1.20 *Cue selection*
Identification of the cue or cues, association of them with the task to be performed, and grouping of them in terms of past experience and knowledge. Cues relevant to the situation are selected as a guide to action; irrelevant cues are ignored or discarded.

1.30 *Translation*
The mental process of determining the meaning of the cues received for action. It involves symbolic translation, that is, having an image or being reminded of something, "having an idea," as a result of cues received; insight; sensory translation; and "feedback."

2.00 Set
A preparatory adjustment or readiness for a particular kind of action or experience.

2.10 *Mental set*
Readiness, in the mental sense, to perform a certain motor act. This involves, as prerequisite, the level of perception already identified. Discrimination, using judgments in making distinctions, is an aspect.

2.20 *Physical set*
Readiness in the sense of having made the anatomic adjustments necessary for a motor act to be performed, including sensory attending and posturing of the body.

2.30 *Emotional set*
Readiness in terms of attitudes favorable to the motor act's taking place.

3.00 Guided response
The overt behavioral act of an individual under the guidance of the instructor. Prerequisite to performance of the act are readiness to respond and selection of the appropriate response.

3.10 *Imitation*
The execution of an act as a direct response to the perception of another person performing the act.

*Adapted from Simpson, E. J.: The classification of educational objectives in the psychomotor domain. In Contributions of behavioral science to instructional technology; the psychomotor domain, Mt. Rainier, Md., 1972, Gryphon Press.

PSYCHOMOTOR DOMAIN: A TENTATIVE SYSTEM—cont'd

3.00 Guided response—cont'd

    3.20 *Trial and error*

        Trying various responses, usually with some rationale for each response, until an appropriate response is achieved.

4.00 Mechanism

    Learned response has become habitual. The learner has achieved a certain confidence and degree of skill. The act is a part of his repertoire of possible responses to stimuli and to the demands of situations where the response is an appropriate one. The response may be more complex than at the preceding level; it may involve some patterning of response in carrying out the task.

5.00 Complex overt response

    Performance of a motor act that is considered complex because of the movement pattern required. A high degree of skill has been attained, and the act can be carried out with minimum expenditure of time and energy.

    5.10 *Resolution of uncertainty*

        Performance of a complex act without hesitation.

    5.20 *Automatic performance*

        Performance of finely coordinated motor skill with a great deal of ease and muscle control.

6.00 Adaptation

    Altering motor activities to meet the demands of new problematic situations requiring a physical response.

7.00 Origination

    Creating new motor acts or ways of manipulating materials out of understandings, abilities, and skills developed in the psychomotor area.

---

siderably by situation.[16] This development would be important because patient educators are regularly faced with having to predict an individual's behavior from one occasion to another over a period of time. Because no taxonomy exists in this area, individual differences are presently emphasized when comparative statements are made about probable performance of many individuals.[16] A second taxonomy that would be useful is one of social skills. I have observed that social skills are the least well taught component of patient education; however, for patients with chronic illnesses, those skills are crucial. The patient with chronic obstructive pulmonary disease may have physiologic difficulties that result from the effects of strong frustrating emotions on the reactive respiratory tract.[15] Voysey speaks of "impression management"—the skill of managing social encounters learned by parents of disabled children. She describes specific skills as: distinguishing true sympathy from mere curiosity,

PROPOSED TAXONOMY OF PERCEPTUAL DOMAIN*

I. *Sensation*

Behavior that demonstrates awareness of the informational aspects of the stimulus energy.

A. Detection and awareness of change. Detection threshold measures in all sensory modes.
   1. Ability to specify the attribute that has changed.
   2. Ability to specify the direction of change.
   3. Ability to specify the degree of change.

II. *Figure perception*

Behavior that demonstrates awareness of entity.

A. Discrimination of unity; discrimination threshold measures in all sensory modes.
   1. Ability to judge brightness as a property of the stimulus under varying illumination.
   2. Ability to judge distance and location of light and sound.
   3. Ability to judge tactile form qualities such as hardness, sharpness, etc.

B. Sensory figure-ground perceptual organization.
   1. Awareness of the relationships of parts to each other and to the whole.
   2. Awareness of relations between the parts and the background, matrix, or context.

C. Resolution of detail.
   1. Response to detail within the sensory (visual and auditory) world.
      a. Ability to judge size as a property of the stimulus at various distances.
      b. Ability to judge shape as a property of the stimulus regardless of orientation.
      c. Tests of field-dependence.
      d. Tests of spatial orientation.
      e. Other.
   2. Response to detail within the sensory (visual and auditory) field.
      a. Ability to discriminate symmetrical figures.
      b. Ability to discriminate asymmetrical figures.
      c. Ability to perceive rapidly successive bits of information.
      d. "Nonsensory" figure-ground segregation.
      e. Other.

III. *Symbol perception*

Behavior that demonstrates awareness of figures in the form of denotative signs when associated meanings are not considered.

A. Identification of form or pattern and relation of discrete information into visual, auditory, and tactile forms; recognition thresholds in all sensory modalities.
   1. Ability to distinguish curves from rectangles.
   2. Ability to distinguish triangles from squares.
   3. Ability to identify letters and digits.
   4. Ability to respond appropriately to gross facial expressions.
   5. Ability to distinguish tones in a musical chord.
   6. Ability to abstract a melody line from its variations.
   7. Ability to distinguish color components of a visual spectrum or composition.
   8. Ability to respond appropriately to verbal directions.
   9. Ability to respond appropriately to written directions.
   10. Other.

*From Moore, M. R.: The perceptual-motor domain and a proposed taxonomy of perception, Audio Vis. Commun. Rev. **18:**379-413, 1970. Used with permission.

PROPOSED TAXONOMY OF PERCEPTUAL DOMAIN—cont'd

  B. Naming classification of forms and patterns.
    1. Ability to recognize faces and identify people by name.
    2. Ability to identify simplifications and schematic drawings.
    3. Ability to name complex objects, pictures, places, melodies, tastes, odors, etc.
    4. Ability to read and comprehend concrete nouns and verbs denoting physical activity.
    5. Ability to indicate similarities and differences between visual, auditory, or tactile forms or their representations and to classify them.
    6. Other.
IV. *Perception of meaning*
  Behavior that demonstrates awareness of the significance commonly associated with forms and patterns and events and the ability to assign personal significance to them; interpretive ability.
  A. Mental manipulation of the identified form or pattern.
    1. Ability to reproduce forms, tunes, or syllables by memory.
    2. Ability to overcome the constancies of brightness, color, size, and shape.
    3. Other.
  B. Ability to attach significance to a symbol and to relate symbols to achieve a significant synthesis.
    1. Understanding of the various parts of speech; comprehension of language.
    2. Ability to make simple associations in all sensory modalities: for example, clouds mean rain, smoke means fire.
    3. Ability to understand verbal imagery, similies, metaphors, analogies, and other figures of speech—connotative meanings.
    4. Other.
  C. Ability to attach significance to a series of events occurring over a period of time.
    1. Insight into cause and effect relationships.
    2. Discovery of new relationships.
    3. Ability to generalize, understand implications, and make simple decisions.
    4. Other.
V. *Perceptive performance*
  Behavior that demonstrates sensitive and accurate observation, ability to make complex decisions where many factors are involved, and ability to change ongoing behavior in response to its effectiveness.
  A. Demonstration of a successful analytical or global approach to problem solving in all areas of endeavor.
  B. Diagnostic ability with respect to mechanical or electrical systems, medical problems, artistic products, etc.
  C. Insight into personal, social, and political situations where awareness of attitudes, needs, desires, moods, intentions, perceptions, and thoughts of other people and onself is indicated.
  D. Demonstration of artistry and creativity in any medium.
  E. Other.

defining some categories of others' actions as insignificant, and predicting the others' responses.[41] Other skills in managing the impression follow on the basis of the assessment. The necessity of those with rheumatoid arthritis to learn to deal with the uncertainty of the disease course results in skills such as pacing activities over time and walking as if they were not suffering.[43] Persons with ulcerative colitis have been found to use "front men," who know about the patients' situations and work in collusion with them to explain or justify their unconventional behavior or to conceal their disability. These patients have to learn strategies for scheduling time, with backup people who can take over their activities if they are indisposed.[35]

Use of the taxonomies

The ultimate usefulness of taxonomies of this type depends on the unique instructional procedures of each category; there is no assurance that most of the taxonomies presently available are that far developed.

Classifying a group of objectives according to the taxonomy can be helpful in three ways: First, if an objective is difficult to classify, it may be that the behavior is not stated precisely enough. This is particularly true for objectives in the cognitive domain, which is most completely developed. Second, in trying to find the correct classification, the teacher is forced to compare the level of complexity of behavior that is being sought with the learner's present behavior. The teacher is then in a better position to compare this distance with the amount of time, the motivation, and the quality of teaching that is available. Third, if a group of subobjectives is at widely variant levels, the teacher may either have misjudged the learner's ability or have stated the behaviors poorly.

The objectives in the learning plan for the patient with the newly diagnosed case of diabetes can be used to illustrate these considera-

tions. "To use aseptic technique in caring for equipment and giving the injection" is difficult to classify. The use of aseptic technique in psychomotor activities is implied, but the objective is not stated precisely enough to determine its cognitive aspect. If the objective read, "To follow the prescribed procedure in maintaining asepsis in caring for equipment and giving the injection," it would imply cognitive level probably at knowledge, whereas "To apply principles of asepsis in administering insulin" specifies the application level of the cognitive domain—a more complex behavior. "To assume responsibility for insulin administration, without fail" is clearly in the middle level of the affective domain, for it requires at least an acceptance on the part of the learner that this regimen is important.[26]

Something must be known about the learners in order to judge the goals. The description of Situation 2 on p. 72 presents little information about the learners. Several factors determine whether or not the objectives are realistic for these particular learners. What is the relationship between the wife and her daughter? Is the daughter available much of the time when help is needed? If the wife is forgetful and overwhelmed with the care of her husband, how much responsibility can she take? Are the two physically able to turn the husband? How much do they know about the care of skin, about massage, about turning and positioning, and how motivated are they? Considering the patient's need, the nurse must be concerned that someone in the home can reach the objectives in one teaching session.

Given that the learners are capable of reaching the goals planned for them, it should be noted that within each set of objectives for the two situations there is consistency in level; that is, in no instance are there behaviors in the higher levels as described in the taxonomy. Had an objective in the second set read, "To determine a nursing regimen for prevention of decubitus ulcers,'' this would be at the level of synthesis and would be quite incongruous with the rest of that set of objectives.

Various combinations of words may be used to express a given intent. Thus there would be differences between teachers and in the same teacher at different times as to the wording of objectives for a particular situation. Consider the alternative ways in which objectives in the case of the bedfast patient in Situation 2 could be stated. "To reposition the patient . . ." could read, "To turn the patient. . . ." "To recognize any evidence of tissue breakdown . . ." could read, "To identify. . . ." The content may also be stated differently. "To massage vigorously, at every turning, the skin that has been receiving pressure from body weight" may be stated, "To massage skin areas on which the patient has been lying, at least every 2 hours, or more often if signs and symptoms of breakdown occur."

The content of any main objective may be divided into subobjectives in several ways. Another teacher writing the objectives about giving insulin might choose not to consider "using asepsis" in a separate objective but would incorporate it along with other safety measures in an objective, "To administer insulin in a safe manner, using asepsis. . . ." The subobjectives should represent logical groupings. For the psychomotor domain these are primarily tasks such as identifying injection sites, drawing solution into a syringe, and so forth. For cognitive areas, the organizing factor is often a concept such as "tissue breakdown" or "responsibility." Each subobjective ought to be of somewhat equal importance in order to communicate to the learner those things that are the major topics of his effort. Consider a situation of imbalance. Instead of the single objective about injecting the solution into tissues, there might have been three objectives: one dealing with the angle of insertion, one with the rate of injection, and one with avoiding the bloodstream. In the total list of objectives, this would place more emphasis on injection than it actually deserves.

The material on pp. 85 and 86 has been prepared in order to give the reader an opportunity to relate the taxonomy to behaviors that are being taught. The material on p. 87 suggests behavioral terms for stating specific learning outcomes by categories of the cognitive and affective taxonomies of educational objectives.

I know of no comprehensive study that describes the behaviors that nurses most commonly try to teach patients. The most common sources of information about teaching are descriptions of programs that exist, but it is sometimes difficult to determine from them the learning goals. Since particular behaviors are often taught better by one method than by another, further examples of objectives in patient teaching will be discussed in the following chapters on teaching and learning.

OBJECTIVES AS CONTENT AND RELATIONSHIP POLICY IN HEALTH

Perhaps too much of this chapter has focused on objectives as tools within the process of teaching. Formal objectives, of course, contain policy regarding health; moreover, health actions on the part of client and practitioner always carry implicit objectives. This is inevitable, since objectives are the goals of purposeful action.

Some authors take exception to the general trend of goals in health education or suggest significant new goals. For example, Kastenbaum thinks that definitions (and therefore our goals) of mental health selectively focus on a small range of phenomena as constituting the total human condition. He notes that it is seldom considered "healthy" for individuals to go through life with a measure of sorrow and other heavy affects in consequence of a severe interpersonal loss that has been suffered. According to Kastenbaum, a person can both sorrow and be "mentally healthy" over a prolonged period of time.[24] Franz Halberg suggests widespread

EXAMPLES OF HEALTH TEACHING OBJECTIVES ACCORDING TO THE TAXONOMIES OF EDUCATIONAL OBJECTIVES

COGNITIVE DOMAIN

Knowledge	To describe three main purposes of the cough, turn, deep-breathe regimen following surgery
	To state why the mother's diet may affect breast feeding
Comprehension	When changing a surgical dressing, to recognize when something has been contaminated
	To translate instructions on a medicine bottle into appropriate action
Application	To apply principles of asepsis to washing a wound with pHisoHex
	Given a general knowledge of safety, to plan how to rid a house of safety hazards
Analysis	To identify factors causing one's bowel upsets
	To distinguish how a quack's argument differs from scientific reasoning
Synthesis	To design an ileostomy bag that suits one's needs better than do available commercial ones
	To interpret to others the feelings one experiences during illness
Evaluation	To assess the health care that one is receiving in terms of its completeness, one's satisfaction with it, and the results obtained

AFFECTIVE DOMAIN

Receiving	To be aware that others are available to help
	To tolerate having a retention catheter
Responding	To cooperate with the insertion of a nasogastric tube
	To feel some satisfaction in caring for one's baby
Valuing	To accept many of the limitations in life imposed by heart disease
	To desire positive health rather than mere absence of disease
Organization	To relate to others in a manner consistent with rehabilitation goals
	To regularly choose those alternatives of action that are consistent with good parenting
Characterization by a value or value complex	To develop for regulation of one's life a code of behavior consistent with respect for the health of oneself and others

PSYCHOMOTOR DOMAIN

Perception	To recognize the "feel" of holding a baby with good balance
	To recognize the difference between systolic and diastolic blood pressure sounds

---

**EXAMPLES OF HEALTH TEACHING OBJECTIVES ACCORDING TO
THE TAXONOMIES OF EDUCATIONAL OBJECTIVES—cont'd**

Set	To demonstrate a well-balanced stance with crutches
	To demonstrate correct placement of sphygmomanometer and steth-oscope
Guided response	To discover the most efficient method of diapering a baby through trial of various procedures
	To imitate the blood pressure measurement procedure after demon-stration
Mechanism	To give oneself an intermittent positive pressure breathing treatment
	To control the fall of mercury in the sphygmomanometer at 2 to 3 mm. per heartbeat
Complex overt response	To skillfully pass a tube through the nose into the stomach with a min-imum of discomfort or danger to the patient
	To measure blood pressure within 1 minute, accurate to ± 5 mm. mercury, in comparison with an expert
Adaptation	To perform one's own design for turning, moving, and transferring a hemiplegic person, weighing 100 pounds more than oneself, in a home environment
Origination	(Rarely used in patient education)

---

implementation of self-measurement procedures regarding one's physiologic and psychologic functioning. Only a small fraction of men and women who suffer from hypertension are aware of their condition, and an even smaller fraction receive correct or adequate treatment. Halberg suggests a program of self-measurement that could alter this situation. It is easy to learn the procedures of taking and recording the measurements, and people with hypertension could continue them over long enough periods to gain information on individualized "usual range" of values for themselves.[21] Others are concerned about learning goals in areas basic to our relationships with patients—such as informed consent. The trouble with informed consent, Ingelfinger says, is that it is not educated consent. He believes that efforts to promote educated consent

are in order. The difference lies in the patients' better ability to comprehend themselves more accurately within the broad context of the situation and to weigh the inconveniences and hazards they will have to undergo against the improvements a research project may bring to the management of their disease in general and to their own case in particular. According to Ingelfinger, patients cannot be given complete information—all the possible contingencies and extensive details may confuse them.[22] Although the present level of patient understanding may not be sufficient, it is difficult to make a precise judgment of how much improvement is enough.

Discrepancy in patient and staff objectives is not uncommon. One study of adult patients in a New York hospital found nurses and patients agreeing that patients should be informed about what is wrong with them, how long the illness

ILLUSTRATIVE BEHAVIORAL TERMS FOR STATING
SPECIFIC LEARNING OUTCOMES*

COGNITIVE DOMAIN   TERMS

Knowledge   Defines, describes, identifies, labels, lists, matches, names, outlines, reproduces, selects, states

Comprehension   Converts, defends, distinguishes, estimates, explains, extends, generalizes, gives examples, infers, paraphrases, predicts, rewrites, summarizes

Application   Changes, computes, demonstrates, discovers, manipulates, modifies, operates, predicts, prepares, produces, relates, shows, solves, uses

Analysis   Breaks down, diagrams, differentiates, discriminates, distinguishes, identifies, illustrates, infers, outlines, points out, relates, selects, separates, subdivides

Synthesis   Categorizes, combines, compiles, composes, creates, devises, designs, explains, generates, modifies, organizes, plants, rearranges, reconstructs, relates, reorganizes, revises, rewrites, summarizes, tells, writes

Evaluation   Appraises, compares, concludes, contracts, criticizes, describes, discriminates, explains, justifies, interprets, relates, summarizes, supports

AFFECTIVE DOMAIN   TERMS

Receiving   Asks, chooses, describes, follows, gives, holds, identifies, locates, names, points to, selects, sits erect, replies, uses

Responding   Answers, assists, complies, conforms, discusses, greets, helps, labels, performs, practices, presents, reads, recites, reports, selects, tells, writes

Valuing   Completes, describes, differentiates, explains, follows, forms, initiates, invites, joins, justifies, proposes, reads, reports, selects, shares, studies, works

Organization   Adheres, alters, arranges, combines, compares, completes, defends, explains, generalizes, identifies, integrates, modifies orders, organizes, prepares, relates, synthesizes

Characterization by a value or value complex   Acts, discriminates, displays, influences, listens, modifies, performs, practices, proposes, qualifies, questions, revises, serves, solves, uses, verifies

*From Gronlund, N. L.: Stating behavioral objectives for classroom instruction, New York, 1970, Macmillan Publishing Co., Inc. Used with permission.

Table 4. Sample contract between nurse and client for teaching-learning

Situation: Wife learning to give home care to husband who has had CVA. This is only one element of the contract that would need to be developed with this wife.

Elements	Specific contract
What is goal?	To learn to give husband an enema.
What does client expect of nurse?	Demonstration of safe procedure adapted to the home and to this patient, with rationale explained and practice supervised.
What does client have to offer?	Motivation to learn in order to keep husband at home and in good physical condition.
What does nurse expect of client?	Willingness to learn from instruction and practice on her own after initial instruction.
What does nurse have to offer?	Expertise in determining when enema is needed, adapting it to individual needs, evaluating its effectiveness, and teaching others how to give the enema.
How do we go about working together?	As patient needs his next enema, nurse will explain basis for this decision to wife, plus how to obtain and prepare equipment and give and evaluate enema. Subsequently, wife will begin to make these judgments and do the skills with nurse's help and in 2 weeks will perform independently.
Contract to be renegotiated:	At the end of fourth home visit—2 weeks from date of contract initiation or at earlier time if patient's condition or care regarding enema changes or if the nurse or wife believes care is inadequate.

is likely to last, how they can participate in their own care while in the hospital, and what symptoms to expect. Nurses and patients also disagreed, with patients much more interested in details about how they were rather than in what would be done to or for them.[14] These findings are very difficult to interpret; they may be related to patients' desire for information about prognoses that nurses felt they could not give. The point to be made is that in particular situations, there will be certain discrepancies in the patients' and staff's ideas of education, as well as other goals. They are worth considering since they may adversely affect the teaching relationship. In one rehabilitation setting, the staff has developed a full list of goals—physical, educational, vocational, and psychosocial—a patient can learn in that setting. The patient and family are interviewed separately,

each choosing goals. This provides a basis for early identification of conflicts, enhances family-staff-patient interaction through negotiation about goals, and encourages the patient and family to be active. The goals are later used as bases for follow-up evaluation to see if the patient is still using those skills in his home.[5]

The use of contracts with patients does operationalize principles basic to learning and the use of objectives into a clinical tool. A sample contract may be seen in Table 4. Blair reports on the use of contracts in a public health setting. The contract is a mutual understanding of the reason for the service and the problems or areas that will be discussed during the visits. It results from the nurse's discussion and clarification with the patient as to what he actually wants and what services can be provided. Blair suggests that it is best to set a limit either in length of time to be expended or in given number of visits and the conditions for renegotiation. Care plans are then based on the contract.[6]

A problem apparently of some magnitude is that people often do not maintain initial behavior changes over a long period of time. The factors that influence a patient to adopt a new behavior are apparently not necessarily the same as those required to maintain it, which require continually confronting and resolving problems caused by personal and environmental factors, such as work schedules, social situations, and family conflicts. Short-term training influences are usually no match for the multitude of factors that affects the person's behavior in weeks, months, and years to come. Smoking is a case in point. Most high cessation rates begin to deteriorate rapidly as soon as treatment is terminated, and the vulnerability of ex-smokers to factors that encourage smoking is well established. Even adopting an antihypertension medication regimen, an act that seemingly requires little change in life style, poses a serious maintenance problem. It appears that goal-focused intervention methods and a health care system responsive to individual needs over an extended period of time are of assistance.[44]

SUMMARY

All that is known about producing efficiency of learning is of no use unless the direction that the learning should take is clearly defined. Thus, the focus of this chapter has been on determination and communication of desired behavior changes. Taxonomies of educational objectives define and order behaviors in terms of complexity, thereby aiding in communication of goals and decisions regarding teaching and evaluation.

STUDY QUESTIONS

1. The following sentences occur in statements of philosophy and objectives for the nursing services of health agencies. What are their implications for patient teaching in nursing?

   a. A goal of nursing is to recognize the patient's need for independence.

   b. A goal of nursing is to recognize the patient's desire for self-awareness in relation to his illness.

   c. We recognize the worth and dignity of each individual.

   d. The patient and the family are to participate in setting realistic goals for themselves in the maintenance of health.

2. You are a public health nurse. You have received a physician's order to teach the husband of a woman with Parkinson's disease to care for her indwelling urinary catheter. You are to change the catheter and visit when necessary. The husband is highly motivated. In conversing with him, you find that he does not know where the catheter lies after it enters the body, although he does know it drains urine into a container.

   a. Write in correct form the main objectives and the subobjectives.

   b. Designate the priority and sequence of objectives.

   c. Classify the objectives according to the taxonomy of educational objectives and indicate implications of the resulting classification for instruction.

3. Write the objective, "To design an ileostomy bag that suits one's needs better than do available commercial ones," at the knowledge and application levels of the cognitive domain and the valuing level in the affective domain.

4. You have just completed a postpartum study of patients who delivered in your unit. Of the 67 mothers, 56 reported deviations from health in their babies at 10 days of age. What implications does this study have for objectives in the teaching program of the unit?

5. One author tells of a patient she saw in the outpatient department. The patient had been discharged from the hospital with a diagnosis of hypertension, for which he was taking reserpine. He was also receiving ferrous sulfate. During a discussion, the patient indicated that he just could not understand what the nurses were trying to do, since he had been told that one of the pills he was taking was to build his blood up and one was to bring his blood down. For someone who does not understand what is meant by hypertension and anemia, this is rather confusing.[39] Suppose that the patient is fulfilling the objective of taking his medication. What would you as the nurse do about his lack of understanding described above?

6. Provide a critique and suggestions for improvement of the following objectives:

   a. The patient will measure his own intake and output and record it as instructed.[37]

   b. When requested, the patient will list in writing, from memory, those foods that are not appropriate on a low-sodium diet.[37]

c. Each morning the patient will circle, from a list of foods, those that are appropriate on a low-calorie diet.[37]

d. (1) After discussing the drug handouts with the pharmacist, the patient will know the following information about his medication:

   (a) The visual identity of each drug.
   (b) The name of each drug.
   (c) How each drug works with respect to the disease being treated.
   (d) Any special instructions regarding administration where appropriate.
   (e) Any ancillary information, such as storage or expected side effects, where appropriate.
   (f) The common adverse reactions of each drug.

   (2) Having learned the above information concerning his medications, the patient will comply intelligently with the medication plan provided him.*

---

*Jinks, M.: The hospital pharmacist in an interdisciplinary inpatient teaching program, Am. J. Hosp. Pharm. **31:**570, 1974. Copyright © 1974, American Society of Hospital Pharmacists, Inc. All rights reserved.

REFERENCES

1. Amend, E. L.: A parent education program in a children's hospital, Nurs. Outlook **14:**53-56, April 1966.
2. Auerbach, A. B.: Parents learn through discussion, New York, 1968, John Wiley & Sons, Inc.
3. Auerbach, A. B., and Rabinow, M.: Parent education groups for unmarried mothers, Nurs. Outlook **14:**38-40, March 1966.
4. Barnard, K.: Teaching the retarded child is a family affair, Am. J. Nurs. **68:**305-311, Feb. 1968.
5. Becker, M. C., and others: Goal setting; a joint patient-staff method, Arch. Phys. Med. Rehabil. **55:**87-89, 1974.
6. Blair, K. K.: It's the patient's problem—and decision, Nurs. Outlook **19:**587-589, 1971.
7. Bloom, B. S., editor: Taxonomy of educational objectives; the classification of educational goals. Handbook I: Cognitive domain, New York, 1956, David McKay Co., Inc.
8. Campbell, C.: Nursing diagnosis and intervention in nursing practice, New York, 1978, John Wiley & Sons, Inc.
9. Cogswell, B. E.: Self-socialization: readjustment of paraplegics in the community, J. Rehabil. **34:**11-13, 35, May-June 1968.
10. Collins, R. D.: Problem solving a tool for patients, too, Am. J. Nurs. **68:**1483-1485, July 1968.
11. Conte, A., and others: Group work with hypertensive patients, Am. J. Nurs. **74:**910-912, 1974.
12. Daniels, A. M.: Reaching unwed adolescent mothers, Am. J. Nurs. **69:**332-335, Feb. 1969.
13. Delehanty, L., and Stravino, V.: Achieving bladder control, Am. J. Nurs. **70:**312-316, Feb. 1970.
14. Dodge, J. S.: What patients should be told; patients' and nurses' beliefs, Am. J. Nurs. **72:**1852-1854, 1972.
15. Dudley, D. L.: Psychophysiology of respiration in health and disease, New York, 1969, Appleton-Century-Crofts.
16. Frederiksen, N.: Toward a taxonomy of situations, Am. Psychol. **27:**114-123, 1972.
17. Freeman, R. B.: Community health nursing practice, Philadelphia, 1970, W. B. Saunders Co.
18. Gebbie, K. M., and Lavin, M. A., editors: Classification of nursing diagnoses, St. Louis, 1975, The C. V. Mosby Co.
19. Golodetz, A., and others: The care of chronic illness, the "responsor" role, Med. Care **7:**385-394, 1969.
20. Gronlund, N. L.: Stating behavioral objectives for classroom instruction, New York, 1970, The Macmillan Co.
21. Halberg, F., and others: Reading, 'riting, 'rithmetic—and rhythms; a new "relevant" "r" in the educative process, Perspect. Biol. Med. **17:**128-141, 1973.
22. Ingelfinger, F. J.: Informed (but uneducated) consent, N. Engl. J. Med. **287:**465-466, 1972.
23. Jinks, M.: The hospital pharmacist in an interdisciplinary inpatient teaching program, Am. J. Hosp. Pharm. **31:**569-573, 1974.
24. Kastenbaum, R.: . . . Gone tomorrow, Geriatrics **29:**127-131, 1974.
25. Kelly, C.: Health care in the Mississippi delta, Am. J. Nurs. **69:**759-763, April 1969.
26. Krathwohl, D. R., Bloom, B. S., and Masia, B. B.: Taxonomy of educational objectives; the classification of educational goals. Handbook II. Affective domain, New York, 1964, David McKay Co., Inc.
27. MacDonald-Ross, M.: Behavioural objectives—a critical review, Instruc. Sci. **2:**1-52, 1973.
28. McCaffery, M. S.: An approach to parent education, Nurs. Forum **6(1):**77-93, 1967.
29. Mager, R. F.: Preparing instructional objectives, ed. 2, Palo Alto, Calif., 1975, Fearon Publishers.
30. Moore, M. R.: The perceptual-motor domain and a proposed taxonomy of perception, AudioVis. Commun. Rev. **18:**379-413, 1970.
31. Mumford, E., and Skipper, J. K., Jr.: Sociology in hospital care, New York, 1967, Harper and Row, Publishers.
32. Newcombe, B.: Care of the patient with head and neck cancer, Nurs. Clin. North Am. **2:**599-607, 1967.

33. Nuttelman, D.: Instructional objectives, Supervisor Nurse **8**(11):35-44, 1977.

34. Perry, S. E.: Some theoretic problems of mental deficiency and their action implications. In Philips, I., editor: Prevention and treatment of mental retardation, New York, 1966, Basic Books, Inc., Publishers.

35. Reif, L.: Beyond medical intervention; strategies for managing life in the face of chronic illness. In Davis, M. Z., Kramer, M., and Strauss, A. L., editors: Nurses in practice; a perspective on work environments, St. Louis, 1975, The C. V. Mosby Co.

36. Simpson, E. J.: The classification of educational objectives in the psychomotor domain. In Contributions of behavioral science to instructional technology; the psychomotor domain, Washington, D.C., 1972, Gryphon Press.

37. Skiff, A. W.: Programed instruction and patient teaching, Am. J. Public Health **55**:409-415, 1965.

38. Smith, D. M.: Writing objectives as a nursing practice skill, Am. J. Nurs. **71**:319-320, 1971.

39. Straub, K. M.: The implication of nursing care plans to the concept of continuity of patient care. In Straub, K. M., and Parker, K. S., editors: Continuity of patient care; the role of nursing, Washington, D.C., 1966, The Catholic University of America Press.

40. University Hospital Nursing Services: The philosophy of the nursing services; objectives of nursing services, Seattle, 1978, University of Washington Hospital.

41. Voysey, M.: Impression management by parents with disabled children, J. Health Soc. Behav. **13**:80-89, 1972.

42. Wiedenbach, E.: Family-centered maternity nursing, ed. 2, New York, 1967, G. P. Putnam's Sons.

43. Wiener, C. L.: The burden of rheumatoid arthritis; tolerating the uncertainty, Soc. Sci. Med. **9**:97-104, 1975.

44. Zifferblatt, S. M., and Wilbur, C. S.: Maintaining a healthy heart; guidelines for a feasible goal, Prev. Med. **6**:514-525, 1977.

CHAPTER 5

Learning

■ Instructional practices are based on the psychology of learning and, when that field lacks clear application to teaching, on what has seemed to produce results for practitioners. Although it is true that individuals, particularly those who are motivated and bright, learn a great deal without a teacher, their efforts can be quite inefficient. Individuals who need to learn health information and skills, even if they are motivated, often do not have sufficient orientation to health matters to attain the goal alone.

It is hoped that after studying this chapter and the following chapter, the reader will be able to (1) state how general findings from learning research are useful in teaching; (2) state the rationale for use of particular methods and techniques in a lesson in terms of their basis in learning psychology and practicality; and (3) evaluate to what degree a lesson plan is internally consistent. (Do objectives reflect readiness? Are content and teaching actions adequate to meet the objectives? Does the evaluation test whether the objectives were met?)

LEARNING THEORY RELATED TO INSTRUCTION

Learning theories in themselves do not present an adequate basis for understanding or managing the many variables associated with learning in social settings; nor do present theories of instruction provide such a basis. No single theory of learning has yet emerged that is applicable to the wide array of outcomes in the many different settings in which learning occurs.[32] Beginning in 1950 the field of learning theory changed from comprehensive learning theories, such as those of Gestalt and Hull, to what may be thought of as miniature models—attention, perceptual learning, imitation learning, short-term memory, long-term memory, concept learning, discrimination learning, and problem solving. Learning theory–related instructional theories include behavior modification approaches, cognitive construct instructional approaches (primary theorist is Bruner), principles of learning instructional theories, task analysis instructional theories (primary theorists are Gagne and Briggs), and humanistic psychology instructional theory (primary theorist is Carl Rogers).[52]

Two general approaches to learning are information processing through a symbolic medium (for example, words and pictures) and experiential learning. A mix of information processing and experiential learning seems most profitable.[16] The two follow different sequential patterns and possess different strengths and weaknesses (Tables 5 and 6). It is not to be assumed that the phases over time automatically unfold.

PRINCIPLES OF LEARNING USEFUL TO TEACHING

Knowledge about learning has yielded some guidelines for teaching, even though they are not comprehensive. Ausubel, a prominent psy-

Table 5. Sequence of learning phases: information processing and experiential learning*

General approach to learning information	Phases over time			
Information processing learning	Reception of information through symbolic medium	Understanding the general principle	Particularizing	Acting†
Experiential learning	Acting	Understanding the particular case†	Generalizing	Acting in a new circumstance

*Information from Coleman, J. S., and others: The Hopkins game program; conclusions from seven years of research, Educ. Researcher **2**:3-7, Aug. 1973.
†Represent weak points; instructional help may be needed.

Table 6. Strengths and weaknesses of information processing and experiential learning*

General approach to learning information	Strengths	Weaknesses
Information processing learning	Can enormously decrease time and effort to learn something new	Is a cost to the compression of experience through language—incompletely understood language; defects in chains of associations and in the processing of information; dependence on prior learning of a complex set of symbols "Cultural disadvantage" lies largely in linguistic and verbal skills required Depends on artificial and extrinsic motivation because action comes at end, not beginning, of learning
Experiential learning	Motivation intrinsic since action is at beginning of chain Less easily forgotten than learning through information processing	Time consuming, involves actions repeated frequently and in enough circumstances to allow development of a generalization from experience Is not effective when consequence of action is separated in time or space from action itself

*Information from Coleman, J. S., and others: The Hopkins game program; conclusions from seven years of research, Educ. Researcher **2**:3-7, Aug. 1973.

chologist, feels that in applying a given psychologic principle to any particular teaching situation, one must exercise professional judgment: that is, weigh the claims of one pertinent principle against another; consider relevant aspects of one's own personality and preparation; evaluate the momentary situation with the learner's personality and preparation, including state of readiness, fatigue, and current understanding; and appraise the adequacy of ongoing communication.[5] For example, the principle that parents learn best what they are motivated or interested in learning may be implemented by presenting the group with no set curriculum and having it develop its own "agenda" in the first meeting and as sessions progress.[2] In making a decision about this approach, one needs to use other principles in conjunction with the one cited above, such as the degree to which the parents posses the experiential readiness to learn in this way and the ability to receive satisfaction and not feel excessive anxiety in such a program. A similar weighing of principles is involved in the following decision: Since learning is most significant when the subject matter is closely related to the parents' own immediate experiences with their children and with one another in relation to their children, parent members are encouraged to be specific when they pose their questions or concerns and to describe in some detail the immediate occurrences that brought the issues to the fore.[2] What possibly conflicting principles need to be considered? (For further clarification of this idea, see study question 3 at the end of the chapter.)

The complexity of variables in the learning situation has made the learning process difficult to study. The results of experiments with animal learning or with human beings in controlled laboratory situations are not necessarily applicable to students in school situations or outside of schools. Little is known about their applicability to the subject matter of health, with the wide variety of abilities, backgrounds, and stress levels of persons learning about health. For these reasons, principles will be stated for only those facets of learning in which there is considerable available evidence. In addition to general principles applicable to all domains, there is information available about cognitive, affective, and psychomotor learning.

General principles of learning

The notion that learning is more effective when a student is ready to learn has already been introduced. This readiness includes both experiential readiness and motivation, although the motivation may be developed considerably during the process of instruction. The principle that moderate anxiety is beneficial to learning and low or severe levels of anxiety detract from learning has already been introduced.

A major purpose of stating objectives specifically is to help the learner understand them and become self-directive. Self-direction is also served by having the teacher explain the goals and provide a model of the correct behavior, as in demonstrating catheter care and indicating what the learner should be able to do and when. After seeing how well the learner is doing (feedback), the teacher provides reinforcement for desired behavior and makes efforts to correct errors promptly. Thus, self-direction is guided so that time and energy are not wasted.

In order to maintain motivation and be truly self-directing, an individual must also receive satisfaction from learning. The teacher maximizes this by setting realistic goals with the aid of the learner. If the learning steps are too easy, motivation lags; and if they are too difficult, the learner feels overwhelmed and discouraged. The teacher constantly assesses evidence of the learner's progress and his feelings regarding it, so that goals can be reset if necessary. This means that if Mrs. Clawson can already perform mouth-to-mouth resuscitation adequately, she may be bored with the class on this topic and can be told that she need not attend it.

Material meaningful to the individual is

learned more readily and remembered longer than material that is not meaningful. It is generally assumed that differences in meaningfulness reflect variations in the frequency of prior experience: if there was a greater degree of prior experience, there is higher meaningfulness.[26]

The "what is it, what is it for" aspect of a concept or skill can be indicated by the teacher's presenting the object or a model or picture of it, describing it, and relating it to things or ideas the learner already knows. Thus the behavior of a mentally retarded child (not understood) may be likened to normal behavior for a child some years younger (generally understood). Or the way in which a woman in labor should push down against the perineum (unknown) can be likened to pushing as if having a bowel movement (known). Some concepts, such as honesty, are not easily visualized but may be explained through a story or a case that is like an experience the learner has had. Other associations that might be made in explanation of mental retardation would include the relationship between one individual's behavior and the generalization that retarded persons have basic needs in common with all human beings and the notion that the intelligence of these people forms a continuum just as there are very bright and less bright normal people. Thus, meaningfulness consists not only of relationships between facts and concepts but also of their link with generalizations, rules, and principles.

For material to become meaningful to him, the learner must also be able to discriminate one concept, skill, or attitude from another. If he does not clearly understand differences between things that are similar, such as sterility and cleanliness, he will be confused. Therefore it is helpful to point out to him differences as well as similarities—for instance, cleanliness and sterility both refer to the relative absence of microorganisms and differ by the degree of absence. Indeed, interference with correct interpretations from inadequately suppressed wrong interpretations appears to be the principal source of forgetting.[6,58]

Another device used to increase meaning is an "advance organizer" introduced in advance of the material to be learned and presented at a higher level of abstracion, generality, and inclusiveness.[3] For explaining menstruation to a group of teen-age girls, the statement "Menstruation is a natural shedding of the lining of the womb," made at the beginning of the lesson, could serve as an advance organizer. Specific details that follow are then viewed within the framework of the organizing statement, which thus gives them meaning.

The depth of meaning that the learner has attained can be tested by asking him to restate an idea in his own words, answer a question using the information, or give examples of a principle. These experiences show what connections he has made between the new idea or object and the old. If all he is able to do is to repeat the words in which the idea was originally expressed, the teacher should immediately realize that he has learned by rote and has little understanding of the meaning of the idea.

Strengthening associations between ideas to make them meaningful enhances the ability to transfer knowledge or skill from a known situation to a new one. Transfer can be defined as the effect of prior learning on subsequent learning and is one of the most important products of education, since no learner can practice all situations he will meet. It is more efficient if an individual can learn general information, skills, and ways of thinking and apply them to many situations rather than learn specifically for each situation. Teaching for transfer is based on evidence that individuals forget nonsense material and isolated facts but do remember general ideas, attitudes, ways of thinking, and skills that are meaningful to them. Also, in order for the transfer to occur, the person must recognize the new situation to be similar to other situations for which a specific behavior has been appropriate.[18] Therefore, a mother who has learned to be cautious when dealing with allergic reactions in her children will probably be cautious (transferring the attitudes) when her husband shows signs and symptoms that she interprets to be caused by allergy.

It is desirable to foster an individual's learning to transfer; however, some people do not have the necessary background. The nurse-teacher has to be constantly aware that he or she cannot just assume that transfer will take place. It is for this reason that the author of a prominent public health nursing textbook suggests that the procedures of public health nursing should be adaptable by the family without change: the nurse should, for example, use household soap instead of green soap. There is apparently little information about how generalization or transfer develops during learning practice or how it varies from one problem to another.

Development of meaning for the learner and of his ability to transfer is really aimed at helping the learner remember and problem solve. Stated in another way, the more interconnections a piece of learning has with a person's experience and the more active he has been in using the learning in different situations, the deeper the impact will be on his memory.

Forgetting learned material is one of the banes of our existence. Explanations for why it occurs include disuse of what was learned, interference from other learning, loss during reorganization of ideas, and motivated forgetting, which may be subconscious. Ideas are remembered for a long time, whereas facts are not. Ways to increase retention include fostering intent to learn and remember, finding meaning in material to be learned, applying newly learned material to a practical situation (practicing), and learning over a period of time.[32]

To some extent, different classes of behavior require different conditions for learning, as explained now in succeeding sections.

Cognitive learning

Cognitive learning involves thinking. Acquiring and developing concepts are basic learning tasks in the cognitive domain, since concepts are the vehicles of thought.[28] A concept may be defined as the label of a set of things or ideas that have something in common.[1] Concepts vary widely in terms of inclusiveness and abstractness. "Tube" is a more inclusive concept than is "catheter," which is a special kind of tube. Both are more concrete than "sterility," for sterility cannot be seen or experienced by any of the senses. These abstract concepts may have multiple meanings, more or less clear, more or less agreed on by users. For example, "support" as it is commonly used in nursing today has multiple meanings with less than complete agreement among users.

All organisms desire to simplify and establish order in their complex environments. People create concepts to help do this by using symbols to transform, compress, and organize sensations. Since reasoning is done by associating and rearranging verbal symbols, precise thinking requires precise meanings for concepts.[18]

A teacher can help individuals develop concepts by a controlled introduction of discontinuity into the learner's environment in the form of new objects, events, or information.[41] The development follows a process of introduction from those concepts that are relatively concrete to those that are more abstract, with increasing differentiation of one idea from others. At the beginning level, the teacher can show an object, such as a syringe. For objects that are difficult to obtain, such as a placenta, a model or picture may serve as an example. For concepts that are not concrete things, the teacher can give an example of an action that embodies the concept. The teacher may explain severe anxiety in words that accompany observation of someone severely anxious in real life or in a film, as a means of making the concept more real. The instructor may also set up other experiences that help the learner to differentiate anxiety from related concepts, such as fear. These experiences allow the learner to obtain a fairly complete notion about anxiety—its various causes, degrees, and effects. The learner begins to be able to make these comparisons verbally, without examples of behavior or objects being presented. He now has a better-developed concept than he had, one that can be useful in classifying the behavior he sees in himself and others.

The less mature an individual is as a learner—whether child or adult—the more he needs concepts presented in concrete ways rather than abstractly. He must see, touch, smell, hear, and taste whenever possible rather than discuss something or read about it. This may be true of persons of the lower class but is also the case with any person of limited intellectual or educational background. Some lower-class people have been described as having had limited experience with certain aspects of the world, so that they have few mental images from which to draw. Development of language, as in labeling objects and actions in the environment, is retarded or not encouraged. Interaction between parent and child tends to be in brief sentences and commands, with much of the communication gestural.[19] There is little reading material available in the home. Moreover, these people seem less able to reason things out, to solve problems. Attention span is short, and motivation to take action is often based on immediate rather than long-term goals. Broad characteristic elements of cognitive style of a variety of low-income groups have been described as physical and visual rather than aural; content centered rather than form centered; externally oriented rather than introspective; problem centered rather than abstract centered; inductive rather than deductive; spatial rather than temporal; slow, careful, patient, persevering in areas of importance, rather than quick, clever, and facile; one-track thinking rather than other-directed flexibility; words used in relation to action rather than word-bound orientation.[45]

The nurse deals with many individuals who have these learning handicaps to some degree. She must be prepared to develop ways of presenting concepts to them and to substitute other experiences for reading. I recall a 15-year-old mother of limited formal education who seemed most interested, when talking with the nurse, in learning about her infant but totally ignored even simply written printed materials. To the nurse the written materials contained delightfully presented and usable information that the mother had requested. With questioning it became obvious that the mother lacked the ability to translate the words into actions and meanings; therefore, the pamphlet was useless. For most learners, a combination of sense experiences and conversation or reading serves to develop a concept.

A concept, then, is a mental construct, an idea. It is not a word or an object but the meaning an individual attaches to the word or object. Teachers cannot give students concepts but can organize verbal descriptions and sense experiences that greatly aid students in acquiring them. How to obtain and produce materials that will help the student develop concepts is considered in Chapters 6 and 7.

Limitations in research on concept learning hamper instructional activities. There is little knowledge about the best ways to sequence instruction, to distribute instruction over time, and to introduce part of a concept initially and then the whole, as well as about when to introduce these concepts (and when not to). There is also limited research on how questioning used in instruction shapes the character of the knowledge acquired.[25,47]

Much more is known about how to know or comprehend concepts than about how to learn to apply, synthesize, and evaluate them, which are the higher mental activities described in the taxonomy of educational objectives in Chapter

4. One cannot engage in these activities until he knows a great deal about a subject, or in other words has a well-developed system of concepts. For example, in order to design an improved cannula for use in hemodialysis (synthesis), one must comprehend the purposes of hemodialysis, the body's reaction to a foreign body in the blood vessels, and the pressure relationship between the blood and the cannula. Developing such a level of thinking is a long-term goal of educational systems. However, the basic thought processes cannot be substantially developed in most of the health-teaching situations the nurse will encounter, although some individuals already have highly developed reasoning skills and may also have lesser skills that can be used with some help from a teacher. Problem solving provides such an opportunity.

The learner may need help at any of the stages of problem solving. The teacher may need to help him recognize a problem, for unless he does so, he is not likely to act to solve it. The patient often needs help in interpreting his feelings of distress in order to focus on and state a problem. The nurse often has information needed to solve problems regarding health matters and can be a sounding board in helping him to think through the problem and a support as he arrives at solutions and tests them.

The results of research give additional guidance on how to help an individual solve a problem. Problem solving is characterized by serial processing, small short-term memory (up to seven items), and infinite long-term memory with fast retrieval but slow storage.[50] Thus an individual's ability to solve the problem with little assistance depends on how much he already understands of its elements. A conceptual framework or a linking of the problem to conceptual spaces of the learner helps him to deal with the small short-term memory and may allow him to retrieve information he already has (since he did not know the problem space was related to the present problem). Other implications for practice may no doubt be deduced.

Following is an example of the nurse helping the patient solve his problem: An elderly gentleman who lives alone has had heart damage and is about to be discharged from the hospital with permanent limitation of activity. He will therefore have a problem in caring for himself as he did before his illness. Although he recognizes the situation as a problem, he needs help in defining its breadth—the extent to which this restriction will affect his daily pattern. The nurse is a source of information to clarify what is meant by the activity restriction. She also has knowledge of the energy the patient will have to expend in different activities and can help him to consider how he can economize on it. The patient, with the help of the nurse, concludes that he can meet the restrictions and remain living alone by having his groceries delivered and allowing a daughter to do his cleaning, washing, and ironing. It is agreed that these new living arrangements will be judged by the amount of energy he must expend, by how tired and how contented he is, and by the physician's opinion about his state of health. The patient then goes home and tries out the hypothesized solutions, evaluating them as determined. At this stage he again needs the nurse's help, best given in his home, in assessing his subjective feelings of tiredness and the total amount of energy he expends. By visiting the home, the nurse is able to think of new solutions that need to be tried. Of course, the situation in this example may be altered slightly or considerably by such factors as the patient's ability to understand the situation, his emotional readiness to deal with it, a decrease in income, the daughter's moving away, or a change in health status. This example is not meant to imply that each patient has only a single problem, although a set of such difficulties is often interrelated.

When there are many problems, reaching a solution is not so straightforward. Considerable compromise may be required, as in the plight of an older person with no financial resources and no family but with a fierce desire for independence. There also are times when people are quite incapable of making decisions, either because they are incapable of this level of thinking or because they experience difficulty in advancing through the steps. The former condition may be seen in the case of a person who has had considerable brain damage from a stroke and must be moved from the home. The family, nurse, and physician solve the problem for this person if he is incapable of reasoning. Difficulty in advancing through the steps of problem solving may be seen in the example of the mother who was distressed because her 2½-year-old daughter was not toilet trained. The mother expressed to the nurse her disgust with this state of affairs and appeared eager to try solutions. After the nurse and the mother discussed what desirable behavior was, the mother formulated hypotheses: she would consistently praise the child for desired behavior and gently reprimand her for undesired behavior. The mother was never able to test these hypotheses, for it became evident that she had such hostile feelings toward the child that she could not control her reactions, as when the child had a bowel movement on the kitchen floor. A situation of this severity occurring more than temporarily would seem to require emotional help. It could be seen in retrospect that the statement of the problem was too limited, so that the hypotheses were unrealistic. This example shows that emotions are sometimes intertwined with problems that may at first seem to be largely a matter of reasoning.

As in any other learning, readiness plays an important part in problem solving. When a family faces a stressful event, their life style and past experience place at their disposal a range of problem-solving possibilities, from which the family members individually or collectively may choose according to their perception of the situation. This is true also for individuals. When the nurse teaches new problem-solving strategies or aids people in further development of those they have used, both the nurse and the learner need to be concerned with how the strategy fits the client's abilities and life style.

Although providing learners with practice in solving problems is important, it is also most useful to label the parts of the process they are using and to talk with them about the process as a method. In the following example, parts of the process are labeled and were later discussed with Mrs. B.

The B. family were basically a "well" family who were experiencing the stresses of normal family development. Separated from her family by a recent move, Mrs. B. first met the public health nurse at an immunization clinic. She eagerly used the nurse's subsequent home visits to increase her understanding of child growth and development and to test out her own ideas about mothering and family life. Johnny, the only child, was 20 months old.

During one home visit the nurse applied the problem-solving method to a developmental question. Mrs. B. had referred to toilet training previously; she picked up the subject again in the following visit.

PROBLEM-SOLVING STEPS
Identification of the problem

MOTHER: I wonder if I should start to do something about toilet training for Johnny.

NURSE: What are some of your ideas about this?

MOTHER: Well, I could let it go for a while, but . . .

NURSE: You're not sure if you want to wait?

MOTHER: Well, no, after all, he's almost two. I don't want him in diapers until he's three! We bought him a little potty chair last month. He climbs all over it. (Sighs)

Determination of possible actions and their probable results

NURSE: What had you thought about doing with the little chair and Johnny?

MOTHER: I could start him on a planned schedule. His B.M.'s are fairly regular. (Discussion follows about schedule, amusements while sitting, possible reactions of child.)

NURSE: You've mentioned two things you might try. First, to let go for a while until Johnny seems more interested; second, to set up a schedule and try to get him into it. There's another idea you might want to consider. Let Johnny get used to sitting on the chair first, and then gradually establish a schedule if he seems ready. (Discussion of probable consequences of this alternative.) All of these are possibilities. Which do you want to check out first?

Selection of one action

MOTHER: Well, maybe he'd be happiest if I first got the idea across to him that he is to *sit* on the potty chair, not climb over it or crawl under it. The schedule could come next. (More discussion as to details of the plan.)

NURSE: You've got some good ideas. Why not try this one idea out? Would you like me to stop by in two weeks or so to see how you're doing?

MOTHER: Okay. We might need a little encouragement. Right, Johnny?

NURSE: Don't forget that there's often more than one right way. I'll see you two weeks from today. Bye.*

The steps of action and evaluation of the action took place after this interaction.

Attitude learning

Although attitudes pervade all spheres of learning, there are times in health teaching when change of behavior in the affective domain constitutes the major task. Acceptance, an emotional adjustment to illness, is a common task. Attitudes of responsibility are called for in taking health action for oneself and in caring for others. A feeling of courage in illness will be recognized by the nurse as frequently important.

An attitude is a learned, emotionally toned predisposition to react in a particular way toward an object, an idea, or a person.[54] Values are similar but more permanent.[32] These feelings are expressions of how an individual believes an object or relationship affects him. Over the years, feelings are gradually developed, become well established, and are reflected in behavior. Often the individual does not realize he is acquiring these attitudes. Membership in groups, particularly primary ones, seems to influence acquisition of attitudes more than it does acquisition of concepts or skills. The influence of these groups is logical, since identification, imitation, and conditioning play an important part in attitude learning.[32] Thus, as an individual is growing up in close contact with the primary group, the family, he is likely to imitate their responsible behavior and be rewarded for it. This becomes a consistent feeling of how he ought to behave—a value.

Although numerous definitions of attitudes have been used, most contemporary definitions can be classified as either probability conceptualizations or intervening variable conceptualizations (an underlying mechanism by which consistency occurs, although the exact content of the mechanism is often ill-defined).[35] There are by now a large number of studies of the relationship between attitudes and behavior, and they do not demonstrate marked correspondence between attitudinal and behavioral measures: product moment correlations are seldom more than .30 and often fall near zero. There is a lack of correspondence between these measures because: they are often "single shot"; attitudes can be general (such as dignity of man) and difficult to express consistently; a person may lack the necessary knowledge to connect his attitude to the relevant behavior; or the behavior may be highly unpleasant. The effect of other attitudes and motives and of the situation is often not known.[34] Thus, predicting behavior from verbal expressions of an individual's attitudes is no longer justified.

Suggestions for teaching attitudes follow directly from knowledge about how they are learned. These include providing someone whose attitudes the learner can view and imitate. This model may very well not be a nurse but another patient with whom the learner seems to be able to identify. This is a basic reason for the establishment of colostomy and ileostomy clubs and other such groups. The use

---

*Collins, R. D.: Problem solving; a tool for patients, too. Am. J. Nurs. **68:**1483-1485, July 1968. I have added the headings for these problem-solving steps.

of the club idea is also one of the most potent ways to reinforce desired attitudes, because it is through successful membership in such groups that these beliefs are reinforced.[18] Another way of influencing attitudes is to provide satisfying experiences, so that the person develops a positive response to ideas or feelings associated with the experiences.[32] For example, personnel in a health clinic should try to provide experiences of the sort that help the patient to have positive feelings toward the clinic.

One of the most severe problems in changing attitudes is that those reinforced in one part of the individual's life may be extinguished in another. This may be true of health attitudes, as in the case of the young unwed mother who showed signs of developing a responsible attitude toward her infant but lost these feelings when she was back with her peer group, which was irresponsible toward all of life.

Understanding also is pertinent to attitude change, particularly when the feeling is not firmly established.[32] However, this relationship may not be predictable: Learning facts about epilepsy may not help a mother to accept an epileptic child. Learning how to do many health-oriented things for themselves and how to work with community health organizations may or may not increase a family's attitudes of self-confidence. The impotence of facts and reasoning in changing attitudes is particularly true with the person with psychiatric problems, for his attitude may be based on strong emotional needs and may be protecting him from anxiety-producing stress.[38]

The body of research from which role playing is drawn is considered to be the most reliable in the area of attitude change. Active participation is more effective than passive exposure to persuasive communications. The minimal requirement of the role-playing technique is that the individual become involved in the attempt to present, sincerely and convincingly, the attitude position of another person. All techniques of attitude change rely on the assumption that change comes out of conflict, discrepancy, inconsistency, or discontent with the status quo. Group pressure techniques make the individual aware that his behavior is in disagreement with the norms of the group. Another technique is social imitation of a model's behavior. Audience participation (group discussion and decision making) helps to overcome resistance. Persuasion is more successful if the persuader has high credibility based on expertise and trustworthiness.[68] Action is both motivational and informational and plays a vital part in attitude change.[31]

Feelings may reflect attitudes or may be more fleeting expressions of affect. In either case, they are constantly present during learning and must be incorporated into the learning process. For example, parent group education is seen as an emotional experience as much as an intellectual one; therefore, expression of feelings that relate to parent-child and family living is encouraged. Those feelings that are close to the surface of consciousness and easily expressed represent an essential part of human existence, even though they are not always recognized as such. The expression of these feelings, since it is not usually a part of social communication, often causes some anxiety in group members but is appropriate for an educational program.[2] A general guideline for every teaching episode might be to assess the learner's feelings about the topic, validate them with him, set up objectives utilizing this knowledge, encourage the expression of conscious feelings, and if necessary try to influence them by using teaching methods such as outlined in this section. Feelings are ever-present when the focus of learning is health and illness, since this whole area of experience relates to threat to one's existence. It is inevitable that nurses who have not learned to communicate with patients about feelings will be less than successful as health teachers.

Learning of psychomotor skills

Everyone can recall the awkwardness of a puppy or child, the unsteadiness of an old man, and the sure coordination of a skilled artist. Motor skills vary with strength, reaction time, speed, balance, precision, and flexibility of tissues.[32]

In order to perform a skill, a person must first possess a neuromuscular system that is capable of performing the skill and then have a mental image of how it is performed. This mental image is provided by a demonstration, which should show the skill and point out relevant cues for successful performance. These are often muscular cues of balance and pull, such as the typist uses to sense where the fingers are and the horn player uses to feel the correct lip placement.[18] Cues may also be seen or heard. When learning to walk with crutches, a person is guided by seeing the floor or objects he might run into, hearing people approach him from behind, and feeling whether he is balanced. To the beginner, the cues must be obvious and are often not noticed much in advance of the action. The mother who is learning how to diaper is so concerned with getting the pin in without sticking the baby that, until she is finished with the job, she is not aware of the cue that the diaper does not fit snugly. The person experienced in doing the motor skill can use many cues rather than just the obvious ones, is not confused by irrelevant cues, attends to them with less conscious concentration, reacts faster, and can take advantage of cues far in advance of action.[18] A person experienced in diapering can do the skill without concentrating on it, is not confused if the edges do not meet exactly, and can see before the pin is in that the diaper will not be snug, so that he pulls it together. This produces a smooth, coordinated sequence of action with minimal expenditure of energy.

In order to develop toward a proficient performance, the learner practices. He uses the mental image as a guide, but he may need at first to have the teacher guide his body so that he experiences the physical sensations that accompany correct motions, as when the nurse holds her hands over the child's as he learns to drink from a cup. For efficiency in learning and maximizing of transfer, it is best for the person to practice in a situation that provides cues similar to those provided where he will use the skill. The colostomy patient is taught in a setup that can be used in a bathroom at home. During the practice, feedback (knowledge of what he is doing right or wrong) is important. This is particularly crucial in the early stages, so that bad habits are not formed. Learners often need help in judging their own performance, even though they do pretty well at judging someone else's. Eventually, the student gets feedback from his own physical sensations and from observing whether the objective of the action is met.

For determining length and frequency of practice sessions, the research results are tentative. In general, short, widely spaced practices are recommended. This means short and infrequent enough to avoid fatigue, which can cause a decrease in function, with resulting frustration. The practice period is too short if it does not allow the learner to complete a whole performance or if it does not extend beyond the period needed to loosen muscles. Intervals between practice are too long if there is excessive forgetting.[18]

After a motor skill is once learned, it can be quickly recaptured even after an interval of many years. It is not possible to make such a clear statement for intellectual learning.[18]

To summarize, there appear to be three phases to skill learning. It begins with a cognitive phase, usually of relatively short duration, during which the learner does not practice much but does cognize the nature of the skill by observing a model and listening to instructions. Only the more obvious cues are differentiated; feedback is elementary and errors many, speed and coordination low, and responses not stable. During the organizing phase, the skill becomes automatic; there is less emphasis on the cognitive and more on the motor. In the perfecting phase there is continuing improvement over a long period of time. Larger behavior units replace the single and intermediate units of the earlier phases.[32]

Training programs to reestablish functions disrupted by nerve damage are developed on the basis of specialized assessments of physiologic readiness. Examples are bladder, voluntary muscle, and speech reeducation, which may be needed for those with varying kinds of damage to the neuromuscular systems. The process of teaching is the same for these programs as for others, but the nurse is less likely to be the primary teacher and will often be functioning as part of an instructional team in which a physical therapist, speech therapist, and others play major roles. As a result of brain injury, the hemiplegic patient may be a poor observer of his environment, fluctuate in mental ability, have a short attention span, and be highly suggestible. Furthermore, it appears that the person with left hemiplegia has greater difficulty with perception. In one teaching method, the patient is instructed to turn his head frequently toward the neglected side to see what is there. The person may also be helped by simple cue cards that list the steps in a procedure or by talking himself through the procedure. Color coding of clothing and other objects can be a guide in placing them correctly. An environment with proper stimulation is important, as is simplicity. It has been found that patients with left hemiplegia do best if they receive instructions verbally and those with right hemiplegia do best if they receive instructions through patomime or demonstration. Routine, repetition, and consistency are essential to learning for these patients.[14]

Social learning

Although probably not a separate kind of learning, social learning occurs in a social setting and focuses on socially relevant tasks, such as dealing with dying and pain. Perhaps several examples will help to clarify the perspective.

Studies of patients on a burn unit focused on pain work and on how patients learned to deal with pain. Dimensions of pain work included diagnosing the meaning of pain, minimizing or preventing it, enduring it, handling pain expression, and getting relief. On the burn unit, enduring pain was emphasized.[53] The patients represented a group who were in various stages of the burn and pain trajectories, in open view of each other, and who spent a rather long period together in an enclosed space. These conditions gave every patient a chance to rehearse and interpret his own illness and its pain trajectory and to compare his state with that of others. The rate of learning differed according to the patient's physical placement on the unit (patient one was next to) and the composition of the patient group at the time. Patients were said to constantly make comparisons among themselves on the trajectory and to measure how much pain expression was legitimate and allowable. Patients said that when they tried to control their own expression of pain and anxiety, excessive or inappropriate expression on the part of other patients was demoralizing. So they taught newer patients to control their expressiveness.[20] This study team found that the staff was not really accountable, in the explicit organizational sense, for the information they provided and the actions they took regarding the patient in pain.[53] Several points can be made as a result of this study: the goals were set by the group for individuals; the open ward provided a range of models to imitate; the staff and other patients provided direct instruction through conversation and reinforcement of various kinds. Whereas the goal was primarily affective at a fairly high level, it had cognitive components (understanding the pain trajectory).

Another example of such learning can be seen in the study of socialization for impending death in a retirement village. The study is based on the notion that an individual is able to view his own identity as nonproblematical if it can be incorporated within shared, taken-for-granted reality and viewed as a typical life in a typical situation. In this village, death appeared to be successfully legitimated for most participants. Approximately 90% of the residents felt that it was better to plan for death than to ignore it, and a similar proportion had already made plans for their own deaths. A high level of social interaction was encouraged and it allowed for the conversational process necessary for legitimization. The resident had role models in the death of his fellows. The milieu was one of support and defined death as appropriate and not a cause for great disruption in the lives of others.[36] The author indicates that these residents did not come to the village already having legitimated their impending deaths. The point of relevance to this discussion of learning theory is the kind of social learning that can occur and the mechanisms that comprise and support the learning.

Learning in children

The field of growth and development is a complex one and includes study of individuals at all ages, of which childhood is one. Readiness to learn depends on maturation, and since a great deal of maturation occurs in childhood, readiness to learn in childhood changes considerably, beginning with visual, auditory, and motion stimulation of infants. The general principles and comments about learning outlined in previous sections of this chapter are applicable to children within their readiness level.

Intellectual development moves from concrete to abstract. Although during the preschool years children can use language to represent objects or experiences, they solve problems by direct manipulation of physical objects.[4] Young children are egocentric and interested only in what affects them. They want explanations for everything but are not concerned about proving the validity of the reason.[67] During the elementary school years, although children need a background of direct nonverbal experience, they can manipulate relationships between ideas verbally without having the objects present. As adolescents and adults they become capable of understanding and manipulating relationships between abstractions without any reference to

concrete reality and eventually can formulate hypotheses based on possible combinations of several ideas and test them.[4]

The developmental tasks of various ages encompass motor skills and development of feelings as well as intellectual growth. The development of trust is crucial until the age of about 2 years. At this point children become more autonomous, learning to walk, run, jump, and feed themselves. The years from 3½ to 7 are described as a time for imagination and learning initiative; the school years, for industry and turning attention to the outside world; and adolescence, for development of identity.[51,61]

This knowledge of growth and development suggests that teachers determine realistic objectives and explain in a way that the child can understand. Allowing the child to manipulate equipment, such as an intermittent positive pressure breathing mask, seems to encourage acceptance of the treatment, especially during the years when direct nonverbal experience is important. The egocentricity and fear of body injury of the child under 5 years of age indicate that he will need to know how a procedure will affect him. It may be explained that during a chest x-ray he will just have to stand still and hold his breath and he will not feel anything. It has been suggested that, if a child is less than 4 years of age, explanation of anatomy and physiology is not useful, because the child does not have the necessary understanding and is prone to develop undesirable fantasies. Since in this age group separation anxiety is a primary problem, teaching should stress continuity of care by the same person and encourage the mother to help care for her child. Preschool children are familiar with the human action or motivational model of causation (people make things happen) and are unaware of invisible physical and mechanical forces. It is suggested that when one talks to these children it is useful to dwell on the physical and mechanical causes of illness and rationales of treatment and help

them set in perspective the probability of psychologic and moral causation.[44]

For children more than 7 years old, more sophisticated language and drawings can be used.[42] Children of school age also benefit from tours of hospital playrooms and wards and from discussion in which they can learn about their illnesses, their origins, and proposed plans of treatment. With a more mature concept of causality, they have the capacity to understand that neither illness nor treatment is imposed on them because of their own misdeeds. They can cooperate with treatment because they can think before they act. They can express their feelings in words and have greater grasp of time sequences and therefore can better tolerate separation.[12]

Third grade is seen as the critical period of change in children's health attitudes and behaviors. Third-graders demonstrate the ability to make a decision of whether to report illness or injury based not only on cognitive abilities but also on learning of the social rules that govern illness and seeking care. By the sixth grade, there is a refinement of these abilities rather than another major change.[40]

Only after the ages of 9 to 11 years, when children begin to be able to relate ideas, do they understand class relationships,[67] so that they can follow the explanation of their pill as a part of the class of objects called medications. The adolescents' task of developing sexual identity makes them ready for learning about mental health in boy-girl relationships.

During school age and adolescence, when the individual is involved in establishing himself in the outside world and developing his identity, the immobilization that often accompanies illness is thought to increase anxiety by restricting patterns of behavior used in the past to relieve frustration and discharge aggression. Even when the rationale for treatment has been shared with the young person and he is able to involve himself in preparation for it, he will retain fear of the unknown until he slowly

learns coping devises to deal with the new tasks facing him. Some of these tasks are as follows:

1. Learning new ways to cope constructively with frustration and with his feelings about the treatment regimen and the persons who implemented it.
2. Doing the grief work necessary to cope with changes in his self- and body-images and the loss of pleasure from activity, self-direction, and independence.
3. Learning the new role of being immobilized. This requires adjustment to new and possibly more rules and regulations than he is accustomed to and dependence upon others for bodily care, age-appropriate stimulation, and privacy which he formerly sought and provided for himself.
4. Establishing patterns of interaction with his environment which provide gratification, control over helplessness and restoration of self-esteem and feelings of self-direction and independence.
5. Readjusting to the "well" role and preparing for going home and back to school when the immobilizing treatment is ended.*

These tasks are made more difficult because children and many early adolescents have not acquired the capacity to project their vision into the future, as adults have, and because mobility is an important tool of communication.[11]

Adolescents need opportunity for dialog with health professionals prepared to deal with the complexity of their questions. An alliance with the professional can assist the adolescent in exercising and experimenting with independence in the management of problems of health or of illness. Health education that is theoretically based and that casts advice in the form of scientific rationales for action rather than imperatives is acceptable and inoffensive to the adolescent mind and ego.[44]

The relevance of this information for teaching is severalfold. First, maturational readiness affects what can be learned and so determines objectives and suggests teaching strategies that

*Blake, F. G.: Immobilized youth; a rationale for supportive nursing intervention, Am. J. Nurs. **69:**2364-2369, Nov. 1969.

might be successful. An example is a study of the understanding that 50 children hospitalized in an isolation unit had of the rationale for gowning, segregation, and confinement. Seventy-one percent of the 3½ to 6 years age group gave incorrect responses, whereas 75% of the 7 to 11 years age group and 92% of the 12 to 17 years age group gave correct responses.[43] Second, since illness and hospitalization can deprive children of activities central to their growth, it is necessary to think in terms of substitute experiences that might be provided to protect the growth potential.[12] It is also important to relieve the anxiety produced by normal developmental crises and by illness and hospitalization, which yield fear of the unknown.

Application of learning principles in operant conditioning

Operant conditioning, also called behavior modification and contingency management, is an application of reinforcement theory, also called operant theory or operant learning theory, and is based on the knowledge that satisfaction motivates learning and that events occurring together are associated. Reinforcement theory is the predominant theoretic orientation of most of a realm of techniques called behavior modification. Contingency management—the rearrangement of environmental rewards and punishments, which strengthen or weaken specified behaviors—is one of many techniques of behavior modification.[55] Its basic tenets are as follows: A positive reinforcement (a smile from the nurse) immediately following a response (using the toilet) can increase the probability that the response will be made again. Also, the removal of an unpleasant stimulus (hunger) can strengthen the action that led to its removal (eating with a spoon). Behavior such as tantrums may be extinguished by ignoring that which has previously received attention (withdrawing positive reinforcers) or by immediate negative reinforcement, such as placing the child's hand under the table and saying

"no" when he throws his spoon.[63] Thus an individual's response can be shaped or gradually changed to meet a goal. Similar techniques are used by everyone in interpersonal relationships, particularly in the parent-child relationship. When they are used by someone trained to do operant conditioning, there should be more objective and knowledgeable analysis of the behaviors and a consistently carried out plan for shaping them. The behavior modification approach may work well in situations where more traditional teaching fails. Perhaps it is particularly effective in situations where there is a "motivation" problem; in those situations, there may be a great deal of reinforcement of present behavior.

Construction of a plan begins with a realistic goal based on the learner's readiness for the activity. A mentally retarded child is ready for finger feeding if he can sit fairly well and place his fingers or toys in his mouth.[30] One observes the behavior in question to see how often, when, where, and with what people it occurs and also catalogs inappropriate behaviors such as kicking, twisting in the high chair, and grinding teeth.

This provides a baseline against which to compare the behavior after nursing intervention; it also yields information about what the individual likes and dislikes and about what is reinforcing his present behavior. One also needs to choose a reinforcer to use in the program. What a person likes to do (for example, watching TV) is likely to prove an effective reinforcer by which to increase the rate of a low-strength behavior (doing chores around the house). It must be something the therapist can control.[9] A 10-year-old child may be observed to have a tantrum lasting 10 minutes every morning after breakfast, during which time the mother and father both hover over him, expressing concern. If this pattern is seen consistently, it is hypothesized that the child likes the parental attention that is presently reinforcing the undesirable behavior of tantrum. One would wonder whether more desirable behavior was receiving this much reinforcement or whether it might be extinguished through lack of reward. Similar patterns were noted regarding fluid intake of a group of patients with spinal cord injuries. Patients often found it difficult to drink sufficient amounts of fluids to yield 2,500-ml. urine outputs, and when this happened, staff became upset and communicated this to the patients. This meant that staff attention often reinforced not drinking. The contingencies were reversed by having each patient make a daily intake record or graph on a clipboard, which was made public. Staff called attention to the increases and praised the patient, whereas decreases were simply ignored.[23]

Nurses know that not all stimuli control behavior and that they have different effects at various ages with different persons. Therefore they observe that a particular child responds with a grin when spoken to or touched. An individual child may also be observed to like a particular toy or a privilege such as going out to play. Food is a commonly used reinforcer, particularly for developing eating skills, and using a lower-calorie diet or withholding food for a period increases the strength of the reinforcer.

After the learner's readiness has been determined and a goal has been established, a plan is then set up. This plan is the program outlining the behavioral steps to be shaped, the schedule of reinforcement, the reinforcers, and the person to carry out the program. Depending on how ready the learner is, it may be necessary for him to acquire the skill in sequence—looking at a spoon, reaching for it, grasping it, dipping it into food, and putting it into the mouth—in order to finally develop the behavior of feeding himself.[59] For others who are already able to do large portions of the skill, one or two steps will suffice, taking perhaps 3 weeks rather than 2 months. At the beginning of training, each desired response may need to be reinforced; later, the reinforcement should be needed less and less, with the schedule of re-inforcement perhaps increased temporarily as more precise and difficult behaviors are required. Thus at the start the nurse may say ''good boy'' and hug the child every time he gets the spoon to his mouth, whereas later this reinforcement is needed only every third time and even later only once a meal. Finally, feeding himself becomes satisfying in itself and requires no external reward. Behavior is learned faster with continuous reinforcement, but that acquired through intermittent reinforcement, once it is learned, is more resistant to extinction.[33] The length of training session depends on the learner's attention span: for a young retarded child learning to feed himself, 20-minute sessions were reported.[8]

Several techniques are used to break tasks into small steps for teaching. Shaping involves successive approximations until the desired behavior is attained—starting with a small element of the behavior and then gradually demanding more complex behavior. An example of a shaping program for teaching feeding to an 18-month-old retarded child may be seen in the box on p. 108. Modeling involves demonstration of the skill so that the learner knows what to do. Fading is a technique of going through a desired activity with the learner and gradually withdrawing teacher participation. At first, the nurse's hand over the child's may be providing actual lifting force to get the spoon to his mouth. Gradually the child's strength is used completely, and the nurse merely prompts him by touching him on the wrist, the elbow, and last, the shoulder and then removes all support. Chaining is a technique used to teach behaviors that normally occur in a fixed sequence, such as washing, toileting, dressing. One teaches the tasks backwards, doing first the last step and then backing up in each training session. Often, all three techniques (shaping, fading, chaining) are used together.[56]

The nurse may do the beginning teaching with a family member or someone else taking over, or the other person may be taught to carry out the process with the nurse providing only consultative services. Which route is taken depends on the ability of the lay person to interpret behavior and consistently give the correct response, on his acceptability to the learner, and on the amount of time he will be with the learner.

Throughout the training period, counts are made of the desired and undesired behaviors, and comparison is made with their incidence at the time the baseline counts were taken. For this comparison, it is useful to make charts: one of desired behavior and one of undesired behavior, with training session number as the abscissa and frequency of behavior as the ordinate. (See reference 8 for example.) The success of the program is evaluated, and modifications may need to be made, including switching of techniques. Shaping proved to be ineffective for Stevie, the little boy mentioned in the box below. Fading was found to be more effective, possibly because reinforcement is delayed less in this technique. It is possible to misjudge a person's readiness level or what is reinforcing his be-

---

SHAPING FEEDING PROGRAM*

. . . we established a program to develop spoon feeding by successive approximation. His mother was included in the planning from the initial collection of baseline data. Sharing the data with the parents is important to foster their cooperation and a sense of trust in you.

The mother was given the following instructions as we began the sessions to teach Stevie to feed himself:

1. When Stevie does something that is part of the activity of spoon feeding (such as looking at or touching the spoon), immediately give him verbal praise and a bit of food (assumed to be positive reinforcers).
2. The most important aspect of reinforcement is immediacy and consistency. Immediately reinforcing his behavior each time he does what you want enables him to associate his actions with getting food and praise.
3. Progressively, he will have to do more and more to get food and praise.
4. When Stevie does something undesirable, immediately say, "No, Stevie," remove the bowl and spoon, and turn away from him for about five seconds or until he stops. Again, the effectiveness of negative reinforcement depends upon immediacy and consistency.
5. At the end of each session, we will look at the data that have been recorded.

Stevie was seated in his high chair with his mother seated at the end of the nearby kitchen table. The mother was facing him and had the food to her side on the table. She held a bowl of cereal with a spoon in it in her right hand. With her left hand, she tapped Stevie's spoon on the tray of his high chair. The instant he looked at his spoon, she praised him, "Good boy, Stevie," and gave him a spoonful of cereal using her left hand. Spoon-feeding behavior was being developed by successive approximation. The shaping sessions were held two consecutive mornings each week. Mrs. S. agreed to feed Steve as usual—at all other times.

This meant that the mother's use of reinforcement and the child's responses could be closely evaluated and changes made as necessary to make the teaching most effective. The progress would have been more rapid had the sessions been at each meal. Visits could not be made that frequently, and we decided to apply reinforcement only when the observer was present, so that bad behaviors would not become established.

---

*Barnard, K.: Teaching the retarded child is a family affair, Am. J. Nurs. **68:**305-311, Feb. 1968.

havior, or a new source of anxiety may disturb the learning process and require revision of the plan. Nurses have an important role in the evaluation of progress; they not only check on the success of the learning process but also make sure the parents see the progress, which may be slow.[8]

Using behavior modification, Berni and others developed a care plan for Billy (below).

The theory and techniques of operant condi-

PLAN FOR BILLY'S CARE*

WEEK 1

Overall goal: To teach the patient appropriate behavior in preparation for discharge by discontinuing attention to his excessively "sick" behavior and by reinforcing "well" behavior.

1. *Goal:* To reinforce ambulation and independence.

   Inappropriate behavior by patient: Refusing to walk, wanting to be carried, and wanting to use wheelchair.

   Negative reinforcers or removal of positive reinforcers: Removing the wheelchair; reducing nurses' social contact, talking, and playing with Billy.

   Appropriate behavior by patient: Walking.

   Positive reinforcers: Nurses smiling and joking with Billy within his physical capabilities.

2. *Goal:* To teach verbal communication and extinguish pointing, grunting, and whining.

   Inappropriate behavior: Grunting, pointing, whining, and not talking.

   Negative reinforcers or removal of positive reinforcers: Nurses refusing to comply with Billy's nonverbal requests after explaining the program to him; reducing nurses' social contact, talking, and playing with him.

   Appropriate behavior: Talking.

   Positive reinforcers: Complimenting his efforts to talk; smiling, talking, and playing with Billy when he talks.

3. *Goal:* To reinforce "well" behavior by deemphasizing bad health and emphasizing positive factors.

   Negative reinforcers: Deemphasizing questions and remarks about his health status, not commenting in front of Billy about his condition, refraining from pointing out his blue nailbeds whenever this occurs.

   Positive reinforcers: Pointing out improvement in his activity, praising him for involvement in the occupational therapy program, praising him when he eats or drinks fluids well.

WEEK 2

Overall goal: To make Billy's daily living experience as happy as possible by providing a feeling of security for him and by teaching him "well" behavior within his physical capabilities.

1. Omit ambulation as a goal for the present.
2. *Goal:* Verbal communication.

   Negative reinforcers: (add) Requesting verbal responses before complying with Billy's requests when he is not talking as he should, going about necessary tasks in silence.

   Positive reinforcers: (add) Taking time to read to Billy.

---

*Billy is a 5-year-old who has ataxia telangiectasia. Adapted from Berni, R., Dressler, J., and Baxter, J. C.: Reinforcing behavior, Am. J. Nurs. **71:**2180-2183, 1971. *Continued.*

PLAN FOR BILLY'S CARE—cont'd

WEEK 2—cont'd

3. *Goal:* To reinforce "well" behavior.
4. *Goal:* To maintain adequate fluid intake.

Negative reinforcers: Responding neutrally when Billy refuses the prescribed fluids.

Positive reinforcers: Placing a plastic translucent cylinder at Billy's bedside, filling it with colored water equal to the amount that Billy drinks, and complimenting Billy as the level of water rises.

WEEK 3

Overall goal: To make Billy feel worthwhile and needed, with "a place in life," in addition to the goals of the first and second weeks.

1. *Goal:* Wheelchair ambulation.

Positive reinforcers: Arranging for portable oxygen tank, and praising patient when he goes to the activity room.

2. *Goal:* To establish verbal communication.
3. *Goal:* To reinforce "well" behavior.

Negative reinforcers: Reacting neutrally to signs of health fluctuation.

4. *Goal:* To maintain prescribed fluid intake (500 cc.).
5. *Goal:* To maintain good nutrition.

Negative reinforcers: Ignoring his refusal to eat.

Positive reinforcers: Commenting when he eats well, giving him attention and choice at the time his menu is made out, making sure that he is served small portions, scheduling meals after pulmonary therapy, and praising him for what he does eat when he has a poor day.

tioning can be used to shape new behaviors, to increase low rates of behavior, to reinstate behavior once exhibited but no longer present, or to eliminate avoidance behavior or so-called anxiety responses.[62] In nursing, operant conditioning has been used to guide learning of self-help skills in retarded persons and to accelerate them in normal children; these skills include spoon feeding, cup drinking, dressing, play skills, ambulation, speech, and toilet using.[59] The technique has been used to extinguish in children such undesirable behaviors as throwing food, undressing,[63] tantrums, and vomiting[65,66] and to reduce such behaviors as spitting, hoarding, upsetting chairs, and scraping walls in patients in mental hospitals, thereby making them more acceptable socially.[7]

In the Patton State Hosital experiment, a token system was used as reinforcement for desired behavior in individual psychiatric patients, for whom the tokens might buy privileges, privacy, food, and other items. Descriptions of how various undesirable psychiatric patient behaviors might be dealt with are available.[49] A similar system was reported to be in operation with moderately mentally retarded patients to develop their learning and social skills to the point that they could live in the community.[13] Another program used was an operant conditioning program to modify behavior of psychotic children 3 to 7 years old and to teach parents and other family members how to interact with the children. Two very interesting case studies have been described.[57] Another account describes successful operant conditioning, by a patient peer, of verbal behavior in a withdrawn patient whose characteristic behaviors included a low rate of initiating verbal behavior with others.[15] An unsuccessful attempt was made to modify incontinent behavior in a group of long-term neuropsychiatric geriatric patients (those with organic dysfunctions in the brain and elsewhere were included in the study) with use of social or material reinforcement.[27] These short summaries of programs and general uses for operant conditioning are not exhaustive of those that have been tried and suggested.

Parents have been taught to use behavior modification with their children, and there does not appear to be any class of overt child behaviors that parents cannot be taught to modify. There are three approaches in training parents: educational groups, individual consultations, and controlled learning environments, such as a situation where professionals observe through one-way mirrors and direct behavior of parents with earphones. (This last approach can also be used in the home.) The training program may involve general or specific steps for a particular behavioral change. Programmed instruction texts are often used to present basic behavioral principles and applications. Instructional techniques include modeling after demonstration by the professional or another parent. Videotape feedback for analysis and correction of procedures is useful.[39]

Operant conditioning would seem to have considerable relevance in achieving learning goals for many clients. Recently, its focus has become more cognitive, since all behavior is seen to be cognitively mediated and affected by expectancies. Guidance in this research and practice should be sought from psychologists who have depth of preparation in learning theory and the interpretation of behavior, with the counsel of physicians who understand the behavior of illness. A major concern about the use of operant conditioning has been that it may merely change surface behavior without getting at its basis, both psychologically and physiologically. Thus, treating pain, vomiting, or anxiety by operant conditioning requires considerable judgment regarding other possible causes of the behavior.

The intent is certainly not that the learning model should replace the medical model but that each should complement the other to provide more comprehensive management. With regard to pain, it is believed that, although the medical model has much factual support, there is not enough to justify universal application of that model to phenomena of chronic pain. Some aspects of chronic pain may also be conceptualized in learning terms—that much of the behavior occurring subsequent to presentation of a presumed noxious stimulus may be accounted for and modified by principles of learning, whatever the original cause of pain. The problem's becoming chronic is evidence that it has not been entirely resolved by medical approaches, and the opportunities for learning pain behavior patterns by operant mechanisms are increased.[21]

The usefulness of operant conditioning theory is exciting and promising; full management of it as a therapeutic tool requires special training. An excellent book by Berni and Fordyce describes its practice in an interdisciplinary health setting.[9] Nurses can learn a great deal from this theory that helps them to analyze learning environments wherever they may be. For example, one father said that when the physician diagnosed his son's disease as diabetes, he gave information about the disease, which the father in retrospect said was accurate. However, the explanation occurred in a very short period of time without reinforcement, and subsequently neighbors gave all sorts of contrary information and advice. The result was confusion, forgetting of what the physician had said, and doubt that he had given true information. This represented extinction of the original learning. One of the concerns about mental hospital environments has been that they frequently disrupt the social relationships of the patient without replacing them, or else replace them with a social milieu inadequate as a relearning device.[55] Indeed, there is growing doubt that the process of reinforcement can be legitimately separated, as it has been in the past, from the concept of motivation.[26]

COMMON AND COMPLEX LEARNING SITUATIONS

Learning has been viewed as an exceedingly complex activity; therefore, the strategy of study of small units of behavior in controlled situations has become common. In real life, very complex interrelationships of factors affect learning, and behavior change in many domains is occurring simultaneously. Presentation and analysis of such real-life situations should help to place use of knowledge about learning in a perspective.

Follow-up support for learning

Very little seems to be known about the general effectiveness of health teaching and about subsequent retention of health knowledge and attitudes. It can be hypothesized that much of the teaching, especially about illness, occurs in situations not especially conducive to learning and retention. These could include hospitals, physician's offices, and clinics. The weight of evidence and logic suggests that learning is typically a gradual (continuous) rather than an all-or-none (discontinuous) phenomenon.[5] However, from reports available, one would question whether the continuity in teaching over a period of time is long enough to result in the necessary learning. In addition, during hospitalization and at other times when individuals are seeking medical care, they may not feel well enough to learn or may be in a stage of psychosocial adaptation not conducive to learning the skills and knowledge they later need. The dependence that is often involved in hospitalization can make it difficult for the patient to envision what posthospitalization independence will require. In many of these situations, family members are not with the patient, and so they miss what is being taught. As a result, patients have no one readily available with whom to check their memory of what was taught or to reinforce it in the home situation. In addition, for ex-patients of the highly focused short-term institution, no posthospital structures exist through which the experience may be collectively reviewed and given meaning; therefore, these patients cope with it on their own. This might be especially pertinent for patients who have undergone alterations that distinguish them markedly from other persons in the community, such as radical facial surgery.

Whether learning is not retained because of the natural forgetting that occurs over time, the nonreinforcement in home environments, or incomplete learning initially, follow-up teaching seems needed for patients, especially those on long-term regimens. In two follow-up studies of diabetic patients, it was found that the longer they had the disease, the more insulin errors they made.[60,64] In one of these studies, large numbers of the patients had what were considered unacceptable daily routines in insulin administration, urine tests, and diet management. The question asked is whether patients with diabetes try what is considered by professionals to be adequate control and then find that the errors do not affect them seriously and so become careless. What part should reinstruction and supportive attention play in this situation to improve performance? To what extent can retention be improved by alteration of the conditions under which the original learning took place? What influence can reteaching have, and how and when might it best be accomplished? What kinds of reteaching and supportive services do patients want, since they have a right not to comply if they do desire?

Complexity of learning situations

Just as the conditions that affect necessity for follow-up teaching are complex, so also are many other learning situations in which the nurse is involved.

Frequently, patients who have had cerebrovascular accidents need to accomplish learning in all three domains, whereas their capacity to learn has diminished in several possible ways. In addition, nurses are often dependent on others with special skills in assessing learning deficits and in developing programs of teaching, but they may not have access to this expertise. Deficits may include poor balance so that these patients lean heavily or fall toward one side but show no awareness of what is happening, difficulty in dressing because they cannot comprehend shapes and designs, and difficulty in judging distance and the passage of time.

Patients with brain damage often have a short retention span and, if given too many long messages, can be overwhelmed and confused. Although they may have good memories for old information, they may have difficulty in generalizing; thus they are sensitive to any change in their environment. Memory jogs, such as written steps or pictures, are helpful. There is often a decrease in ability to judge the appropriateness of their own behavior. They can be helped by information or feedback about their social errors if corrections are made in a matter-of-fact, pleasant manner.[22]

Basically, the task of aiding learning is to utilize principles of learning within patients' altered states of readiness. In the case of perceptual deficits, patients are taught conscious movements to correct them, such as turning the head to compensate for alteration in field of vision or looking in a mirror and shifting one's weight to avoid leaning. Verbal or pantomimed instructions can help patients judge distance. They need an environment that will stimulate them to learn but that is not too complex—one in which people will talk with them and require them to perform some tasks but make directions brief, concrete, and free of abstractions with one idea or command being expressed at a time. Routine, repetition, consistency, and practice are essential for learning for these patients.[12] In rehabilitation of stroke patients, teaching and learning are pervasive in staff interactions with the patient, with many goals being sought at once and direction of patient learning coming from various team members.

A different kind of complexity is involved for teachers when they are trying to effect learning in clients whose education and life style are different from their own. Although the general principles of learning still apply, tactics and approaches need to be altered to meet the client's readiness. Nurses need a view of the breath of ways in which learning can occur, some faith and skill in the use of the nursing process and the process of teaching, and a view of their role as service to the client; otherwise they may find themselves demanding that patients learn in what is essentially a middle-class way—highly verbal, teacher oriented, and future oriented. Although the teaching-learning relationship must be reciprocal, often the teachers bear responsibility for initiating it, and their expectations regarding acceptable ways to learn and teach soon become evident to the client. For example, in teaching low-income groups whose low level of educational achievement and susceptibility to day-to-day crises tend to make them preoccupied with tangible immediate problems, health educators have found it difficult to organize and sustain interest in groups for discussing and learning about noncrisis matters. The majority of these families would probably do best with health education directed toward defined problems that they have recognized and toward a specific course of action they see as reasonable and possible. Teaching goals for food selection need to be realistically related to welfare budgets and local shopping facilities and are likely to be more successful if explained in terms of essential foods rather than food elements. The nurse is advised to use constant reality testing, "Do you think this will work?" or "Will your family drink powdered milk if you fix it?" In addition, an aggressive, "reaching out" kind of recruitment is also suggested.[24]

In their daily practice, nurses and other health workers constantly encounter situations that require analysis of patient learning. For example, a nutritionist was concerned that a diabetic patient, whom she was trying to teach diet restrictions, immediately wanted to know which foods he could eat, when her intention had been to first teach him basic information about food elements and principles of diabetic diet restrictions. The perspective that learning theory can give to an educator in such a situation is that some people learn more easily inductively (from concrete facts to abstract principles) and others deductively (from principles they deduce specific actions). Other possibilities are that the patient is excessively anxious about his diet and that this might be relieved by the information he wants. No doubt there are other possible hypotheses.

Analysis of learning problems in terms of known principles and theory is useful; however, nurses also have a role and responsibility for extending knowledge about how patients learn. Rubin's work on maternal acquisition is illustrative. She describes distinct operations involving mimicry and role playing, fantasy and introjection-projection-rejection, and grief work in letting go of former roles incompatible with the new role and of the part played by the woman's own mother and later by peers, as models for each phase.[48] This research, which needs to be extended, has obvious potential for teaching interventions.

SUMMARY

Since fulfillment of particular objectives is the purpose for educational efforts, the teacher draws on a core of knowledge about learning, including growth and development, in order to guide the change. For cognitive behaviors an important consideration is establishing a bridge of meaning between old and new understandings; for attitude learning opportunity for imitation of a model; for motor skills, practice with feedback. Operant conditioning involving discriminative use of behavior reinforcers has already been shown to be significant for nursing.

Nurses are commonly involved in complex situations in which multiple classes of learning are occurring simultaneously and in which multiple principles of learning are applicable. Teaching then is based on judgements about priority and tactics, which are checked by evidence of goal attainments.

STUDY QUESTIONS

1. It has been stated that for natural childbirth, the patient is a member of the birth team. Information should be given freely to her about her progress, since such information serves as a guide in her method of breathing, in conservation of energy, and in her sense of security in labor. The patient's role is active, and she needs to be treated as a responsible adult.[25]
   a. What principles of learning support the above statements?
   b. What guidance do learning principles give in setting the limits to the amount of information given to the patient?
2. Following are sequential responses of patients who had suffered coronary occlusions. Indicate possible rationale for the behavior, in terms of theory about readiness and learning.
   A first response to this illness was anxiety and a frantic search for a "cause" of the illness, as a way to control the disease by excluding this activity.
   Some patients had an urgent need for rigid definition by the physicians about the correct way and extent of exerting themselves during convalescence and later, which is a kind of bargaining for control of the symptoms.
   Some patients wished to remain confused about their understanding of the illness.
   Other patients sought to identify with others whom they knew had suffered a coronary occlusion. This helped

to decrease the ambiguity they experienced in the early stages of the illness because, by following the pattern of convalescence of their colleagues, they were able to structure some expectations for their own future.[37]

3. An assumption on which parent group education can be based is that parents learn best when they are free to create their own response to a situation. At no time does the leader pressure toward group consensus or conformity.[2] What possibly conflicting learning principles are involved in the decision to function according to this assumption?

4. Some findings suggest a relationship between feelings of guilt on the part of parents of handicapped children and the adequacy of their knowledge.
   a. What could explain this relationship?
   b. How would you use this information?

REFERENCES

1. Archer, E. J.: The psychological nature of concepts. In Klausmeier, H. J., and Harris, C. W., editors: Analyses of concept learning, New York, 1966, Academic Press, Inc., pp. 37-63.
2. Auerbach, A. B.: Parents learn through discussion, New York, 1968, John Wiley & Sons, Inc.
3. Ausubel, D. P.: The psychology of meaningful verbal learning, New York, 1963, Grune & Stratton, Inc.
4. Ausubel, D. P.: Stages of intellectual development and their implications for early childhood education. In Neubauer, P. B., editor: Concepts of development in early childhood education, Springfield, Ill., 1965, Charles C Thomas, Publisher.
5. Ausubel, D. P.: Educational psychology; a cognitive view, New York, 1968, Holt, Rinehart and Winston, Inc.
6. Ausubel, D. P., and Blake, E., Jr.: Proactive inhibition in the forgetting of meaningful school materials, J. Educ. Res. **52:**145-149, 1958.
7. Ayllon, T., and Michael, J.: The psychiatric nurse as a behavioral engineer, J. Exp. Anal. Behav. **2:**323-334, 1959.
8. Barnard, K.: Teaching the retarded child is a family affair, Am. J. Nurs. **68:**305-311, Feb. 1968.
9. Berni, R., and Fordyce, W. E.: Behavior modification and the nursing process, ed. 2, St. Louis, 1977, The C. V. Mosby Co.
10. Berni, R., and others: Reinforcing behavior, Am. J. Nurs. **71:**2180-2183, 1971.
11. Blake, F. G.: Immobilized youth; a rationale for supportive nursing intervention, Am. J. Nurs. **69:**2364-2369, Nov. 1969.
12. Blake, F. G., Wright, F. H., and Waechter, E. H.: Nursing care of children, ed. 8, Philadelphia, 1970, J. B. Lippincott Co.
13. Bourgeois, T. L.: Reinforcement theory in teaching the mentally retarded; a token economy, Perspect. Psychiatr. Care **6:**116-136, 1968.
14. Burt, M. M.: Perceptual deficits in hemiplegia, Am. J. Nurs. **70:**1026-1029, May 1970.
15. Cockrill, V. K., and Bernal, M. E.: Operant conditioning of verbal behavior in a withdrawn patient by a patient-peer, Perspect. Psychiatr. Care **6:**230-237, 1968.
16. Coleman, J. S., and others: The Hopkins games program; conclusions from seven years of research, Educ. Researcher **2:**3-7, Aug. 1973.
17. Collins, R. D.: Problem solving; a tool for patients, too, Am. J. Nurs. **68:**1483-1485, July 1968.
18. Cronbach, L. J.: Educational psychology, ed. 3, New York, 1977, Harcourt Brace Jovanovich, Inc.
19. Deutsch, C. P.: Learning in the disadvantaged. In Klausmeier, H. J., and Harris, C. W., editors: Analyses of concept learning, New York, 1966, Academic Press, Inc.
20. Fagerhaugh, S. Y.: Pain expression and control on a burn care unit, Nurs. Outlook **22:**645-650, 1974.
21. Fordyce, W. E., and others: Some implications of learning in problems of chronic pain, J. Chronic Dis. **21:**179-190, 1968.
22. Fowler, R. S., Jr., and Fordyce, W.: Adapting care for the brain-damaged patient, Am. J. Nurs. **72:**2056-2059, 1972.
23. Fowler, R. S., Fordyce, W. E., and Berni, R.: Operant conditioning in chronic illness, Am. J. Nurs. **69:**1226-1228, June 1969.
24. Freeman, R. B.: Community health nursing practice, Philadelphia, 1970, W. B. Saunders Co.
25. Glaser, R.: Concept learning and concept teaching. In Gagne, R. M., and Gephart, W. J., editors: Learning research and school subjects, Itasca, Ill., 1968, F. E. Peacock Publishers, Inc.
26. Glaser, R.: Learning. In Ebel, R. L., editor: Encyclopedia of educational research, ed. 4, New York, 1969, The Macmillan Co.
27. Grosicki, J. P.: Effect of operant conditioning on modification of incontinence in neuropsychiatric geriatric patients, Nurs. Res. **17:**304-311, 1968.
28. Harre, R.: The formal analysis of concepts. In Klausmeier, H. J., and Harris, C. W., editors: Analyses of concept learning, New York, 1966, Academic Press, Inc.
29. Hoff, F. E.: Natural childbirth; how any nurse can help, Am. J. Nurs. **69:**1451-1453, July 1969.
30. Holtgrewe, M. M.: A guide for public health nurses working with mentally retarded children, Washington, D.C., 1964, U.S. Government Printing Office.
31. Kelman, H. C.: Attitudes are alive and well and gainfully employed in the sphere of action, Am. Psychol. **29:**310-324, 1974.

32. Klausmeier, H. J., and Ripple, R. E.: Learning and human abilities; educational psychology, ed. 4, New York, 1975, Harper & Row, Publishers.

33. Layton, Sister M. M.: Behavior therapy and its implications for psychiatric nursing, Perspect. Psychiatr. Care **4:**38-52, 1966.

34. Lemon, N.: Attitudes and their measurement, London, 1973, B. T. Batsford, Ltd.

35. Liska, A. E.: Emergent issues in the attitude-behavior consistency controversy, Am. Sociol. Rev. **39:**261-272, 1974.

36. Marshall, V. W.: Socialization for impending death in a retirement village, Am. J. Sociol. **80:**1124-1144, 1975.

37. Martin, H. L.: The significance of discussion with patients about their diagnosis and its implications, Br. J. Med. Psychol. **40:**233-242, 1967.

38. Matheney, R. V., and Topalis, M.: Psychiatric nursing, ed. 6, St. Louis, 1974, The C. V. Mosby Co.

39. O'Dell, S.: Training parents in behavior modification; a review, Psychol. Bull. **81:**418-433, 1974.

40. Palmer, B. B., and Lewis, C. E.: Development of health attitudes and behaviors, J. Sch. Health **46:**401-402, 1976.

41. Patterson, E. G., and Rowland, G. T.: Toward a theory of mental retardation nursing; an educational model, Am. J. Nurs. **70:**531-535, 1970.

42. Petrillo, M.: Preventing hospital trauma in pediatric patients, Am. J. Nurs. **68:**1469-1473, 1968.

43. Pidgeon, V. A.: Children's concepts of the rationale of isolation technique. In American Nurses' Association: ANA clinical sessions, San Francisco, 1968, Meredith Publishing Co., pp. 21-27.

44. Pidgeon, V. A.: Characteristics of children's thinking and implications for health teaching, Mat. Child Nurs. J. **6**(1):1-8, 1977.

45. Riessman, F., Cohen, J., and Pearl, A.: Mental health of the poor, New York, 1964, The Macmillan Co.

46. Rosengren, W. R., and Lefton, M.: Hospitals and patients, New York, 1969, Atherton Press, Inc.

47. Rothkopf, E. Z.: Two scientific approaches to the management of instruction. In Gagne, R. M., and Gephart, W. J., editors: Learning research and school subjects, Itasca, Ill., 1968, F. E. Peacock Publishers, Inc.

48. Rubin, R.: Attainment of the maternal role. II. Models and referents, Nurs. Res. **16:**342-346, 1967.

49. Schaefer, H. H., and Martin, P. L.: Behavioral therapy, New York, 1969, McGraw-Hill Book Co.

50. Simon, H. A., and Newell, A.: Human problem solving; the state of the theory in 1970, Am. Psychol. **26:**145-159, 1971.

51. Smart, M. S., and Smart, R. C.: Children; develop-ment and relationships, ed. 3, New York, 1977, The Macmillan Co.

52. Snelbecker, G. E.: Learning theory, instructional theory, and psychoeducational design, New York, 1974, McGraw-Hill Book Co.

53. Strauss, A., and others: Pain; an organizational-work-interactional perspective, Nurs. Outlook **22:**560-566, 1974.

54. Summers, G. F., editor: Attitude measurement, Chicago, 1970, Rand McNally & Co.

55. Tharp, R. G., and Wetzel, R. J.: Behavior modification in the natural environment, New York, 1969, Academic Press, Inc.

56. Thompson, T. I., and Grabowski, J., editors: Behavior modification of the mentally retarded, New York, 1972, Oxford University Press.

57. Turner, R.: A method of working with disturbed children, Am. J. Nurs. **70:**2146-2151, 1970.

58. Underwood, B. J.: Interference and forgetting, Psychol. Rev. **64:**49-60, 1957.

59. Vevang, B., Leonard, P., and Pierson, L.: Experience in mental retardation for basic nursing students, Nurs. Forum **6**(2):183-194, 1967.

60. Watkins, J. D., and others: A study of diabetic patients at home, Am. J. Public Health **57:**452-459, 1967.

61. Whipple, D. V.: Dynamics of development; euthenic pediatrics, New York, 1966, McGraw-Hill Book Co.

62. Whitney, L.: Operant learning theory; a framework deserving nursing investigation, Nurs. Res. **15:**229-234, 1966.

63. Whitney, L. R., and Barnard, K. E.: Implications of operant learning theory for nursing care of the retarded child, Ment. Retard. **4:**26-29, 1966.

64. Williams, T. F., and others: The clinical picture of diabetic control, studied in four settings, Am. J. Public Health **57:**441-451, 1967.

65. Wolf, M. M., and others: A note on apparent extinction of the vomiting behavior of a retarded child. In Ullmann, L. P., and Krasner, L., editors: Case studies in behavior modification, New York, 1965, Holt, Rinehart and Winston, Inc.

66. Wolf, M., Risley, T., and Mees, H.: Application of operant conditioning procedures to the behavior problems of an autistic child. In Ullmann, L. P., and Krasner, L., editors: Case studies in behavior modification, New York, 1965, Holt, Rinehart and Winston, Inc.

67. Wu, R.: Explaining treatments to young children, Am. J. Nurs. **65:**71-73, July 1965.

68. Zimbardo, P., and Ebbesen, E. B.: Influencing attitudes and changing behavior, ed. 2, Reading, Mass., 1977, Addison-Wesley Publishing Co., Inc.

CHAPTER 6

Teaching: definition, theory, and interpersonal techniques

■ Although nurses have actually been teaching while assessing readiness and defining objectives, they now arrive at the point where they try to produce behavior change. The common notion of teaching as giving information to a class disregards other very important facets of the task. It also presents a very limited view of the variety of teaching methods and techniques available and of the kinds of behavior changes possible.

There are a number of learning tools available: printed material in books and pamphlets, programmed instruction, pictures and other visual aids including television and motion pictures, certain situations and environments, and individuals and groups. Depending on the learner and the material, these tools more or less provide self-instruction for the learner. Although individuals learn many things without a teacher, most need a teacher part of the time. Today the teacher is less a dispenser of information, that is, of factual material, than a programmer and designer of many kinds of learning experiences, who reaches toward particular goals and uses a combination of tools, including the relationship with the learner. Teachers who are less knowledgeable and skilled in teaching tend to be rigid in their responses, often limited to giving the learner information they think he needs. More skilled teachers are more flexible

in that they can alter their teaching according to the learner's responses and are capable of using many techniques and tools in appropriate ways. These behaviors fall on a continuum; determine where your own present teaching behaviors fall.

OVERVIEW OF INSTRUCTIONAL FORMS

The reader will recall from the last chapter that the theory of instruction concerned with optimizing the learning process is not yet well developed. In the meantime, it would be useful to have an overview of instructional forms, of their differences and common elements. Having considered learning in terms of its broad classes—direct experience through reinforcement, observation of a model, and symbolic systems including natural language—we may now examine the instructional side of the situation. Reinforcement has the limitation of being ambiguous because it does not indicate the critical alternatives the learner faces in making a decision but only the consequences of the formal performances. Teachers can make the situation less ambiguous by immediately reinforcing the learner's positive behavior and by making clear the feature of the stimulus that is to be attended. Language is an instructional device par excellence because a word indicates not only a perceived referent but also the excluded set of alternatives, and language coding is less ambiguous. Its major limitation in instruction is not only that it demands literacy but that instruction in it is limited to rearranging, ordering, and differentiating knowledge or information that the learner already has available from other sources, such as modeling or his own experience. Modeling is graphic but does not always reveal reasons for actions.

According to one point of view, all of these instructional forms, which seem to have widely different topographies, can lead some learners to the same terminal performance and to some extent convey the same information. All of them increase in the amount of information conveyed (information density), from reinforcement, to modeling, to language.[41] Obviously, research is not complete; although this chapter will point out reasons for choosing one approach or form rather than another, it is important to remember that various instructional forms overlap in their degrees of efficiency.

KNOWLEDGE ABOUT CONTENT TO TEACH

For the most part, decisions about content to teach are made by inferring what a patient needs to know from an established body of thought. It is rare to have research verifying content; most research deals with process of teaching and either avoids consideration of content or standardizes it. Several studies of persons undergoing threatening procedures (gastroendoscopy, removal of children's orthopedic casts) have found that those told about typical physical sensations showed less distress than did those told about the procedure or those not given preparatory information. The messages focus on what is felt, tasted, heard, seen, and smelled during the procedure (about which there is high agreement) but not on the intensity, which tends to vary among individuals. Note that the sensation content describes the event from the patient's point of view, whereas the less effective description about how and

where a procedure will be done represents the provider's point of view.[27]

THE TEACHER-LEARNER RELATIONSHIP

To a varying extent, the teacher-learner relationship is one between an authority and a subordinate or is one between two equals. Which relationship is more predominant depends on the difference in knowledge of subject matter between teacher and learner and on other cultural factors such as age, sex, and social status. Although it is essential for nurses to understand thoroughly what they are teaching, they relate to the learner as less of an authority if he or she has a good general knowledge of the subject or is generally well educated. The social status of the nurse, particularly the student nurse, is considered to be subordinate to positions of physician, professor, businessman, lawyer, matron, and many others. Sometimes these social positions are accompanied by an attitude of superiority that is communicated to the nurse.

Therefore, it is not unusual for students of nursing, and often older nurses also, to view themselves as subordinate in knowledge and social status to the clients for whose learning they are responsible. It becomes easy to assume that patients are in such a strong position that they need no teaching, or, even if one sees evidence that they do, to be afraid to approach them. This may be illustrated in the case of the nurse needing to teach a middle-aged successful businessman how to care for his colostomy or to discuss his bladder operation. A frequently encountered example is the young student who is just learning about maternity or the care of children and is dealing with women who are older and have been mothers for some time. Feelings of hesitancy are natural but can be overcome by gaining a thorough understanding of material before trying to teach it and by constructing a relationship that might be expressed as, "I'll learn from you and perhaps you can learn from me." There is no doubt that nurses will feel more comfortable in their teaching role as they gain maturity and a better understanding of the subject matter. However, in patient teaching, as in all other activities, inexperienced nurses must become comfortable with themselves as learners, seek supervision, and accept their errors as the basis for improvement.

Entering into a teaching relationship with a prospective learner requires a commitment to seeing that the individual or group of learners receives teaching until the goals are reached or until instruction is no longer profitable. This does not mean that nurses take on the responsibility for solving the problems, although they do use knowledge of them in setting goals. The relationship should be interpreted to the client in terms of how it may assist him, when the nurse will be available without interruption, and how long the relationship will last.[21]

This commitment is made as part of a professional relationship, with the nurse-teacher knowing full well that the reactions of learners to teachers can be quite hostile and that, even in individuals who are eager to learn, motivation sometimes falters. Changes in behavior, which learning must create, may be difficult for the learner because they remove his security in familiar ways of acting; or, when a person recognizes a need for change but does not know how to accomplish it, he may go through a demoralizing experience.[49] There are, on the other hand, many persons who express appreciation for instruction. Although these expressions are heartwarming and the hostile ones can be threatening, they both must be viewed with equanimity. The teacher must attain a perspective not only of competence as a teacher of many persons but also of the experiences people go through in order to learn to deal with health needs.

The difficulty professionals face in dealing with hostility is suggested in a study of 14 Baltimore families in which a child had bulbar polio. Parents were not informed that their children would have residual disability from the disease until long after physicians and other medical workers knew for certain what the effect would be. Physicians hedged, and since the parents were not given bad news, most of them remained more hopeful than they should have been. From private interviews carried on for the study, it was found that physicians did not wish to contend with the emotional reaction that the parents would have had to knowledge of residual disability. With a number of the parents, this lack of information had the unfortunate effect of diverting them from taking full advantage of available rehabilitation therapies.[14] If the consequences can be so adverse, it would seem wise for professionals to examine their desires to so control this expression of feeling toward them.

TECHNIQUES AND METHODS OF INSTRUCTION BY INTERPERSONAL INTERACTION

Much of teaching occurs by interpersonal interaction, more or less formal or structured in form. Lack of formality or of a high degree of structure does not imply lack of planning. For some it is a conscious choice of a more acceptable learning style, because the give-and-take is desirable for motivation or for learning that requires consistent, complex feedback. A great deal that the nurse does day by day in helping a patient understand how he is coping with a health stress is often done in an unstructured way in an informal atmosphere. It has been suggested that, if nurses encourage their patients to respond to questions such as "What did you notice?" "What happened? Can you describe it?" "What did you think?" "What did you say?" "What did you feel?" they convey interest in the patient's expressiveness, and that, if patients respond, they learn and also provide themselves and the nurse with data from which meaning can be abstracted.[43] The outlining of such a description sequentially can relieve confusion and help a person gain perspective and objectivity in distinguishing between action and feeling and their relationship to each other.[6]

The lecture and discussion, widely known in school settings, are really basic forms of teaching that are applicable as well to teaching of patients. Each of these methods emphasizes particular characteristics, including structure. A lecture implies a person presenting a discourse, often highly structured, usually to a group of learners. Discussion suggests a focus on exchange of ideas between persons, usually not highly prestructured, often in a small group so that individuals can be actively involved. These methods are often not found in their pure form: in a particular teaching interaction, the predominant form may be a teacher's presenting information, but there also may be considerable exchange between teacher and student (or students) and between students. Each of these forms of instruction can be used by someone teaching one learner or a number of learners. By its very nature, each provides conditions better for certain learning goals than for others.

A major way in which these interpersonal interaction techniques vary is in their directness. Direct behavior may be defined as emanating from the teacher and often requiring a particular response from the learner. In indirect behavior the roles are more blurred; much more of the interaction is initiated by the learner; and the teacher focuses on maximizing this by reflecting the learner's feelings and thoughts. Direct teaching is generally considered to be most useful when the learner is anxious, when he needs to learn rapidly, or when reflective thinking or attitude alteration is not necessary. Appropriate times for direct or indirect approaches can be illustrated by patient teaching during labor. There is a sociability in the first stage, during which the patient can be oriented to the environment and the pattern of labor to come can be reviewed in an easy give-and-take manner (indirect).[15] A classic characteristic of transition from the first to the second stage is confusion.[25] In the second stage, it becomes important for the patient to surrender control and mastery of her body, and she should not be harassed with lengthy explanations but should be given firm suggestions as to position and directed to breathe deeply with contractions. This directness of teacher approach will need to continue as the task at hand consumes all of the patient's energy.[15] At presentation of the head, the nurse should pant with the patient so that she can stop pushing.

The lecture at its best is an efficient and interesting way to learn about something. It can be a means for giving information, for showing relationships among concepts, for demonstrating higher-level intellectual skills, and for influencing attitudes not yet strongly formed. Its weaknesses are that it does not allow students to ask questions and that it does not ensure that they are actively thinking about the material being presented.

The lecture can be strengthened for many learning outcomes by allowing or requiring some exchange between learner and teacher and between learners. A nurse teaching at the bedside of a patient, helping him to comprehend the effects of his surgery, will probably give as part of the lesson an explanation that could be considered a lecture. During the explanation, the nurse might illustrate the need for surgery by drawing from the patient information about his symptoms. The nurse ought to be interested in what he wants to know about the entire experience and is likely to discuss with the patient his feelings about having the surgery. This kind of easy give-and-take, a combination of information giving and discussion, is often motivating and quite useful for assuring that the patient comprehends.

Lecture and discussion, as general teaching methods, can be adapted considerably for persons, including those of lower socioeconomic status, who seem not to be able to understand a "lecture." These persons may have poor vocabularies and limited verbal ability, but they probably are also reacting to a lecture as a symbol of school, in which they may not have been successful. Nurses in a maternity clinic of a large municipal hospital with many patients of lower socioeconomic status set up unstructured conferences, purposely not called classes, in the clinic waiting area, which the women were free to come to, move about in, and leave at will. The invited four or five patients were the core for a group, which grew with each session. In general, demonstrations of self-help measures and audiovisual aids created lots of interest. Patients were encouraged to talk about some of their own experiences, and, when they did, their descriptions often vividly stimulated the group, with the group leaders interrupting only to praise a mother's knowledge or handling of a situation or to correct false information.[5]

Other techniques developed clinically have the purpose of giving, rehearsing, and confirming information and perspective. Predischarge family conferences were instituted on a cardiology service when staff discovered that many patients became more anxious or depressed before discharge and could not recall the information that had been provided to them during their hospitalization. The predischarge conference offered an opportunity for the patient and members of his family to review his medical problem, his posthospital care, and his psychosocial status and encouraged asking of questions that needed further clarification. Subjects reviewed were emotional responses, adjustments, stresses, patient and family methods of coping with the illness, and detailed explanation of activities, including return to employment.[26]

Rehearsal of learning through a trial situation is an effective teaching technique as well as being evaluative. Following is such an interaction with a patient who has had coronary artery surgery:

NURSE: Suppose you are gardening and you get angina. What would you do?

PATIENT: I would stop gardening, rest, and take a nitroglycerin (NTG).

NURSE: The chest discomfort continues. What would you do next?

PATIENT: I would take another NTG, and my doctor told me also to take a Librium.

NURSE: Your angina persists. What now?

PATIENT: I would take a third NTG, but I'm not supposed to take more than three for each attack. If this NTG doesn't help in about five minutes, I call my doctor.

NURSE: Good. You are doing what is best. Where is your doctor's phone number?

PATIENT: It's right by the phone. But my wife knows it by heart.

NURSE: Suppose your doctor is not available?

PATIENT: Then I would go to the emergency room. But I would feel silly if it turns out to be nothing.

NURSE: Maybe the doctor will tell you it's nothing but indigestion, to take an Alka-Seltzer and go home. Remember, though, he had to examine you, take a cardiogram, and do other tests to be sure. He couldn't tell just from your symptoms. I doubt any physician would say you were foolish to come in. As you know so well, chest discomfort, not promptly relieved by rest and NTG, can be serious—the sooner you get to a doctor, the better.*

Group instruction

Group instruction involves consideration of purposes and advantages as well as techniques for developing a group and managing it for instruction. One may ask why special consideration is given to groups. This question is probably asked because health services have mostly been provided with individuals as the unit of service, and constructing "unnatural" groups for instruction requires checking that the services are not harmed.

Reasons for teaching groups

Groups may be used in patient teaching for two reasons: this may be an economical way to teach a number of individuals at one time, and the experience of being part of a group may be the most likely way to meet the objectives. In

---

*From Winslow, E. H., and Macvaugh, H. III: Coronary artery surgery, Nurs. Clin. North Am. **11:**371-383, 1976.

the former instance, the presentation may be much like a lecture and the number of learners considerable. Smaller numbers are necessary for discussions, which are most useful in meeting objectives regarding development of attitudes or partially developed concepts. Indeed, in one case, discussion was deliberately chosen for teaching expectant parents because it was found that a significant part of their interest lay in the area of feelings about becoming parents.[52]

In making a decision to use discussion, consideration must be given to cultural values. Although discussion may be a workable method with middle-class Americans embracing democratic self-help ideals, it may not be workable with groups that embrace other values, as in rural Japan, where respect for authority is a built-in value.[42] Nursing students working with Puget Sound Indians found that asking a direct question forced the Indian woman to violate her anonymity value. These people would not speak of themselves and their needs but would express the feelings and thoughts of their friends. The students found this opposed to their professional orientation to speak directly to the person and not to gossip about those present.[1]

Four descriptions of group education programs show how this type of program has been used for economy in teaching and for its special effects on motivation and attainment of certain objectives. Haar described a program she began when she was giving individualized nursing service to a number of families with children with phenylketonuria (PKU) and noted that many mothers were unable to bring their children's diets under optimum control and that this was unrelated to the mothers' intellectual understanding of the dietary regimen. Most of them also felt isolation with their problem because of the rarity of the disease. These families seldom met or knew of one another. Haar set up a study in which one group of ten mothers attended six 1½-hour meetings at 1-week in-

tervals. The mothers were matched according to the child's age at initiation of diet and length of time on diet with other mothers in a control group who received individualized education from the public health nurse at home. The goal was to help the mothers gain insight into their problems, feelings, and reactions through verbalization. The leader of the experimental group used nondirective methods of group discussion; the bulk of the discussion centered on daily management problems, clarification of facts about PKU, child development, and parent-child interaction and feelings. Before the group sessions, no one in the control group and only one of the experimental group were in optimum dietary control (as measured by the child's serum phenylalanine level), whereas, after the group sessions, one in the control group and six in the experimental group were in optimum dietary control (significantly different at the .05 level).[22]

Group learning has been utilized extensively in health education for prenatal care, postpartum and infant care, child care, management of diabetes, as well as other types of care. Preoperative instruction is usually given individually, but Mezzanotte has described how she utilized group education for this purpose, hoping to capitalize on the theory that, in a group, individuals have a tendency to identify with others having similar goals or problems and thus gain moral support and encouragement through this identification. Six groups of patients having elective abdominal surgery, averaging four patients each, were given a 30-minute class the day before surgery that focused on preparation for surgery and suggestions for the control of pain and for activity that would promote satisfactory recovery. In an interview 5 to 7 days postoperatively, all patients said the instruction had been beneficial, and 11 said they liked meeting with other patients scheduled for surgery. When asked to state a preference for either group instruction or a shorter period of individualized instruction, 20 (of 24) said they preferred the group session.[38] Both Haar and Mezzanotte were apparently able in these instances to meet the needs of a number of patients effectively, with savings in time.

A Seattle public health agency's decision to use groups was not made primarily to increase effectiveness; rather, it was a response to the economic crunch in that city. At the same time, the agency participated in a research study about mothers' intended actions for childhood symtoms. New mothers, after a visit from the nurse during the month after their child's birth, were assigned to group or to control treatment, which would be continued during home visits. On the measure of intended actions for childhood symptoms, the mothers in groups did significantly better, and this system of providing care required less than one-third as much in public health nursing time.[35]

At the Kaiser-Permanente Medical Center in San Francisco, pediatric nurse practitioners did a pilot study of cluster visits and found them highly rated by mothers, more economical of the nurse practitioners' time, and worthy of a larger, controlled study. Four mothers with babies of the same age were chosen at random. Each cluster visit lasted 1½ hours; during the first 40 minutes infants were examined one by one, and during the next 40 minutes the nurse and the mothers talked about child rearing. For the baby's first year, four cluster visits, alternated with three solo visits with the same pediatric nurse practitioner and one with the pediatrician, were planned. The solo visits took care of highly individual problems. The informal interaction among the mothers while they were waiting for individual exams was also instructional. This system of using groups can accomplish a special kind of learning—demonstration over a period of time of three other babies' growth and development and more than a superficial comparison and learning of new mothering patterns from each other.[17]

The potential for groups in patient education is just beginning to be tested. This topic must receive high priority since it can lead to cost containment and more economical use of the public's funds. Of special importance also is testing of service to groups that have not received it. An example is remotivation groups with aged, mentally retarded, or mentally ill patients. Techniques and topics for this kind of group teaching are well described in an article by Lyon.[33] The teaching of "natural" groups such as families is also part of this service. A course designed to teach families of in-patients on a psychiatric unit was motivated by the realization that the family has been expected to bridge the therapeutic gap between the hospital and home but often without clear-cut training or instructions. The unit of intervention is the family of a patient; in this program, they are taught how to use basic behavior modification techniques, that is, to reinforce desirable behavior and ignore undesirable, or negative, behavior. Families had apparently not been learning to discriminate between ignoring behavior and ignoring a person.[51]

Constructing and implementing teaching with groups

Obtaining members, developing purposes, and planning and carrying out interaction strategies require somewhat different knowledge and skills than does work with individuals. Teachers must at least be aware of the composition and size of the group even if they do not control them, for these factors can have a considerable effect on learning. Although nurses are not as likely as health educators to be responsible for planning strategies for educating whole communities and other large groups, they may be asked to address community groups. They must be cognizant of the possible impact of their messages and realize that the organized groups they are addressing may be composed of and controlled by a relatively small portion of the total community.[12]

In clinics, schools, and classes for parents and diabetic persons, the nurse-teacher is apt to have more control over the composition of the group. An obvious consideration is how far advanced an individual is in meeting the objectives of a class, so that he is neither bored with relistening to something he already knows nor overwhelmed by an advanced class. Although variation in ability and experience is desirable, large differences should be detected by a pretest related specifically to the objectives of the course or lesson or by an intake interview, which should also serve to explain the group to the individual and to assess his motivation for entering it. Then both the teacher and the prospective group member have some basis on which to decide whether the person will fit into a particular group or must receive individualized instruction or some other form of instruction.

Some groups form spontaneously and may be aided by professional help. For example, the parents of hospitalized leukemic children sought out one another in lounge areas and formed spontaneous groups. They had a number of concerns, and a group was formed with a health professional. As is usual with this kind of group, the tasks involved demand a combination of counseling and teaching. Their concerns included: how to deal with baldness, manipulation of parents by children, discipline, the child's anger toward staff, how the child dies, and how to solve family interaction problems. Suicidal thoughts in their children generally were not anticipated by the parents. Information dissemination and didactic instruction of parents seemed best undertaken when stresses were minimal.[23]

An example of teaching done by a nurse using group discussion illustrates the kinds of goals and teacher-learner activity characteristic of this method. Meeting at a mental health center, mothers of 6- to 10-year-old children were organized into groups of 18 members. They were told that the sessions would give them a chance to share their concerns as parents, to see the variety of ways there are to look at and handle these concerns, and to discuss the ways in which specific kinds of behavior are interrelated with general areas of child development. The individual learner's goals, as they were expressed, fit into these general statements of purpose: to know if it is normal for 6-year-old children to lie or steal, to know the effect of child placement within a family, to decide when a child should go to bed, and to compare one child's behavior with normal behavior.[7] Because feelings accompanying these topics were strong and mothers needed to attain solutions useful for their particular family, discussion seemed to be a profitable method. The role of the leader was interpreted to the group as having three major functions: to add information to the discussion when needed, to clear up misconceptions that the group did not correct, and to guide the discussion so that the topic could be developed as meaningfully and fully as possible. The desired effect of the sessions was for each group member to inspect her own feelings and motivations as she heard what others thought, felt, and did. She would agree with some, differ with others, and begin to discover what she wanted to do in her own situation. She also should come to learn a way of evaluating an issue, such as a family problem, of looking at its many sides and seeing more clearly implications for all who are involved. There was evidence that such behavior occurred. For example, newer mothers were concerned about not perceiving in their children the inadequate behavior that teachers were seeing. Comments of veteran mothers and consideration of their own school experiences helped them to develop a philosophy of their own about this conflict.[7]

Because group education cannot be group therapy, deep personality changes cannot be expected. It is aimed rather at helping persons whose problems are conscious, although the neurotic person often can gain from group education by developing enough ego strength to function despite areas of conflict. As part of the attitude-learning process previously referred to, it was expected that individuals would have difficulty inspecting their own feelings. These difficulties presented themselves in various kinds of behavior: in expecting to be told how to solve problems, in being angry or defensive, and in squelching every suggestion made by others. It was expected that the progress of the group in meeting the objectives would take many weeks; in this instance, 10 weeks were scheduled. An example of progress can be seen in the group who spent many weeks talking about how to be good mothers: finally, their feelings about their own loss of identity as individuals came out.[7,8] This group was used for information giving and discussion for both cognitive and affective objectives. The description indicates that at least some individuals were active and involved in their learning.

Perhaps the clearest definition of group education has been written by Auerbach in the field of parent education. Auerbach's book contains clear delineation of goals of groups for education, differentiated from groups formed for other purposes, and a wealth of information about implementation of parent group education. In terms of definition and goals, the class for parent group education stresses primarily the need to understand the meaning of behavior within a family, so that parents may respond more effectively. It deals with the capacity available to learn by experience. It usually is offered on a nonselective basis to all who choose to attend, unless a parent is clearly not able to learn because of acute emotional difficulties. No attempt is made to explore forgotten or unconscious material. The group primarily focuses on helping the members develop validity, or ''reality,'' for their opinions, independent thinking, and individual decision making. Becoming a good group member is a secondary goal.[4]

Groups are usually set up for parents of children of specific ages because this enhances their identification with each other and free sharing of experiences. Parents often come to these groups with considerable awareness of the difficulties in their family relations, so that it is not unusual to find a preponderance of negative feelings closely tied to a sense of failure. In addition, parents may initially be suspicious and may fear seeming ''gossipy'' or talking about private affairs not usually shared with others, and they may need, with the leader's help, to learn how to use the experience. These groups commonly last for 8 to 12 sessions. The leader does not lead in any predetermined channel but follows the group's lead, using knowledge and skills to clear up their confusion and expand their understanding—partly by opening up new aspects of the issue for their consideration and by underscoring or interpreting comments. When the group falls into a pattern of repeating the same content again and again or there is a mood of self-pity, of wallowing in their common misery, it is time to move on. The discussion should end on a corrective note.[4]

In places such as community centers, many kinds of groups are used. In the center described by Milio, there were the usual instruction groups but also groups that were taught how to use the ''system'' through role playing and direct action techniques.[39]

Many varieties of interaction techniques can be used in group teaching, and there are many sources to consult for information about them. Leadership interventions may include: outlining and interpreting group objectives, increasing interaction among members, encouraging the sharing of common problems, superimposing a theoretical framework, and summarizing the group's progress toward its goals.[36]

One report provides a variety of strategies and the kind of content that can be forthcoming from a group. In a preoperative teaching program for women about to have hysterectomies, the nurse used the following comment with a quiet group: ''There are a lot of old wives' tales about hysterectomies. People say you're going to gain 40 pounds, or your hair will fall out, or you'll lose all interest in sex. What have you heard?'' Later one patient asked, ''But how can you enjoy sex if there is nothing there?'' The nurse had seen the women individually before the group sessions to screen their emotional status and knowledge of impending surgery and disease process and arranged individual conferences with those who seemed unduly anxious. Sometimes signs of extreme stress were not at first apparent but became evident during the discussion, in which case the patient was counseled individually following the group meeting.[37] This example is not meant to imply that stress in a member should not be dealt with by the group, only that it is common for the nurse to screen out the level of disruption that might interfere with the learning of the rest of the group.

Role playing

Role playing is an excellent technique for diagnosis of readiness and also for teaching ideas and attitudes. A person is assigned to play himself or another person, often within a situation that the teacher has described in order to elicit the desired behavior. A related technique is to teach by enacting a role that the learner can model. An example would be enacting a positive or desirable parental role in relation to a child's specific behavior and then discussing and labeling the behavior that was portrayed.

Through role playing a desired behavior is rehearsed; thus a person is taught the skills required and made more confident in carrying it out. An example is the nurse and an unmarried 20-year-old woman acting out how to ask the physician questions and how to talk with her family.[54] Reversal of the roles is a technique useful for sensitizing one person to the other's situation. Role playing provides a kind of behavioral and mental rehearsal that is a form of practice and thus a means of increasing retention of learning.

Role-playing techniques have been cited as being useful in teaching the poor from disadvantaged backgrounds. They appear to be congenial in situations that have been described as physical, action oriented, concrete, and problem directed rather than introspective and prefer instruction that is easy and informal in tempo. Role playing has also been thought to reduce the role distance between client and professional and to be a good technique for developing verbal power.[44] The technique would appear to have considerable potential for reducing overintellectualization and for uniting understanding with feeling.

Teaching by environment

The notion that environment affects learning was introduced earlier. The following studies show two ways in which environment influences the learner. Indigenous workers have been used to influence the health actions of the population of which they are members; this is done to maximize the community's contact with individuals who are seen by health agencies as having positive health goals. In one example, this technique was used to increase immunization levels in hard-core areas resistant to previous immunization programs.[48] Spaulding's study of black primiparae of low socioeconomic status describes how an environmental situation influences the learning goals that are attained and retained. Many of the mothers, when discharged from the hospital, lived in an extended family environment in which there were other women experienced in child care. Family members assisted in the care of the infant and were the ones from whom advice was most often sought. Infant care contrary to the family was not likely to be carried out.[46] With these examples in mind, conscientious teachers evaluating the effectiveness of their methods might ask: Does the environment in which the behavior will be used give enough support to it so that the desired learning is really feasible? When can the natural, or immediate, environment or a special environment be used as a major means for teaching?

Environments that originally attract clients for reasons other than learning specific skills or attitudes may hold them long enough for learning sufficient to alter attitudes and motivation to occur.

How many women throughout the world are using maternal and child health services, not necessarily because they have had prior education about their nature or their meaning, but rather because of a certain feeling of trust, a certain feeling of protection, a certain feeling that they are receiving adequate care and also, perhaps, that they are respected and wanted there—a whole variety of reasons indeed which seem just as important as having an intellectual conception of the nature and functions of such services.

Very often in these situations it seems that the information aspect, the facts of the matter, belong at a somewhat later stage in health education rather than as a starting point. We may possibly induce changes in behaviour by means which are not traditionally regarded as educational at all. The placing of services in convenient proximity to the intended user, so organizing them that continuity of relationship between their professional staff and community members is not only possible but encouraged, the building up of warm, mutually trusting relationships, the general satisfaction felt in using a service, may all favourably influence health related behaviour in a variety of ways. Thus, wanting to know more, a readiness to know more, about health and about a service may well emerge from, rather than precede, the use of a service.*

Within hospitals and clinics, many of the day-to-day decisions involving environment seem to have potential for effective learning. This is the basis for the tactic of structuring the interpersonal environment of the convalescing patients with myocardial infarction so that they are thoroughly involved in decision making and planning for the future, the goal being to avoid permanent dependency responses.[19] Assignment of patients to rooms in which they are alone or placed in close contact with other patients may establish learning or fail to establish that which may be needed, and a helping environment in which nurse-patient interaction occurs and is rewarded is a necessary background for teaching. In one setting serving a poor population, the playroom serving as a baby-sitting service for siblings and children waiting to see the physician was altered to serve as a base for a parent-education program to encourage parents to promote the cognitive development of their preschoolers. The physical setting was changed to the "prepared environment" of Montessori to allow children to pursue self-selected activities at their own pace. This mode of operation permitted the staff to invite parents to observe the educational and creative aspects of play while also supervising the waiting children. A structured curriculum emphasizing language, perceptual development, and problem solving was developed with methods that could be transmitted by parents with a wide range of educational backgrounds. An assistant tutored the parent using role-playing techniques, which allowed the mother an opportunity to be both child and teacher. Parents consistently mentioned differences in behavior: children were listening and paying attention better, and they showed gains in cognitive performance. Children's activities previously seen as aimless and "bad" were now viewed as constructive and amenable to modification by the parent.[40]

Since it takes so long in a hospital setting to treat some patients, they may learn and retain new habits of being patients and tend to adopt the role of chronic invalid. It is necessary to alter an environment that reinforces this kind of behavior past a useful point. Milieu therapy points to construction of the environment in such a way that it encourages desirable behaviors. For patients undergoing long-term rehabilitation, it may be necessary to provide over a period of weeks or months opportunity to gain or retain problem-solving, social, and interper-

---

*Steuart, G. W.: The specialist in health education; training for the future, Int. J. Health Educ. **9:**165-169, Oct.-Dec. 1966.

Table 7. Correct and incorrect responses to 50 medical terms by 125 patients*

	Correctness of response					
	D Adequate		B and C Wrong or vague		A No knowledge	
Medical term	Number	Percent	Number	Percent	Number	Percent
Vomit	123	98.4	0	0.0	2	1.6
Relieve	120	96.0	5	4.0	0	0.0
Appointment	120	96.0	4	3.2	1	0.8
Constipated	116	92.8	6	4.8	3	2.4
Rash	110	88.0	10	8.0	5	4.0
Injection	108	86.4	5	4.0	12	9.6
Skull	107	85.6	13	10.4	5	4.0
Amputate	103	82.4	6	4.8	16	12.8
Persistent	101	80.8	15	12.0	9	7.2
Splint	100	80.0	11	8.8	14	11.2
Abdomen	100	80.0	9	7.2	16	12.8
Negative	90	72.0	17	13.6	18	14.4
Sterile	90	72.0	28	22.4	7	5.6
Symptoms	89	71.2	23	18.4	13	10.4
Reaction	88	70.4	22	17.6	15	12.0
Swab	87	69.6	26	20.8	12	9.6
Abortion	87	69.6	11	8.8	27	21.6
Mole	87	69.6	28	22.4	10	8.0
Pulse	86	68.8	37	29.6	2	1.6
Isolate	86	68.8	11	8.8	28	22.4
Nasal	80	64.0	14	11.2	31	24.8
Deformity	80	64.0	24	19.2	21	16.8
Fatal	79	63.2	32	25.6	14	11.2
Autopsy	75	60.0	29	23.2	21	16.8
Routine	75	60.0	34	27.2	16	12.8

*From Samora, J., Saunders, L., and Larson, R. F.: J. Health Hum. Behav. **2:**83-92, 1961, published by the American Sociological Association.

sonal skills needed for functioning in society. The treatment program may attempt to engage the patient in various social encounters with staff and patients that expose him to increasingly challenging problems to provide tests of his skill and judgment. The patient needs these skills and enlightened self-interest in order to deal with rebuff and rejection and with massive physical insult in retaining roles such as work associate, homemaker, friend, and acquaintance.[31] Stanford Hospital reports that, for reha-

bilitation patients, there is a "house" on the grounds where patients live with their families for 3 days. This allows direct practice in a home environment with help close by if necessary.[13]

Oral teaching—using words that communicate

Since teaching is communicating and communicating is accomplished in large part by language, the teacher must be skilled in the use of language. Nurses need special knowledge of

Table 7. Correct and incorrect responses to 50 medical terms by 125 patients—cont'd

	Correctness of response					
	D Adequate		B and C Wrong or vague		A No knowledge	
Medical term	Number	Percent	Number	Percent	Number	Percent
Acute	75	60.0	22	17.6	28	22.4
Allergic	74	59.2	45	36.0	6	4.8
Cavity	73	58.4	24	19.2	28	22.4
Specimen	70	56.0	47	37.6	8	6.4
Sedative	68	54.4	22	17.6	35	28.0
Deficient	67	53.6	36	28.8	22	17.6
Germs	63	50.4	55	44.0	7	5.6
Intern	63	50.4	44	35.2	18	14.4
Bacteria	61	48.8	30	24.0	34	27.2
Cerebral	57	45.6	18	14.4	50	40.0
Nutrition	56	44.8	49	39.2	20	16.0
Digestion	54	43.2	63	50.4	8	6.4
Vitamins	51	40.8	67	53.6	7	5.6
Cardiac	43	34.4	9	7.2	73	58.4
Orally	43	34.4	57	45.6	25	20.0
Tissue	40	32.0	60	48.0	25	20.0
Dilate	40	32.0	43	34.4	42	33.6
Respiratory	38	30.4	24	19.2	63	50.4
Secretions	36	28.8	20	16.0	69	55.2
Appendectomy	35	28.0	28	22.4	62	49.6
Therapy	32	25.6	37	29.6	56	44.8
Nerve	28	22.4	80	64.0	17	13.6
Malignant	22	17.6	35	28.0	68	54.4
Terminal	16	12.8	60	48.0	49	39.2
Tendon	16	12.8	58	46.4	51	40.8
TOTAL	3,608	57.7	1,453	23.3	1,189	19.0

language because of two conditions inherent in health teaching: medical terminology is foreign to much of the public, and individuals with considerable health needs often have poorly developed language skills, resulting in low levels of understanding.

The language skills one develops are related to style of life. Those who have experience in encouraging prenatal care have indicated that literate people who have developed the habit of reading can be reached in many ways, including posters, newspapers, and other written media. The illiterate respond to radio and television, but best to a person-to-person approach.[50] The consequences of language and thought development in terms of client behavior and the ways in which individuals can be reached have significance for the nurse. For example, the unsophisticated tuberculosis patient has been described as so poorly informed or limited in his understanding that he cannot sufficiently appreciate or comprehend what is going on in diagnostic, therapeutic, and preventive activities. Such a patient can readily be confused by alterations in terminology and medical instructions. Also, he may sometimes act on casual remarks of a detrimental or unproductive nature made by neighbors or friends or by paramedical personnel working in a health facility. In contrast, the more sophisticated patient is able to comprehend medical terms and may also be fully cognizant that the management of tuberculosis is being revised constantly. On this basis, he takes initiative in seeking out the optimum treatment and medical care for himself and his family. Unfortunately, tuberculosis is most prevalent in people with depressed standards of living— those who are poor and culturally deprived.[16] For a group of medically indigent black diabetic patients, it was concluded that a very simple teaching program had to be constructed to take into account their inability to understand concepts such as asepsis, to think abstractly about signs and symptoms and physiology principles, and to keep written records for the physician.[3]

In a study done nearly 20 years ago, information about understanding of spoken medical vocabulary was obtained from 125 patients of surgical-gynecologic and medical services in a publicly operated general hospital. This was largely a lower-class sample, heavily weighted with Spanish-Americans and blacks. The terms listed in Table 7 were compiled from patient interviews and from a knowledge of clinic and ward situations and were believed to be those in common use in conversations with patients.[45] It would have been difficult for me to predict which words the patients would not know, which perhaps suggests that one's judgment may be less than accurate about these things. Although not included in this investigation and apparently not documented by a formal study, there is concern that the difference between laymen's slang terms and terms of professionals is acute in the area of mental disease.[30]

In an informal study, hospitalized patients were found to have poor understanding of *NPO,* *ambulate, emesis basin, force fluids,* and *void.*[11] Study has also been done on understanding of patients with rheumatism of terms commonly used in discussing this disease. Half the patients confused *loin* and *groin.* Less than a third of the patients thought *cervical* related to the neck, and many thought the spinal cord was a bone in the back. Rheumatic sufferers often thought "morning stiffness" was an inability to move. Patients and physicians did not agree on definitions of *numbness, sciatica, slipped disc, sciatic nerve, lumbar,* and other terms.[58]

Published reports of terms and concepts that cause comprehension difficulties are very important and are usually accessible to nurses. Sickle cell counseling done as part of a child and youth project with parents of low socioeconomic status and educational background of fourth to twelfth grades found the term *trait* to be a difficult one. It had virtually no meaning to this population, and it probably is not a word found in the vocabularies of many people with elementary or even high-school education. Many of these parents thought they were being told their child had a "trace"; thus they thought it referred to a mild illness.[24]

Common words can take on changed meanings when used in a medical setting. For example, *dirty* and *clean* have more particular meanings in the medical professions than in common usage. *Small* and *large* require something with which to compare size; otherwise, one may not know how to compare a "large incision" with a "small opening" in the abdomen through which bowel contents are evacuated. *Bad* and *good* also need to have explicit meaning, indicating consequences. "It's bad to give oneself an enema when sitting on a toilet" might be misinterpreted as "bad" in a moral sense, but more likely the use of this kind of explanation would merely fail to provide the learner with knowledge of why it is bad.

This information about client comprehension of words and the possibility of a lack of comprehension and its consequences is far from complete. The concern seems to focus on lower-class patients, leaving large populations unstudied. Although the results of these investigations do not allow for an accurate prediction of what words an individual can understand, they should alert nurses to the kinds of words that can be misunderstood and encourage a belief in the value of carefully determining what a patient knows.

Directions to patients can have a similar unfortunate vagueness. Consider the dentist whose directions to the patient after tooth extraction are, "Come back if you have trouble." A half-hour later the packing comes partially out of the socket. Is that trouble? McAtee gives a fascinating account of one patient's ability to follow the directions, "Take one teaspoon of this medicine before every meal." This mother had no teaspoon measures in her house, only plastic spoons collected from the local ice cream stand; she had no concept of a teaspoon as a measurement because she had never learned to cook and had almost no reading or writing skills; she had no clock at home, because this was a luxury item; and her family either ate only one meal a day or ate snacks all day long. This woman would not question the nurse and said, "Yes," to all instructions.[34] What directions would you give this woman?

Not surprisingly, oral directions, in comparison with written, are less definitive; thus they are more likely to be forgotten. What is surprising is the extent to which this obvious fact is ignored in practice. Estimates are that patients remember one half (generously, two thirds) of the statements made by a physician in a given session.[28,56] One study found that the physician gave each patient a little more than ten items of information. None of the patients remembered all he had been told, and the average amount retained was no different if the interview occurred right after the clinical examinations or several weeks later. In this study, amount remembered varied by category—from 74% for information about further investigation to 31%

for explanation about the disease or its treatment, with 45% recall of the instructions. Articulate patients were given more information by the doctor and informed more often, so they remembered more, as did patients with a good prognosis. On the average, the proportion of information forgotten increased with the total amount of information given. Perhaps the need for information should be diagnosed as carefully as the requirements for medications.[28]

The use of written information would no doubt improve patients' retention of information. The use of another device, called advance organizers, showed significant increases in recall. In this study, the advance organizers were category names to organize the material. The material used in the experiment consisted of the following fifteen statements:

1. You have a chest infection.
2. And your larynx is slightly inflamed.
3. But I think your heart is all right.
4. We will do some heart tests to make sure.
5. We will need to take a blood sample.
6. And you will have to have your chest x-rayed.
7. Your cough will disappear in the next two days.
8. You will feel better in a week or so.
9. And you will recover completely.
10. We will give you an injection of penicillin.
11. And some tablets to take.
12. I'll give you an inhaler to use.
13. You must avoid cold draughts.
14. You must stay indoors in fog.
15. And you must take two hours' rest each afternoon.*

Use of the advance organizers went as follows:

> I am going to tell you:
>> what is wrong with you;
>> what tests we are going to carry out;
>> what I think will happen to you;
>> what treatment you will need; and
>> what you must do to help yourself.

---

*From Ley, P., and others: A method for increasing patients' recall of information presented by doctors, Psychol. Med. **3:**217-220, 1973.

First, what is wrong with you . . . (statements 1-3)

Secondly, what tests we are going to carry out . . . (statements 4-6)

Thirdly, what I think will happen to you . . . (statements 7-9)

Fourthly, what the treatments will be . . . (statements 10-12)

Finally, what you must do to help yourself . . . (statements 13-15)*

Notice that the category names are not medical terms; rather they are categories meaningful to patients.

One physician used a taped final interview with his patients as a means of improving understanding and retention. On the average, patients listened to the tapes 3.5 times, and most had spouses or relatives who also listened. Nearly all felt they were helped with this tool.[9]

Analogies are frequently used in teaching, presumably in an attempt to give meaning to medical ideas by relating them to what is commonly known. For example, a film on diabetes explains the body's use of food as being similar to the use of fuel by a car engine. The normal mechanism of blood glucose triggering release of insulin can be compared with a thermostat that regulates a furnace to maintain an even temperature. The tissue of a colostomy stoma may be described as the same type as that inside the mouth, since the mouth is the beginning of the alimentary canal. It has been suggested that this latter explanation will help to remove the mystery and fear of what the stoma looks like before the patient has seen it.[29] A cardiac monitor may be explained to patient and family as being "like having a cardiogram all the time," since the patient is likely to have had that experience. Analogies seem to be very useful in bridging the gap to new experiences; however,

they can be interpreted incorrectly and lead to incorrect action. Besides independently thinking through the strengths and weaknesses of a particular analogy, one should try it on patients and ask what they think it means. Sometimes nurses' thought patterns are so different from their clients that it is difficult to predict client interpretations.

Because of their backgrounds, health professionals may tend to overuse verbal instruction. They often value independence and symbolic learning and may choose a verbal means of instruction to motivate a person, when joining the client in the health action would be more effective. Verbalization can serve as a means of maintaining a professional distance from clients and at the same time creating a student-teacher role hierarchy and a status gap between helper and client; however, it may fail as a teaching technique if used exclusively.

Demonstration and practice

Demonstration involves an acting out for learners, or showing them. It includes showing an intellectual skill or an attitude as well as showing how to do a motor skill. The interpersonal techniques discussed in the previous section are prime ways to demonstrate ideas, problem solving, or attitudes, all of which do need practice in order to be learned. The practice can occur by working through exercises and by functioning in mock or real situations that require use of the skill and attitude.

An example of an idea that might be demonstrated is the relationship between patient activity and alarm and oscilloscope patterns for those patients being observed with cardiac monitors. In one study of 100 patients admitted to cardiac care units with myocardial infarctions, the vast majority of those who noticed static on their oscilloscopes invariably attributed this to serious cardiac dysfunction. They had no idea that static is a frequent occurrence and could be produced with even very simple movements of the

---

*From Ley, P., and others: A method for increasing patients' recall of information presented by doctors, Psychol. Med. **3:**217-220, 1973.

arms or body. Demonstration of this effect and how the alarm can be set off is a possible way to decrease the kind of anxiety seen in one patient who said: "The nurse told me not to move. Whenever I did, the monitor went crazy. It proved that she was right and that when I moved, I was damaging my heart."[10]

Demonstration has most commonly been thought of as a performance of procedures or psychomotor skills, which, combined with practice, is the method most suited to the attainment of skills. Since these skills are not learned separately from attitudes and factual knowledge, the demonstration and practice sessions are usually combined with giving of information (lecture) and with discussion to clarify concepts and feelings.

The purpose of the demonstration is to give the learner a clear mental image of how the skill is performed. Therefore, assurance that the demonstration can be adequately seen is of prime importance. If the motions are small, as in giving an injection, probably no more than a few people can see clearly enough. If there are more learners, the view may be attained only by redemonstration for small groups or by presentation of a prime view by television or motion picture. In some instances, an over-the-shoulder view of the demonstrator is best to provide the learner with a clear idea of how he will do the action. When the demonstrator is removing fluids from a vial and giving an injection, the mirror image that the viewer receives by facing the demonstrator is not entirely realistic.

Since the mental image must be accurate, the demonstration has to be practiced and submitted to critical examination before it is presented. The learner, who is not knowledgeable about the skill, has difficulty in distinguishing irrelevant and incorrect actions from those that are correct and relevant. A demonstration that shows a baby being bathed in a tub without the nurse's testing the temperature in any way pro-

vides an incorrect model, even though the temperature may have been checked before the demonstration began. An irrelevant action might be taking the baby's temperature before the bath, which without an explanation would imply that this always should be done. The teacher must expect that learners will mimic the demonstration down to the tiniest detail; it must be so accurate that they can do so without error. Equipment must be tried out before the demonstration to see that it works. It is disruptive to be showing the Clinitest and find that the test tube is too narrow to let the tablet fall into it or to be showing the procedure of transferring a patient from wheelchair to bed and discover that a lock on the wheelchair is broken. Even if the teacher maintains composure, he or she is still unable to demonstrate how the equipment is to be used, without getting a replacement. This is not to say that a lesson can or should be absolutely error free. An occasional mistake can be useful to show how the teacher goes about correcting it. This may occur when the nurse is ready to dry the baby and finds the towel was left on the other side of the room. Continual errors, however, are confusing to the learner.

Of great importance is adequate visualization of every procedure the learner will be expected to perform; that is, the entire task should be shown. I remember a film demonstrating a baby bath, in which the way to cleanse genitals was talked about but never shown. In addition, the verbal instructions dealt only with cleansing of female genitals. Imagine a new young mother who has been told that "it is very important to wash in these folds." This teaching gives neither information about why "it is very important" nor an adequate notion of how to go about the task.

Since learner practice is so important to development of a motor skill, it must be considered as a part of the teaching plan. When there is sufficient equipment and the group is small enough, practice may begin by the learner's re-demonstrating motions immediately after the teacher does them. Further practice should take place in a setting like that in which the skill will be performed, with the teacher supervising enough to provide feedback for a correct performance and to stimulate motivation if needed.

Patients who are going to use home dialysis programs and their families must learn a series of motor skills as well as develop judgment in carrying out the procedure and feelings of competence and independence. One such instructional program that has been described in nursing literature illustrates some key points in the teaching of motor skills, even though cannulas may no longer be commonly used. A utility room was used for instruction, since it most resembled a bedroom-kitchen situation in a home. The learners were first taught how to care for and clean cannulas, then how to take blood pressure, fill a syringe, assemble equipment, initiate and discontinue dialysis, monitor dialysis, and detect and correct problems.[18] It would seem that the sequence of these skills was planned to move from simple to complex. To give experience in declotting cannulas—a complication that occurs infrequently—mock situations were set up. Patients were also told to come to the hospital when they actually had need for declotting, and they would be taught further at that time. Almost all patients actually had drops in blood pressure during the first dialysis, at which time they were provided with some practice with the real situation. The learners were already highly motivated. After 2 or 3 months of instruction and practice in the training unit, the transfer to home was made, and there was a steadily decreasing need for professional assistance.[18]

To compensate for failing senses, such as vision in diabetes, patients often have to learn how to use special aids for doing tasks. Not only are the materials (tools) different, but the mode of demonstration also has to be altered to compensate for the failing sense. It is reported that diabetic patients often have difficulty in correctly assessing their visual loss and may in addition have neuropathy, which can affect the equipment that should be chosen. When the patient has slight visual impairment, the use of brighter lighting, a white background, and glass rather than plastic syringes can help. There is also available a longer syringe with bolder markings and wider spaces between calibrations, or a magnifying device can be used. There are other aids for needle insertion into the bottle. One can detect when the insulin bottle is empty by taking a marble out of a dish with each dose or injecting air into the vial and listening for the bubbles. Inserting the needle from the skin surface gives better control. Also available is a scale with braille markings. There are a number of other tools and procedures that are described in books on rehabilitation to use with persons who have visual and other handicaps.

Patients are learning new skills for self-care, such as giving transfusions for hemophilia. Such a trend can be expected to continue. Female paraplegic patients are being taught self-catheterization. The patient sits in a semi-Fowler position and with a large magnifying mirror identifies the meatus. She uses sterile gloves, cleanses herself without contamination, and inserts the catheter.[53]

Direct stimulation of receptors

Although long a part of nursing, the direct stimulation of receptors may not have been seen as training, or the full potential of such a technique may not have been appreciated. Gaffney and Campbell report on such a technique to train patients with central nervous system damage to eat as normally as possible, through enhancing lip closure, sucking, and swallowing. Depending on the patient's physiologic readiness, only two to three stimulation methods may be sufficient to accomplish the desired result. They also describe assessment techniques to determine the patient's readiness. For example, in determining whether the patient can open his mouth, his lips can be touched with a spoon; one can apply light pressure on the chin or stroke the digastric muscle beneath the chin.[20]

Practicing skills by microteaching

There are certain skills and strategies used in teaching that can be learned and practiced, and microteaching seems to be an excellent way to do so. Some of these skills include use of statements that focus, statements telling the learner to pay special attention to certain things, and statements of summary or closure; use of reinforcement of skills; use of planned repetition; use of illustration and examples; use of fluency in asking teaching questions; use of planned variation of the stimulus situation to which learners are asked to respond; use of attention to behavior (relaxing and listening to what the learner has to say), including use of eye contact; use of gestures, movements, and posture positions; use of verbal attention in response to the last comment of the client, that is, not introducing new data of one's own; and use of reflection of feeling. Practicing teachers plan and teach a short lesson (perhaps 5 minutes in length at first) aimed at one particular goal, which is videotaped if possible and then played back for them to analyze, preferably with the help of a teaching expert.[2] This provides opportunity for repeated practice until mastery, in a teaching situation that is less complex than the real one and one in which the teacher's primary responsibility is to learn.

STUDY QUESTIONS

1. "Teaching the Patient About Open Heart Surgery" is the title of an article in the October 1965 *American Journal of Nursing*. In explaining to the patient, the nurse uses phrases (quoted in part) such as ". . . you have a defective aortic valve"; "the narrowing is due to calcium deposits . . . left behind by infections such as rheumatic fever"; ". . . lack of atmospheric pressure creates a negative pressure, or a pulling force that keeps the lungs always expanded"; "the chest tubes are connected to a closed system called an underwater seal system"; and others. The nurse compares the two pleura to Saran Wrap in explaining that the outside of the lung and the lining of the chest wall slide over each other with perfect ease.[55]
   a. What level of education would a patient probably need to have to understand explanations in this terminology?
   b. Why is the analogy between pleura and Saran Wrap likely to be confusing? Is the comparison of a leaky heart valve to a warped door less confusing?
2. It has been said that groups—even those with only one staff member—may be more effective than one-to-one teaching, because groups contain a number of helpers. How would you respond to this argument?
3. You are teaching a group of parents of mentally retarded individuals about their children's sexuality. It is clear that they need information, and they also need to face and make decisions in the sexual realm of their children's behavior. What general group teaching approaches would you use?
4. When patients were asked if they had been catheterized, most did not know what it meant. How would you then alter the question?

REFERENCES

1. Aichlmayr, R. H.: Cultural understanding; a key to acceptance, Nurs. Outlook **17**:20-23, July 1969.
2. Allen, D., and Ryan, K.: Microteaching, Reading, Mass., 1969, Addison-Wesley Publishing Co., Inc.
3. Anderson, R. S., and others: Evaluation of clinical, cultural and psychosomatic influences in the teaching and management of diabetic patients; a study of medically indigent Negro patients, Am. J. Med. Sci. **245**:682-690, 1963.
4. Auerbach, A. B.: Parents learn through discussion, New York, 1968, John Wiley & Sons, Inc.
5. Beebe, J. E., and others: Bench conferences in a large obstetric clinic, Am. J. Nurs. **68**:85-87, 1968.
6. Bermosk, L. S.: Interviewing; a key to therapeutic communication in nursing practice, Nurs. Clin. North Am. **1**:205-214, June 1966.
7. Bruce, S. J.: What mothers of 6-to-10-year olds want to know, Nurs. Outlook **12**:40-43, Sept. 1964.
8. Bruce, S. J.: Do prenatal educational programs really prepare for parenthood? Hosp. Top. **43**:104-106, Nov. 1965.
9. Butt, H. R.: A method for better physician—patient communication, Am. Intern. Med. **86**:478-480, 1977.
10. Cassem, N. H., and others: Reactions of coronary patients to the CCU nurse, Am. J. Nurs. **70**:319-325, 1970.

11. Cosper, Bonnie: How well do patients understand hospital jargon? Am. J. Nurs. **77:**1932, 1934, 1977.

12. Cumming, J., and Cumming, E.: Mental health education in a Canadian community. In Paul, B. D., editor: Health, culture and community, New York, 1955, Russell Sage Foundation.

13. Davies, N. H., and Hansen, E.: Family focus; a transitional cottage in an acute-care hospital, Fam. Process **13:**481-488, 1974.

14. Davis, F.: Uncertainty in medical prognosis, clinical and functional, Am. J. Sociol. **66:**41-47, 1960.

15. Davis, M. E., and Rubin, R.: DeLee's obstetrics for nurses, ed. 18, Philadelphia, 1966, W. B. Saunders Co.

16. Deuschle, K., and Hochstrasser, D.: Doctors and patients; some human factors in tuberculosis control, Bull. Int. Union Tuberc. **36:**74-82, 1965.

17. Feldman, M.: Cluster visits, Am. J. Nurs. **74:**1485-1488, 1974.

18. Fellows, B.: Hemodialysis at home, Am. J. Nurs. **66:**1775-1778, 1966.

19. Foster, S., and Andreoli, K. G.: Behavior following acute myocardial infarction, Am. J. Nurs. **70:**2344-2348, 1970.

20. Gaffney, T. W., and Campbell, R. P.: Feeding techniques for dysphagic patients, Am. J. Nurs. **74:**194-195, 1974.

21. Gregg, D. E.: The therapeutic roles of the nurse, Perspect. Psychiatr. Care **1:**18-24, 1963.

22. Haar, D. J.: Improved phenylketonuric diet control through group education of mothers, Nurs. Clin. North Am. **1:**715-723, 1966.

23. Heffron, W. A., and others: Group discussions with the parents of leukemic children, Pediatrics **52:**831-840, 1973.

24. Heimler, A., and Chabot, A.: Sickle cell counseling in a children and youth project, Am. J. Public Health **64:**955-997, 1974.

25. Hoff, F. E.: Natural childbirth; how any nurse can help, Am. J. Nurs. **69:**1451-1453, 1969.

26. Hollingsworth, C. E., and Sokol, B.: Predischarge family conference, J.A.M.A. **239:**740-741, 1978.

27. Johnson, J. E., and others: Easing children's fright during health care procedures, Mat.-Child Nurs. **1:**206-210, 1976.

28. Joyce, C. R. B., and others: Quantitative study of doctor-patient communication, Q. J. Med. **38:**183-194, 1969.

29. Katona, E. A.: Learning colostomy control, Am. J. Nurs. **67:**534-541, 1967.

30. King, S. H.: Perceptions of illness and medical practices, New York, 1962, Russell Sage Foundation.

31. Kutner, B.: Milieu therapy in rehabilitation medicine, J. Rehabil. **34:**14-17, March-April 1968.

32. Ley, P., and others: A method for increasing patients' recall of information presented by doctors, Psychol. Med. **3:**217-220, 1973.

33. Lyon, G. G.: Stimulation through remotivation, Am. J. Nurs. **71:**982-985, 1971.

34. McAtee, P.: Poverty, relevance and program failure, Nurs. Outlook **17:**56-58, Sept. 1969.

35. McNeil, H. J., and Holland, S. S.: A comparative study of public health nurse teaching in groups and in home visits, Am. J. Public Health **62:**1629-1637, 1972.

36. Marram, G. D.: The group approach in nursing practice, ed. 2, St. Louis, 1977, The C. V. Mosby Co.

37. Merkatz, R., and others: Preoperative teaching for gynecologic patients, Am. J. Nurs. **74:**1072-1074, 1974.

38. Mezzanotte, E. J.: Group instruction in preparation for surgery, Am. J. Nurs. **70:**89-91, 1970.

39. Milio, N.: 9226 Kercheval; the storefront that didn't burn, Ann Arbor, 1970, The University of Michigan Press.

40. Morris, A. G., and others: Educational intervention for preschool children in a pediatric clinic, Pediatrics **57:**765-768, 1976.

41. Olson, D. R.: On a theory of instruction; why different forms of instruction result in similar knowledge, Interchange **3:**9-24, 1972.

42. Paul, B. D.: Anthropological perspectives on medicine and public health. In Skipper, J. K., Jr., and Leonard, R. C.: Social interaction and patient care, Philadelphia, 1965, J. B. Lippincott Co.

43. Peplau, H. E.: Professional closeness, Nurs. Forum **8**(4):342-360, 1969.

44. Riessman, F., and Goldfarb, J.: Role playing and the poor. In Riessman, F., and others, editors: Mental health of the poor, New York, 1964, The Macmillan Co.

45. Samora, J., and others: Medical vocabulary knowledge among hospital patients, J. Health Hum. Behav. **2:**83-92, 1961.

46. Spaulding, M. R.: The effectiveness of tape recordings with primiparas of the lower socioeconomic group in coping with mothering tasks. In Batey, M. V., editor: Communicating nursing research; problem identification and the research design, Boulder, Colo., 1969, Western Interstate Commission for Higher Education.

47. Steuart, G. W.: The specialist in health education; training for the future, Int. J. Health Educ. **9:**165-169, Oct.-Dec. 1966.

48. Stewart, J. C., Jr., and Hood, W. R.: Using workers from "hard-core" areas to increase immunization levels, Public Health Rep. **85:**117-185, 1970.

49. Straub, K. M.: The implications of nursing care plans to the concept of continuity of patient care. In Straub,

K. M., and Parker, K. S., editors: Continuity of patient care; the role of nursing, Washington, D.C., 1966, The Catholic University of America Press.

50. Sundberg, A. M.: Influencing prenatal behavior, Am. J. Public Health **56:**1218-1225, 1966.

51. Tarver, J., and Turner, A. J.: Teaching behavior modification to patients' families, Am. J. Nurs. **74:** 282-283, 1974.

52. Thaxton, A.: Teaching expectant parents what they want to know, Am. J. Nurs. **62:**112-114, May 1962.

53. Turgeon, E.: Self-catheterization for female paraplegics, Nurs. '74 **4:**83, July 1974.

54. Underwood, P. R.: Communication through role playing, Am. J. Nurs. **71:**1184-1186, 1971.

55. Varvaro, F. F.: Teaching the patient about open heart surgery, Am. J. Nurs. **65:**111-115, Oct. 1965.

56. Waitzkin, H., and Stoeckle, J. D.: The communication of information about illness, Adv. Psychosom. Med. **8:**180-215, 1972.

57. Winslow, E. H., and Macvaugh, H. III: Coronary artery surgery, Nurs. Clin. North Am. **11:**371-383, 1976.

58. Wright, V., and Hopkins, R.: Communicating with the rheumatic patient, Rheumatol. Rehabil. **16:**107-118, 1977.

CHAPTER 7

Teaching tools: printed and nonprinted materials

PRINTED MATERIALS

■ In using written materials as teaching tools, one must consider more than vocabulary and sentence length. Other factors, such as format, headings, illustrations, line width, type size, and style of writing, affect readability but are not incorporated into the Dale-Chall formula (see pp. 142-143).[47] Also of great importance is whether the information is correct or, if there is a difference of opinion as to what is true, whether it expresses a point of view the nurse wishes to teach. Finally, to be useful the written material must play a part in meeting one of the learning objectives. Precisely what part it should play in meeting which objective should be considered before the material is given to the learner to read.

Printed teaching material can be described as frozen language, selective in its description of reality (which is both a strength and a weakness), providing limited feedback, but constantly available. Print partially relaxes time requirements and is more efficient than oral language (except for those who have not learned to read efficiently) because the reader can control the speed at which he reads and comprehends. Writing does require a sequential presentation. Certain kinds of thinking seem to demand written expression: For example, a complex sequence of thoughts that incorporates definitions, qualifications, and logical constraints is expressed best in writing. It can be formulated with care and often without a strict time limit. Most people who have learned to read well generally prefer to acquire information by reading; it is ideal for understanding complex concepts and relationships. If the learning objective primarily entails skill in dealing with persons or things, then demonstrations, concrete experience with the activity, and oral coaching and guidance would seem to be more effective media than print.[9]

Predicting reading comprehension

Of considerable importance is the reading skill of individuals who need health teaching because learning by reading is economical in regard to teacher time. A study of reading material used in a particular clinic with diabetic patients produced startling results. Three hundred patients—about half the population of this clinic—were chosen by random sample of patient visits for the study. These people had an average of 6.8 grades of schooling. The material, which was primarily on an eighth grade reading level, was probably comprehensible to only 22% of this group. It was found that 43% of the patients studied were unable to profit from any written health materials.[25] Other examples are not uncommon. With four readability formulas, one investigator found the Patient's Bill of Rights to be written above high school and probably at college reading level. In one hospital that she studied, 83% of the patients probably could not fully comprehend the document—54% because their education was below the readability level, and 29% because their condition prevented their reading at the time of the study.[20]

The presumption that individuals read at the level of their completed formal education is not necessarily correct, although that level is probably the best available predictor of reading level. This fact became evident in a study done at the pediatric emergency room at Los Angeles County Southern California Medical Center. Two hundred and fifty-five mothers were chosen randomly from mothers who registered at the desk and were given materials written at the fourth (see below), sixth, and eighth grade reading levels. Of the 45% who could not read at more than sixth-grade level (15% of them were reading at fourth-grade level), 37% were high-school graduates and 27% had attended a college. Thus, one mother in seven probably could not be reached by material written at above the fourth-grade level.

The paragraph on p. 141, written at an eleventh- or twelfth-grade level, is from Los Angeles County Southern California Medical Center's routine written instructions to parents for home care of impetigo. *Parents' Magazine* is written at the eighth-grade level; only a small percentage of the parents that use the pediatric service of this hospital say they get medical information by reading such magazines.[54]

Studies have also been done of readability of directions on non-prescription medications (Table 8). Samples of directions and alteration of them to a more moderate reading level can be seen in the boxes on p. 140.

In order to match the learner to the material, teachers must know something about the factors that determine readability and be able to measure it. When the reading level of material is beyond the skill of the learner, comprehension is decreased, recall is sketchy and inaccurate, and motivation for further instruction from printed sources is reduced.

Readability is predicted by a large number of formulas and more recently by the Cloze method, which removes every fifth word and asks the reader to fill it in. Most of the formulas use two basic variables: complexity of words (using lists of familiar words or counting word length) and complexity of sentences (sentence

---

PATIENT EDUCATION MATERIAL WRITTEN AT THE FOURTH GRADE LEVEL*

DIET INFORMATION

Mrs. Brown's doctor has told her that her daughter, Linda, weighs too much. This is not due to her glands. She weighs too much because she eats too much.

Linda should eat the foods we all need to keep us healthy. These foods are meat, fish, cheese, milk, eggs, fruit and vegetables. These are the foods which have lots of proteins, vitamins and minerals. Linda needs to eat less of the foods that can be taken away safely. These foods are the starches and the extra fats. Then she will use up the extra fat her body has stored.

*From Wingert, W. A., and others: Why Johnny's parents don't read; an analysis of indigent parents' comprehension of health education materials, Clin. Pediatr. **8**:655-660, 1969.

PORTION OF WARNING AND CAUTION STATEMENTS FOR ASPIRIN-TYPE DRUGS*

Original material, written at 11th or 12th grade level: Keep this and all medicines out of children's reach. In case of accidental overdose, contact a physician immediately.

Material rewritten at 4th grade level: Keep this and all medicines out of children's reach. If someone takes too much by accident, talk to a doctor right away.

*From Pyrczak, F., and Roth, D. H.: The readability of directions on non-prescription drugs, J. Am. Pharm. Assoc. **16:**242-267, 1976.

PORTION OF CAUTION STATEMENT FOR ASPIRIN-TYPE DRUGS*

Original material, written at grade 13-15 level: If pain persists for more than 10 days or if redness is present, or in arthritic or rheumatic conditions affecting children under 12 years of age, consult a physician immediately.

Material rewritten at 4th grade level: If pain lasts for more than 10 days or if skin is red, talk to a doctor right away. If children under 12 years of age have signs of arthritis or rheumatism, talk to a doctor right away.

Note: Sentence length was reduced and these difficult words removed: *persists, redness, arthritic, rheumatic, conditions, affecting, consult, physician, immediately.*

*From Pyrczak, F., and Roth, D. H.: The readability of directions on non-prescription drugs, J. Am. Pharm. Assoc. **16:**242-267, 1976.

Table 8. Readability levels of warnings and cautions in directions for selected over-the-counter drugs*

Drug (brand name)	Type of statement	Lowest level at which statement can be read with ease
Bactine Antiseptic	Caution	Grades 13-15 (college)
Ben-Gay Pain Relieving Lotion	Warning	Grades 11-12
Compoz	Caution	Grades 11-12
Compoz	Warning	Grade 16 and college graduate
Coricidin Cold and Hay Fever Tablets	Warning	Grades 13-15 (college)
Di-Gel	Warning	Grades 13-15 (college)
Ex-lax	Caution	Grades 13-15 (college)
Ex-lax	Warning	Grade 4 and below
Nytol	Caution	Grades 11-12
Preparation H	Caution	Grades 13-15 (college)
Vicks Cough Syrup	Warning	Grades 11-12

*From Pyrczak, F., and Roth, D. H.: The readability of directions on nonprescription drugs, J. Am. Pharm. Assoc. **16:**242-267, 1976.

PATIENT EDUCATION MATERIAL WRITTEN AT THE
ELEVENTH OR TWELFTH GRADE LEVEL*

1. Description. Impetigo usually starts with small blisters on a reddened skin and soon begins to ooze watery material and then forms brownish crusts. This may spread rapidly especially if there is itching and the patient scratches. The germs get under the fingernails and everywhere the child scratches a new infection will start.
2. The affected areas should be scrubbed hard with pHisoHex to remove all crusts. Occasionally this causes bleeding.

---

*From Wingert, W. A., and others: Why Johnny's parents don't read; an analysis of indigent parents' comprehension of health education materials, Clin. Pediatr. **8:**655-660, 1969.

length is easily calculated and has a high correlation with complexity). Beyond these two variables, further additions add relatively little predictive power and become cumbersome and unreliable. If one is interested in doing research, a more complex formula may be useful. These two variables do not exactly determine ease or difficulty; they are merely good *indices* of difficulty. Shortening word or sentence length of itself does not necessarily improve readability. The formulas themselves are often validated against reading tests. Direct measurement of the subject's comprehension can be done with a comprehension test covering the material in the passage. Some readability formulas *predict* the reader's ability to comprehend, which of course is different from a comprehension test but much more efficient and more likely to be done.[23]

Perhaps the Dale-Chall readability formula, which uses a list of familiar words, is most widely used. There does not seem to be available a formula specially adapted to medical or health terminology in its list of familiar words. I prefer the Fry formula (Fig. 3), which indicates the grade level of written material, because of its ease of computation, including use of a chart. Practice using it or another formula until you become proficient, which might take 20 minutes. (I found this textbook to be written at

the high college level, almost off the edge of the readability chart!)

Of health education materials the nurse is likely to use, the literature about diabetes seems to have received the most attention with regard to readability. This is attributed to the fact that most diabetic persons must follow a strict regimen and assimilate large amounts of new information for effective control of their disease.[47] The same might be said of many others, such as those on hemodialysis or peritoneal dialysis, particularly at home, or the mother of a child with severe asthma, for whom there is less literature available than for the diabetic patient.

Scholars using the Dale-Chall formula for studying written materials for diabetic persons raised considerable question about the appropriateness of these materials for many learners and suggested ways to improve readability. Twenty-one large teaching hospitals in the United States were asked for the printed material they distributed to diabetic patients to help them understand their disorder. From census data it was determined that the median educational level of citizens 40 years of age or older is about 8 years; for the nonwhite population 25 years of age and older, the level is 6.9 years. The average printed material studied was written for a person with a ninth-grade educa-

A DIABETES WORD LIST OF THE 198 MOST FREQUENTLY OCCURRING UNFAMILIAR WORDS*

insulin	181	ounce	12	accurate	7
diabetic	122	plunger	12	Clinitest	7
diabetes	87	reduce	12	common	7
diet	74	standard	12	complications	7
urine	59	strainer	12	dosage	7
syringe	57	therefore	12	increase	7
patient	47	effect	11	indicate	7
calories	31	examination	11	nondiabetic	7
protein	29	medical	11	obtain	7
injection	26	mixture	11	particularly	7
alcohol	25	occur	11	requirement	7
weight	25	test tube	11	scale	7
disease	24	avoid	10	starches	7
contain	23	mild	10	tissue	7
control	23	pregnancy	10	vial	7
carbohydrate	22	recipe	10	withdraw	7
results	22	regular	10	zinc	7
normal	21	saccharin	10	acetone	7
grams (gm.)	20	solution	10	acid	6
condition	19	supply	10	available	6
physician	19	variety	10	balance	6
percent (%)	18	vitamin	10	collect	6
special	18	determine	9	factors	6
exercise	17	energy	9	immediate	6
inject	17	fluid	9	kidneys	6
necessary	17	method	9	quantity	6
treatment	17	produces	9	relative	6
usually	17	vary	9	replace	6
require	15	average	8	routine	6
specimen	15	cleanse	8	source	6
throughly	15	container	8	sponge	6
clinic	14	example	8	substitute	6
dose	14	frequent	8	successful	6
protamine	14	gelatine	8	unit	6
infection	13	individual	8	actually	5
overweight	13	insert	8	addition	5
pancreas	13	mold	8	advise	5
portion	13	period	8	apply	5
types	13	prescribe	8	approximately	5
area	12	prevent	8	callus	5
develop	12	reaction	8	coma	5

*The words are grouped in order of frequency of occurrence. Unfamiliar words are defined as words that fail to appear among the 3,000 words in the Dale list. From Thrush, R. S., and Lanese, R. R.: The use of printed material in diabetes education, Diabetes **11**:132-137, 1962.

A DIABETES WORD LIST OF THE 198 MOST FREQUENTLY OCCURRING UNFAMILIAR WORDS—cont'd

combine	5	consider	4	per	4
degree (°)	5	constantly	4	permitted	4
desirable	5	convert	4	population	4
diagnosis	5	corns	4	practical	4
dietitian (ician)	5	diabetes mellitus	4	purchase	4
discuss	5	dietetic	4	reagent	4
etc.	5	difficulty	4	recommend	4
forecast	5	easily	4	sample	4
gangrene	5	entire(ly)	4	serious	4
include	5	examine	4	severe	4
injury	5	glucose	4	site	4
margarine	5	grasp	4	soften	4
menu	5	information	4	specified	4
negative	5	instructions	4	stopper	4
positive	5	intermediate	4	strength	4
press	5	invert	4	sufficient	4
pressure	5	laboratory	4	suggestions	4
action	4	lanolin	4	sweetened	4
activity	4	limited	4	sweetener	4
acute	4	lower (ed) (verb)	4	syrup	4
ADA	4	maintain	4	system	4
attach	4	material	4	tube	4
beverages	4	medication	4	U40	4
bladder	4	onset	4	U80	4
carotene	4	Orinase	4	various	4

tion. Therefore, one half of this population probably could not read it.

For the learner who has less than fifth-grade education, approximately one word in five of these materials would be unfamiliar. This is an average; in some passages, because of variance in reading difficulty of as much as four grades, every second or third word would be unknown, a fact that would lead to considerable difficulty in comprehension. This person would probably have to learn about a thousand new words in order to read these materials—a staggering load. It is true that a small percentage of unknown or unfamiliar words occurring many times might be a major source of reading diffi-

culty. By removal of 198 words that appear in these diabetic materials (see opposite page and above), the reading level could be decreased four grades. Notice that many of these are crucial words—syringe, protein, alcohol, saccharin. Besides removal of little-understood words, addition of illustrations or pictures or of synonyms in parentheses (carbohydrate or starch) can improve readability.[47]

There are some limitations to the Dale-Chall formula and to this study. In assessing patients, the nurse must remember that the highest grade completed may not correspond to the reading level of an individual, although it does provide a ready estimate. The results are based on

DIRECTIONS FOR USING THE READABILITY GRAPH*

1. Select three one-hundred-word passages from near the beginning, middle and end of the book. Skip all proper nouns.
2. Count the total number of sentences in each hundred-word passage (estimating to nearest tenth of a sentence). Average these three numbers.
3. Count the total number of syllables in each hundred-word sample. There is a syllable for each vowel sound; for example: cat(1), blackbird(2), continental(4). Don't be fooled by word size; for example: polio(3), through(1). Endings such as -y, -ed, -el, or -le usually make a syllable, for example: ready(2), bottle(2). I find it convenient to count every syllable over one in each word and add 100. Average the total number of syllables for the three samples.
4. Plot on the graph the average number of sentences per hundred words and the average number of syllables per hundred words. Most plot points fall near the heavy curved line. Perpendicular lines mark off approximate grade level areas.

Example

	Sentences per 100 words	Syllables per 100 words
100-word sample page 5	9.1	122
100-word sample page 89	8.5	140
100-word sample page 160	7.0	129
	3) 24.6	3) 391
AVERAGE	8.2	130

Plotting these averages on the graph, we find they fall in the 5th grade area; hence the book is about 5th grade difficulty level. If great variability is encountered either in sentence length or in the syllable count for the three selections, then randomly select several more passages and average them in before plotting.

*From Fry, E.: A readability formula that saves time, J. Reading **11**:514, April 1968.

analysis using the readability formula, rather than on a determination of what patients actually learned from the materials. Revisions of materials should be tested for comprehension, because readability formulas are not designed to take into account certain elements that may reduce comprehensibility, such as ambiguous words or phrases. Also, it cannot be assumed that these hospitals and their teaching materials are representative of others in the United States.[47] Despite these limitations, the starkness of the evidence and magnitude of the problem of teaching all those diabetic persons who need

and want help prick one's professional conscience.

Further evidence of patient difficulty with written materials was found in a study of 31 patients on low-sodium diets. The study evaluated a booklet developed as a reference to help the patient decide whether or not to eat certain foods. The median education level of these patients was ninth grade. They encountered considerable difficulty with use of the index. For example, they could not locate peanut butter in the index, because it was listed under "fats." Since some did not understand the phrase

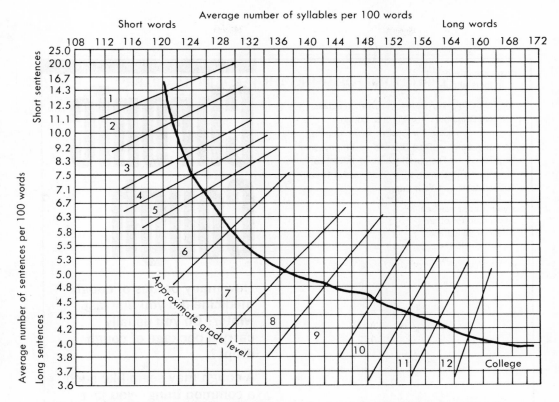

Fig. 3. Graph for estimating readability. Directions: randomly select three 100-word passages from a book or an article. Plot average number of syllables and average number of words per sentence on graph to determine area of readability level. Choose more passages per book if great variability is observed. (From Fry, E.: A readability formula that saves time, J. Reading **11**:514, 577, April 1968.)

"bread and its exchanges," they had difficulty looking up cereals. Descriptions of nutritional components of some foods were listed under the symbols "C," "P," "F," "Na," and "Cal," which had no meaning to many patients. Through interviews with 27 of these persons, it was found that only three knew that sodium occurs in foods as a constituent of salt and also independent of salt. Their confusion was increased because at times professional people tended to refer to "sodium-free diet" as "salt-free diet." Patients, therefore, did not bother to check the booklet for items that they did not

perceive to be salty, such as Alka-Seltzer, bread, milk, and bologna, and a few "killed the salt" in such foods as bacon, ham, and sausage by boiling them.[8]

Analysis of sample instructional materials

A sample of a pamphlet to be used with the lay public is shown in Fig. 4. By means of the study questions at the end of this chapter, the reader is encouraged to make an assessment of what objectives this pamphlet might meet. Its statements do seem to be correct. No pictures are used to create interest or explain content,

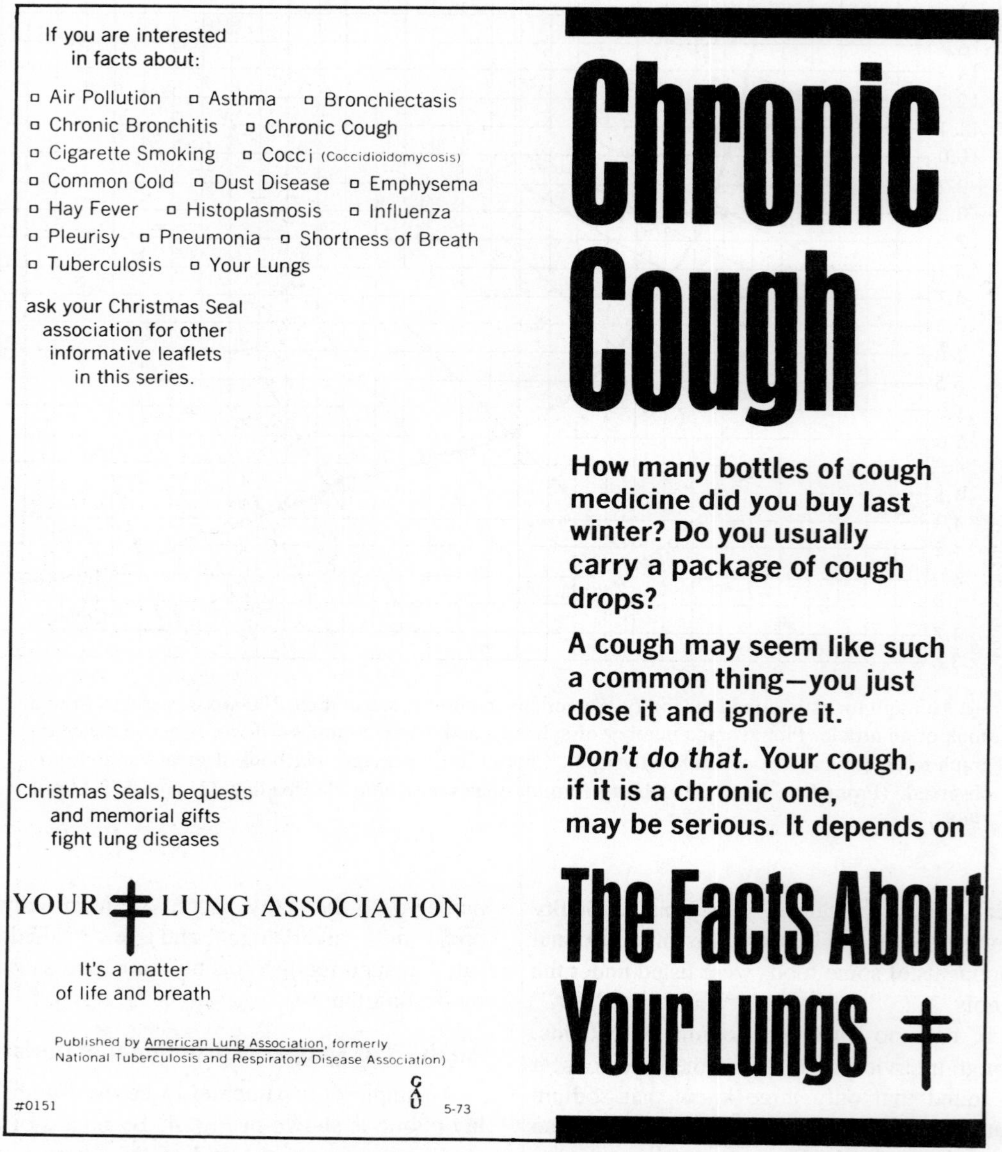

If you are interested
   in facts about:

□ Air Pollution □ Asthma □ Bronchiectasis
□ Chronic Bronchitis □ Chronic Cough
□ Cigarette Smoking □ Cocci (Coccidioidomycosis)
□ Common Cold □ Dust Disease □ Emphysema
□ Hay Fever □ Histoplasmosis □ Influenza
□ Pleurisy □ Pneumonia □ Shortness of Breath
□ Tuberculosis □ Your Lungs

ask your Christmas Seal
   association for other
   informative leaflets
      in this series.

Christmas Seals, bequests
   and memorial gifts
   fight lung diseases

YOUR ✝ LUNG ASSOCIATION

It's a matter
of life and breath

Published by American Lung Association, formerly
National Tuberculosis and Respiratory Disease Association)

#0151   C
                         U   5-73

Chronic Cough

How many bottles of cough medicine did you buy last winter? Do you usually carry a package of cough drops?

A cough may seem like such a common thing—you just dose it and ignore it.

Don't do that. Your cough, if it is a chronic one, may be serious. It depends on

The Facts About Your Lungs ✝

Fig. 4. Sample pamphlet: **A,** back and front. (Courtesy the American Lung Association.)

WHEN A COUGH IS CHRONIC

Has your cough been hanging around for a month or more? Then you have a *chronic* cough. It doesn't matter that you cough only in the morning when you get up, or only at night when you lie down. If you've been coughing for more than a month, your cough is chronic.

Maybe you cough only during winter and feel fine the rest of the year. That cough is a chronic cough.

WHAT ABOUT SHORT-TERM COUGHS?

Just about everybody coughs from time to time. The common cold, for instance, is often followed by a cough that can last as long as two or three weeks. But if your cough following a cold hangs on longer than usual, it may be developing into a chronic cough.

If there is shortness of breath with a cough, or any pain, or blood in the stuff you cough up, you should see your doctor immediately, even though your cough may not have lasted more than a few days.

WHAT ABOUT SMOKING?

Do you smoke a pack or more of cigarettes a day? If you do, you're considered a heavy smoker. Heavy cigarette smoking can cause a chronic cough.

But don't dismiss a cough that hangs on as "just a cigarette cough." That cigarette cough of yours is serious in itself. It means that your excessive smoking has already damaged your breathing passages. In fact, the smoker who coughs is the person most likely to get lung cancer. And more likely to get emphysema.

You may be so used to your cigarette cough that you can't tell when something new has been added. Are you coughing more than you used to? For longer at a time? Or has your cough changed its character? Maybe you're coughing up streaks of blood or more phlegm (mucus). Any of these happenings may be a sign that something is wrong.

CHRONIC COUGH IS A SYMPTOM

A chronic cough is not a disease in itself. It is a sign of something wrong with the breathing system. That's why it isn't smart to take cough medicine for more than a week or two unless your doctor tells you to. Medicine may help with the cough, but meanwhile the underlying illness can be getting steadily worse.

The most likely causes of chronic cough are: lung cancer . . . bronchitis (inflammation in the lung tubes) . . . bronchiectasis (in which pus pockets form along the tubes) . . . tuberculosis . . . other lung diseases.

WHY GO TO THE DOCTOR?

The instant you realize you have a chronic cough, go to your doctor. The doctor can make a number of tests to find out if a lung disease is causing your cough. Then he can start treatment early in the game. That is when most lung diseases can be dealt with successfully.

If you're coughing too much, find out why. It may be something minor or it may be serious. Until you know for sure, it's nothing to fool around with or neglect.

Be sure—or you may be sorry!

B

Fig. 4, cont'd. Sample pamphlet: **B,** inside. (Courtesy the American Lung Association.)

PATIENT INSTRUCTIONS FOR IVP

Description: X-ray visualization of kidneys.
Directions:

Do not take any fluids after your evening meal until the exam is completed.
Unless it is contraindicated, 2 ounces of castor oil will be given to you the night before x-ray.
You may have a dry breakfast, if there is time.
To x-ray when called.

THE INNOCENT MURMUR*

Fact sheet used to instruct parents about the benign nature of the functional or innocent murmur in their child

What is a murmur?

A murmur is merely an "extra" sound heard when the heart is listened to with a stethoscope. It is the sound of blood being propelled through the heart.

What is its significance?

Some diseases of the heart are associated with murmurs as well as with other findings. In pediatrics, approximately 50 per cent of all our patients, well or ill, will have "murmurs" heard. More than 90 per cent of these children have absolutely no heart problem whatsoever. A cardiogram (ECG) and chest film usually rule out heart disease in eight out of ten of the remaining 10 per cent of children with murmurs. Thus, 98 per cent of children with murmurs have the *innocent murmur*.

Why do we tell parents that we hear a murmur if these sounds are mostly innocent?

Because, at a later date, another physician hearing a murmur might think of heart disease and inappropriately treat your child unless he knew that this extra heart sound had been heard before. This is especially true if your child was being seen for an acute illness with fever, joint aches and pains, etc., which mimic rheumatic fever. Please ask any physician who examines your child to describe any findings or treatment to your satisfaction. It is your right to know and our job to inform you.

*From Scanlon, J. W.: Do parents need to know more about innocent murmurs? Clin. Pediatr. **10**:23-26, 1971.

but they would not seem particularly useful for this subject matter. Although the illustration does not show it, red is used on the covers and for the headings of the sections on content in the body of the pamphlet. Color catches attention and helps to make clear the sectioning of mate- rial into topics that follow a train of thought.

The organization of this pamphlet is excel- lent. Note that it centers on a single concept— cough. The sequence begins with definitions, differentiating the concept "chronic cough" from the overall concept "cough" and relating

INFORMATION SHEET GIVEN TO PARENTS ATTENDING HOSPITAL PHARMACY*

Antibiotic treatment for infection

1. Your child has an ear infection. The treatment requires special care to avoid any aftereffects. The antibiotic given will help to cure the infection completely when taken faithfully for the full 10 days. This may seem unnecessary when your child is active again after a few days, but we recommend 10 days of treatment to be quite sure that all the germs have been killed. Finish all the antibiotic.

2. Give 4 times a day, through the hours that the child is awake. Space doses out evenly. If one dose is forgotten in the day, give two doses at once before the child goes to bed at night. Use the measuring spoon to give the antibiotic.

3. Do not give along with food. It is best to give ½ hour before feeding. It may be given at the same time as any other medicine.

4. If there is fever or pain, be sure to continue aspirin in regular doses, as the antibiotic may take 2-3 days to fight the infection before the fever and pain disappear.

5. Do not give any of this antibiotic to another child. It may hide but not cure a serious illness.

6. Report back if severe diarrhea or a skin rash develop. These may be due to the medicine.

7. Store the antibiotic at the back of the refrigerator, out of reach, and shake the bottle well before giving the dose, to make sure that the antibiotic which settles at the bottom gets a chance to be mixed again.

8. Keep the return appointment so that your child's infection can be checked to make sure that no further treatment is needed.

*From Mattar, M. E., and others: Pharmaceutic factors affecting pediatric compliance, Pediatrics **55**:101-108, 1975.

it to symptoms the reader might see in himself. The sequence goes on logically to implications and action. Check the readability level.

Many health agencies prepare some teaching aids of their own, often incorporating schedules or procedures specific to that agency. These written materials must also be viewed with consideration of objectives to be met, correctness of material, and likelihood of patient comprehension. The example of patient instructions for IVP raises many questions, particularly with regard to understanding by patients and objectives to be met. It contains many words or phrases that most people are not likely to know: *IVP, visualization, dry breakfast, contraindicated, cathartic,* and, perhaps, *x-ray* and *kidneys.* It is not specific in discussing points a patient is likely to wish to know, such as

whether or not he will get breakfast, when a cathartic might be contraindicated, when he is likely to go to the x-ray department, and what will happen during and after the procedure. A summary sheet such as this is useful in that it presents factual information for initial orientation and acts as a reminder. It is not a substitute for patient-nurse contact, since it offers no opportunity for questions, no consideration of the patient's feelings about undergoing the procedure, and no opportunity for assessing whether or not the patient understands the directions and is likely to carry them out. These are all important objectives in preparing a patient for a forthcoming diagnostic test.

Reproduced on the opposite page and above are two information sheets given to patients or their parents. The first one was developed in response to the frequent misunderstanding of innocent murmurs. The decision about what contents to include was based on what parents wanted to know and what they actually seemed to understand or had obtained from authoritative sources. Pre- and poststudy with experimental and control groups of parents of well children found the sheet to be instructional, although not for all parents.[41]

Based on these data, logical analysis, and readability estimates, what is your assessment of the fact sheet on innocent murmurs? According to the Fry graph, readability is at the ninth-grade level; considering that these were middle-class parents, most could probably understand it. Note the use of advance organizers (the titles) that categorize the materials and that the categories would be useful to the parents. The title gives an objective, even though the behavior is not very clear. Since the study was done with parents whose children did not have murmurs, it is not clear whether they would have more difficulty using it because of a lack of previous learning on this topic and also whether the fact sheet would leave unanswered too many questions that parents of children with heart murmurs actually have about this condition.

The information sheet on p. 149 was developed in response to poor rates of compliance with antibiotic treatment among parents of children with acute otitis media. Oral instructions and careful filling of the prescriptions by the hospital pharmacy did result in better compliance with antibiotic treatment than was the case with similar families who had their prescriptions filled at their neighborhood pharmacy and may or may not have received careful instruction. Thus, the effect of the written information sheet was not separately assessed.[33] The readability level is at the top of the seventh grade, which is too high if one accepts the suggestion that all handout material should be at the sixth-grade level.[54] The sheet very neatly anticipates all the common questions parents would have,

plus the errors commonly made by parents following this regimen. It meets the contents standards for medication teaching (see Chapter 10) and is firm without implying that parents will knowingly fail to comply.

Availability and impact of materials

Reading materials are widely available from government and private sources, but their suitability and quality must be scrutinized carefully. Teaching aids are also frequently available from such local sources as the social security office, cancer or mental health chapter, or planned parenthood association. *Nursing Outlook* and *American Journal of Nursing* contain descriptions of written and audiovisual materials, and companies that produce medical products may advertise instructional materials more or less specific to their products. Addresses of sources have been gathered together by Lenahan.[26] Wood has compiled a list of booklets to give to patients and families,[55] and Isquith reports of a guide for health-related audiovisual aids for Spanish-speaking audiences.[21] A list of health education literature for parents of handicapped children may be found in the article by VanVechten and co-workers[52] and books for children about death in the article by Aradine.[4]

One highly innovative project developed educational material for family planning in the format of *True Confessions* magazine. Its acceptance among the target population—young women (less than 27 years) with an average of 11 years education and two to three children—was high. They could identify with the people in the stories, which were written with a very specific educational goal in mind and based on premises about family-planning behavior from research. The goal was continuance of contraception for this particular group. The premises were that the woman would be more effective if she could fit the use of birth control into her life in a natural, incidental manner and if she believed that she could control her own life and did not have to be a passive victim of circumstances. The stories made these points in an interesting manner.[13]

One possible effect of misleading literature was described in an account of an educational program for patients with arthritis. Patients' questions revealed that they had read the pamphlets assigned as part of the educational program, but they still had questions, particularly because they had read misleading articles or been told about "cures" by friends. The patients questioned the cures but felt that if they did not try them, relatives would feel they were not trying to get better. Patients felt relieved when the physician indicated which "cures" were not useful.[51]

It is useful to think beyond the individual pamphlet or book to the themes or messages common to a large number of these materials in a particular field. Although there seems to be no clear indication of the impact of such materials, some have been criticized for the unrealistic image they portray, often bound to the middle-class culture. The observation has been made that the stereotype in magazines, baby books, and printed matter distributed free with diapers is of a 24-hour loving, giving mother who, if she is really like this, will produce a mentally healthy and otherwise satisfactory offspring.[32] An analysis of the mental health "message" found in 27 mental health pamphlets showed that approximately 60% of the content was in the middle-class cultural mold and that another 30% consisted of ambiguous platitudes. Examples of this kind of material are: "Mentally healthy people accept their responsibilities," "Being mentally healthy means feeling right about other people," "Such things as a happy childhood spent in a serene household with loving guidance from parents who are themselves well balanced contribute to mental health." The conclusion of this analysis was that the mental health movement is unwittingly propagating a middle-class ethic under the guise of science and that much more research and theoretic de-

velopment is required before the public can be approached with any degree of confidence that what is being offered as the substance of mental health has reasonable validity.[18]

Public information about sickle cell disease was found to contain a number of inaccuracies. Sickle cell trait is frequently classified as a mild form of sickle cell anemia. There is no scientific basis for the classification. Some informational materials on sickle cell anemia state or imply that the patient's status will be improved if certain recommendations, such as nutritional advice, are followed. No published data indicate a correlation between nutritional status and severity of sickle cell anemia. A dramatic medical television show portrayed both an adult and a child with sickle cell anemia having fainting episodes. Although fainting is virtually non-existent in sickle cell anemia, viewers were led to believe that a major disaster could occur while a person with sickle cell anemia was driving a car or crossing a street, because they are prone to lose consciousness without warning. There was also an association made between pain crises and death, creating the erroneous impression that whenever a person with sickle cell anemia had a pain attack, there was a real possibility that death would occur.[53]

The criticisms cited above are not meant to imply that written materials available for health teaching generally present a biased message. Rather, nurses should be alert to the value orientations present in any teaching material and should determine whether they are sufficiently congruent with teaching objectives to be used. For certain patients a great deal of the available material may be inappropriate solely because of the values it portrays. Nurses should also be aware of themes in literature commonly read by patients with whom they work, since these can be a potent influence that either supports or negates their own efforts toward particular learning objectives, and since this awareness helps them to anticipate background knowledge the learner is likely to have acquired, including common misconceptions. Since nurses are involved in production of materials, they can influence the content and try various ways of making them effective.

The Kaiser Health Education Resource Center in Oakland, California includes a patient health library as well as health exhibits. The library is a centralized source to which health professionals may refer patients. A survey of medical staff and plan members indicated they would support the service. There also are mini-libraries to assist instructors and counselors in the various educational and counseling activities offered at the center.[11]

Patient package inserts for prescription medications are a relatively new source of information to consumers. Except for the brief label affixed to the container by the pharmacist, prescription medication information is usually limited to the verbal explanations provided by health care professionals. Isoproterenol inhalators were the first products that the Food and Drug Administration required to have a patient package insert (PPI), and in 1970 a PPI was required for oral contraceptives following the discovery of increased risk of thromboembolic disorders associated with use of birth control pills. Subsequently, labelling has been required for diethylstilbestrol and medroxyprogesterone acetate, a long-acting injectable contraceptive. Consumer groups are indicating that PPI's are necessary for prescription medications since such medications are inherently dangerous and the oral communication about them between physicians and patients is frequently inadequate. The purpose of PPI's is being argued, with concern that it is difficult to make them both patient education and right-to-know documents. Experience with oral contraceptive PPI use is that the overwhelming majority of users state they received and read the insert. PPI's have the potential for negative effects: information about adverse reactions to medication could frighten and confuse people; patients may tend to incorrectly self-medicate without

the supervision of a physician; or PPI's may be used improperly as a substitute for verbal instructions rather than as a reinforcement of directions by the physician or pharmacist.[37] It is believed by some that recommendations appearing in PPI's would become a minimal standard of care for all to follow.[34]

Programmed instruction

Programmed instruction is primarily verbal, although pictures and diagrams also are used. It is a written sequential presentation of learning steps, requiring the learner to answer questions about the material presented and telling him whether he is right or wrong. Examples of portions of programmed materials can be seen on pp. 153 and 154. Some material is used in a teaching machine, which separates a view of instructional materials from a view of correct answers to the questions. The learner controls the speed of presentation by advancing materials through a frame.[29] Programmed material is also presented by computers, which have the added capability of storing response patterns for a particular learner and selecting further lessons based on these patterns. Many units, including the samples on pp. 153 and 154, are presented in book form with answers on another page or in a column to be covered until the student wishes to compare his own answer with the suggested one.

Use of a program takes advantage of learning principles that are often difficult to apply with other teaching techniques, particularly with a group of learners. It requires the learner to be active rather than passive. It provides him with immediate feedback, correcting his answer if it is wrong and reinforcing correct answers with knowledge of success. It allows the student to work at his own pace.

Although programmers essentially agree on these facts, two major philosophies have grown up regarding the effect of errors and the resulting size of learning step and the importance of recognition versus recall. Proponents of the

EXAMPLE OF LINEAR PROGRAMMING, BOOK FORMAT*

knows

11 *Visitors.* No matter how kind hospital personnel may be, they are still strangers to the patient. He is always pleased to see people he _____ .

touch (contact)

12 Even if he can read and watch television, the patient often feels cut off from the outside world, and wonders what is happening at home or at work. Visits from his family and friends will keep him in _____ .

look forward

13 Furthermore, a day in the hospital can seem long and dull to the patient. Visitors can provide a very welcome break in the monotony. When a patient knows that a visitor is coming, he has something to _____ to.

demands

14 Many hospitals restrict the number of visitors a patient may have at one time. A patient usually feels obligated to be pleasant and responsive to his visitors, and too many visitors may place too many _____ on him.

number

noise; disturb

15 Another good reason for restricting the _____ of visitors is that a large group gathered in a small hospital room cannot help making a great deal of _____ . This might _____ others patients nearby.

help (guide)

16 A visitor coming to the hospital floor for the first time may be confused and uncertain. When she sees such a visitor, the nurse offers to _____ him.

speaking

17 Some visitors, on the other hand, come so regularly that they become familiar to the nurses on the floor. When she sees a familiar visitor, the nurse should always make a special point of _____ to him.

bed

chairs

18 When visitors come to your patient's room, they can hardly be expected to stand. However, since they might jar the patient and since they may carry infection, they should not be permitted to sit on his _____ . A considerate nurse makes certain that there are enough _____ for the visitors to sit on.

on her patient,
of course

19 Not all visitors will help the patient, and some may severely upset him. This can present the nurse with a very delicate problem—a problem that she should not try to handle herself, but should refer to the physician or the head nurse. If no help is available, however, the nurse thinks first of the impression she is making *(on the visitors/on her patient).*

*From Anderson. M. C.: Basic patient care, Philadelphia, 1965, W. B. Saunders Co., pp. 199-200.

EXAMPLE OF BRANCHING PROGRAMMING, BOOK FORMAT*

(page 31)

See if you can tell the difference between performances (*doing* words) and abstractions (*being* words). *Circle the words below that describe performances:*

stating	listing
writing	appreciating
valuing	internalizing
drawing	smiling

When you have finished, turn to page 33.

(page 33)

Check your responses with mine. The performances are circled.

(stating)	(listing)
(writing)	appreciating
valuing	internalizing
(drawing)	(smiling)

The circled words describe things that people might do. The words not circled describe internal states or conditions. Valuing, for example, is not something that someone does; rather, it is something that is felt.

Now let's look at some statements and practice recognizing which ones include *performances*. Read the statements below, and turn to the page whose number appears beside the statement containing a *performance*.

Be able to understand mathematics.   *(page 35)*

Be able to sew a seam.   *(page 37)*

(page 35)

You said that "be able to understand mathematics" included a performance. Not for a minute . . .

linear construction (example, pp. 153 and 156) believe that learning should be as nearly errorless as possible and that, in order to accomplish this, steps in the program should be small. Questions require recall (construction of one's own answer) rather than recognition of the correct answer in a multiple-choice type of question. Branching, or intrinsic, programming, shown above, contains more explanation before questioning, in an effort to refrain from fragmentizing the material. Its proponents are not so concerned that learning be errorless; rather, the questions are to assume a diagnostic function to find where learning has not occurred. If he chooses a wrong response, the learner is directed to a branch of the main program for supplemental instruction.[24] It is not unusual to find programs that combine features of both linear and branching techniques.

Choice of programmed materials involves many of the same criteria used for choice of other written materials—correctness of subject matter, appropriateness of values, relationship to the objectives, and readability for various learners. The teacher must be aware that this tool can save him or her a great deal of time and effort and that it can be effective, but some learners have found it to be boring, impersonal, and concerned with minutiae. Moreover, it requires self-direction in learning from written material. It can better be used to teach facts, concepts, principles, and even psychomotor skills than other learning outcomes.[22]

These assets and liabilities were evident in a pilot study of the program for diabetes prepared by United States Industries for use in Auto Tutor Mark II—a teaching machine. The program was tested with 184 diabetic patients at four diabetic medical centers in Boston. These people represented a wide range in age, education, and reading skill. Of the 106 completing the research procedures, 77% showed some gain in information over their pretests. Four fifths of those who completed the program felt that it helped them to learn about diabetes and self-care. It was found that newly diagnosed diabetic patients learned significantly more than did those who had been known to have diabetes for a long time. The aged and low-level readers made more errors and took more time than younger or more advanced readers but could learn the same amount if given the opportunity. There was no attempt to assemble data on retention of learned material or on the effect of learned material on motivation for good self-care. As a group, the 40% who did not complete the program were older, with a median

age of 61 (as compared with 42 years for those who completed), had three grades less education, were more recently diagnosed as diabetic, and were two occupational classes lower than those who completed the program. Fifteen percent of them could not make use of visual-verbal material in English: they were illiterate, had visual impairments, could not read English, or were too physically incapacitated to participate. Thirteen percent were considered to be resistant or showed no interest in the program, and the other 12% did not complete it because of difficulties in scheduling.[45]

Teachers who wished to use this program would want information from the publisher about how well the subject matter was retained and would want to inspect the contents for coverage of the topic and for correctness. However, the results of this study would provide them with the knowledge that many patients can learn from the program, that patients with some combination of older age and low-level reading skill are likely to require more time to complete it, and that certain individuals will be unable or unwilling to participate.

Another formal report of development and testing of programmed instruction materials has been made; these materials were developed for maintaining patients on warfarin sodium therapy (see sample of the linear format of programmed instruction in frame on p. 156*). Apparently, programmed instruction materials have also been developed for teaching dietary principles in renal dialysis. The relative scarcity of these materials is probably because of the amount of effort required to develop them and the high level of verbal ability required of the patient in order to learn from them. At any rate, patients who were taught by the programmed instruction unit on warfarin sodium did signifi-

---

*Sample frame programmed instruction. From Clark, C. M., and Bayley, E. W.: Evaluation of the use of programmed instruction for patients maintained on warfarin therapy, Am. J. Public Health **62:**1135-1139, 1972.

19.

Warfarin should be taken at the same time each day so that you get into the "warfarin habit." Your physician may suggest a time, such as lunchtime or bedtime. By taking warfarin at a specific time, you will maintain a constant level of the medicine in your body, and you will be less likely to forget to take it.

Fill in the blank:
For most effective results, take your warfarin at _____ each day.

(flip over)

The best answer is at "the same time" each day. If you said "at breakfast," or "at bedtime," or "at dinner," you may be correct, but you should ask your physician at what time he recommends that you take your warfarin.

Go to Frame 20

cantly better on a posttest than those taught by written handout or with no specific instructions from investigators. Although all participants were volunteers, individuals were assigned randomly to these three groups. Terminal behaviors desired were: (1) subject could identify the name and action of his anticoagulant medication; (2) he could identify two signs of undesirable effects of his anticoagulant medication; (3) he could calculate the number of warfarin sodium tablets to take for a given dosage and tablet strength; (4) he could differentiate between desirable and undesirable practices relating to safety. As is not unusual to find in such studies, previous experience with anticoagulant drugs had no apparent impact on test scores.[10]

AUDIOVISUAL AIDS

Audiovisual aids, sometimes combining sight and hearing with touch, smell, and taste, represent additional ways to communicate. They take many forms, from which the teacher must choose a form likely to aid in meeting particular objectives. Usually that decision relates to the degree of reality needed to ensure transfer to the real situation. As with written materials, completeness and correctness affect learning. On the basis of available research, the effectiveness of a particular instructional material is more dependent on the nature and quality of the message than on the characteristics of the channel of communication.[50]

One of the reasons this may occur is that such research has not recognized a distinction among three separate design elements: the medium, the presentation form, and the content. Presentation form is the structure by which the information is carried by a medium. For example, a picture of an elephant in a book and verbal description of it by a teacher differ in both media and presentation form. However, a picture of an elephant on a slide and the one in the book have the same presentation form but different media. Consider the presentation form of programmed instruction: (1) its stimuli are presented in verbal or illustrated form; (2) it demands written or selection response; (3) the presentation lasts as long as the learner desires; (4) the learner must make some response before proceeding to the next item. This form is really independent of both content and media. A workbook is an obvious medium, but others, such as slide-tapes, TV–problem books, and peer-tutor scripts, are possible. A classification system of presentation may be seen in Fig. 5. The primary disadvantage of transient presentations is that the learner

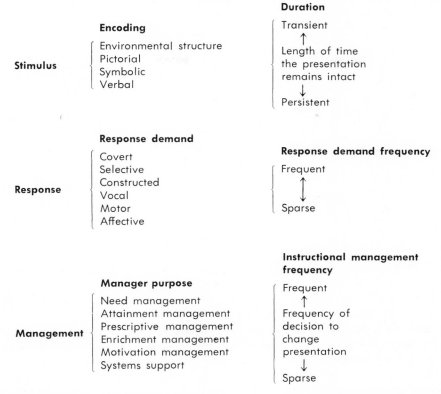

Stimulus

Encoding
- Environmental structure
- Pictorial
- Symbolic
- Verbal

Duration
- Transient
  ↑
- Length of time the presentation remains intact
  ↓
- Persistent

Response

Response demand
- Covert
- Selective
- Constructed
- Vocal
- Motor
- Affective

Response demand frequency
- Frequent
  ↑
  ↓
- Sparse

Management

Manager purpose
- Need management
- Attainment management
- Prescriptive management
- Enrichment management
- Motivation management
- Systems support

Instructional management frequency
- Frequent
  ↑
- Frequency of decision to change presentation
  ↓
- Sparse

Fig. 5. The dimensions of presentation. (From Tosti, D. T., and Ball, J. R.: A behavioral approach to instructional design and media selection, AudioVis. Commun. Rev. **17:**5-25, 1969. Used with permission.)

must store information because it is not available in the environment for a long period of time. This is not important if the presentation is already familiar. For persistent media, the disadvantages are not indicating real time in a behavioral sequence and not requiring response from the learner in a time sequence. It is, of course, possible to combine persistent and transient presentations to overcome their respective disadvantages.

One chooses presentation form by making it congruent with the response form described in the objective. A medium consistent with the response form is chosen, although some media accommodate to several forms (Figs. 6 and 7).

Often there is no one best medium or media mix for a given objective; one chooses an alternative based on costs, availability, and user preference.[49]

Types
Diagrams and charts

Human relationships are not physical objects; however, well-designed diagrams using circles, lines, and arrows can portray the essence of a relationship vividly. For a lay individual a single diagram could summarize and clarify the concept of the health team, more than many a lengthy verbal description. In Fig. 8, Diagram 1, placement of personnel around the circle

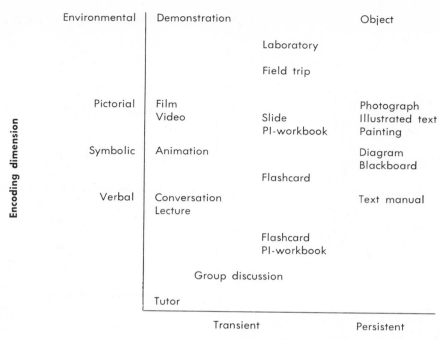

Fig. 6. Media classified by encoding versus duration. (From Tosti, D. T. and Ball, J. R.: A behavioral approach to instructional design and media selection, AudioVis. Commun. Rev. **17**:5-25, 1969. Used with permission.)

Encoding dimension	Transient		Persistent
Environmental	Demonstration		Object
		Laboratory	
		Field trip	
Pictorial	Film / Video	Slide / PI-workbook	Photograph / Illustrated text / Painting
Symbolic	Animation		Diagram / Blackboard
		Flashcard	
Verbal	Conversation / Lecture		Text manual
		Flashcard / PI-workbook	
	Group discussion		
	Tutor		

Duration dimension

Encoding dimension	Covert	Selective	Vocal	Constructed	Motor
Environmental	Demonstration / Field trip	Item sort			
Pictorial	Film / Video / Slide / Painting / Photograph	Multiple-choice teaching machine		Illustrated PI-text	Laboratory
Symbolic	Blackboard / Diagram	Card-sort	Flashcard		Diagram
Verbal	Lecture / Audiotape	PI-workbook	Conversation / Role-playing / Audiotape		
	Text	Tutor	Tutor	Tutor	Tutor

Response demand dimension

Fig. 7. Media classified by encoding versus response demand. (From Tosti, D. T., and Ball, J. R.: A behavioral approach to instructional design and media selection, AudioVis. Commun. Rev. **17**:5-25, 1969. Used with permission.)

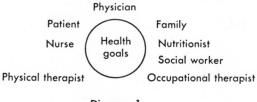

Diagram 1

The health team

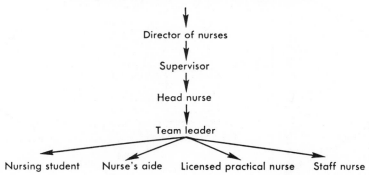

Diagram 2

Structure of nursing services

Coal ——— Fire ➔ Heat

Sugar ——— Insulin ➔ Energy

Diabetes = lack of sufficient amount of available, effective insulin

Diagram 3

Analogy to explain diabetes (Observed at the Diabetes Education Center, Minneapolis, Minnesota)

Fig. 8. Examples of teaching diagrams.

CALORIE AND SUGAR VALUE OF FOOD

Calories (per gram)	Food	Proportion converted to blood sugar
4	Carbohydrates	100%
4	Protein	58%
9	Fat	10%

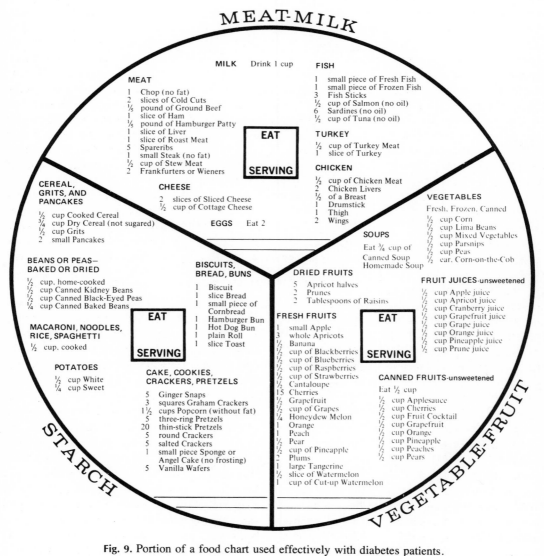

Fig. 9. Portion of a food chart used effectively with diabetes patients.

communicates the relative importance of roles, with the physician at the top, patient and family and nurse next in line, and so forth. The circle indicates that the health team is working toward health goals, but it does not make clear their relationships in doing so. Therefore, its design could be improved to represent the concept more completely and accurately. The concept in Diagram 2 is simpler to portray; it shows the superordinate-subordinate relationship in the structure of nursing services, with arrows indicating flow of power. For some purposes this diagram would not be considered complete, since it does not show the two-way communication that must occur. Many diagrams can be made more attention catching by use of drawings instead of words, but in Diagram 2 it would seem difficult to differentiate the various health workers with drawings. Diagram 3 was first constructed without the words *fire* and *insulin,* which were added in the course of the explanation. This tactic is meant to focus the learner on the essence of the relationship between insulin and utilization of sugar for body energy.

A chart may be seen as an organized group of facts about something. Consider patients undergoing hemodialysis over long periods of time. In one training program, patients not only are instructed what their diets should be but also are taught to understand the significance that their diet has in relation to the levels of blood urea nitrogen (BUN) and potassium (K). A chart can be used that shows the levels of BUN and K, blood pressure on and off dialysis, and weight gains between dialyses. Since these aspects of treatment are directly related to food and fluid taken in, this record can help patients understand their programs in relation to themselves and other patients in the unit. Such a record can create a healthy competition between patients and act as a dietary control.[15] The chart on p. 160 is an arrangement of basic facts that were used as part of an explanation of why carbohydrates are the most rigidly controlled foods in a diabetic diet. It can also form the basis for explanation of why fat exchanges might not need to be distributed so equally over meals as would exchanges containing much carbohydrate and protein.

Fig. 9 is a portion of one chart apparently very effective with diabetic patients. These patients were described as motivated to stay on their exchange plan diet but unable to understand it. The entire chart, which contained all meals and snacks, was used as a teaching tool and placed on the wall. During development, the dietician went to the home with the nurse to determine what numbers to place in the boxes, based on the patient's diet and his preferences, such as a heavy meal in the middle of the day. He was encouraged to talk about his favorite mixed food dishes so they could be fit into food groups. As practice in learning, the patient was asked to write menus before the nurse's next visit. Nurses and sometimes aides now do a lot of the teaching, with planning aids developed by the dietician.[14]

Diagrams such as these can serve as motivators for patients and provide factual knowledge. Provision of all the necessary information in one easy-to-understand form can get their understanding and focus their attention on what to do.

Physical objects

When one teaches about actual physical objects, it is often preferable to use the real thing. Nothing can act like a baby during a bath but a baby. However, models are useful when the third dimension must be retained but the real thing is too small, too large, too complicated, or too expensive; when the real thing is unavailable; when the desired view cannot be exposed; or when the object cannot be manipulated. For example, for explaining about the birth passage, a doll may be advanced through an actual-size model of the bony structure of the pelvis. Many times, anatomy and physiology cannot be adequately visualized with the use of a real person because other tissues are in the way or a body part, such as the eye, is too small and complex. A tracheostomy in the throat of a dummy can be useful for showing its position, removing and reinserting parts of the tube, and practicing general movements with the suction tube. The dummy is clearly limited because it lacks functioning muscles and secretions, and there are teachers who would insist that it would be better to start the learner working with a real tracheostoma. However, if there is none available or if the one that is available is difficult to care for, early practice on a model may be helpful. Since someone whose heart or breathing has stopped is not often available, models in the form of dummies are used to teach resuscitation techniques. Diabetic patients with visual impairment often need to be provided with special physical objects, such as a scale with braille markings, long syringes with bold markings, and so forth.[17] Thus models may be used because they teach better than real objects or because they are more practical to use; at times they are absolutely essential. However, models frequently are expensive and may not be easily available in many places where patient teaching is taking place.

Pictures

The research literature on pictorial learning is sparse in comparison with that on verbal learning; thus theory about how people learn from pictures is immature. Pictorial learning is superior to verbal for recognition and recall. However, when the subject matter is abstract, it is difficult to communicate with pictures. Pictures that vary in rather gross aspects (photos versus simple line drawings, color versus black and white, static versus moving) usually have not been found to create differences in learning. People do prefer color and motion and realistic rather than abstract pictures, but preference may not be highly related to learning.[28] Media used to convey pictures always distort the various visual dimensions—resolution, color fidelity, and size—to some degree. Some as in the case of a painting, may eliminate or exaggerate various parts of an object. These distortions

may or may not be important to a particular learning task.

Photographs and drawings lack the third dimension but are readily available or can be produced by the teacher. The third dimension is not so imperative when one is showing familiar objects or those in which shape and space are not the primary considerations. Examples that fall into these categories and are frequently not available include an infected finger or an abnormal stool in infants, although one must be aware that odor can be important in recognizing abnormal stool. In both of these examples, photographs would be more desirable than diagrams because they more accurately portray the details of the real item. Diagrams are particularly pertinent for removing superfluous detail present in real objects. During an explanation to a patient about diverticulitis, visualization is obviously desirable. Whereas a photograph shows details of the tissue that he does not need to know, a simple line drawing can communicate the concept of a pouch in the intestinal wall. Drawings in the form of cartoons are used to create interest in a topic. Either drawings or pictures have been used in place of real food servings to help diabetic patients visualize combinations of food appropriate to their diets.[12]

Pictures may be presented in many ways, depending on the size of the audience and equipment available. For a single individual, visuals on paper 8½ by 11 inches can be used. For small groups, posters can be prepared; drawings can be done with crayons or felt-tipped pens on flip charts (pads of paper approximately 32 by 26 inches) supported on an easel or chair back; cutouts can be attached by magnets or flannel to metal or flannel boards; or drawings can be done on the blackboard. Suitable for both large and small groups are 2-by-2-inch slides, lantern slides, or filmstrips that can be projected on a screen or wall. An opaque projector can produce an enlarged image of material from a paper or book, retaining the color. Overhead projectors do a similar task with transparencies, which are sheets of plastic, either prepared with diagrams or drawn at the time of presentation. In a situation in which teaching is a regular part of the nursing activities, these materials and equipment may be available; more commonly, the nurse interacts with an individual patient and will use an easily obtained visual, such as the pictures in the *Birth Atlas* or some other book, or will sketch the objects needed for a given lesson.

Some programs based largely on slides are available. An example is a self-instruction unit for stroke patients developed at the University of Rochester. Development included use of tests for aphasia and perceptual problems to determine minimum ability necessary to complete the self-instruction program. Fifteen hundred 35-mm. color slides were used to teach skills such as ambulation, dressing with one hand, and exercises. Each task sequence was presented to the patient twice: the first time he merely observed the sequence; the second time he performed each step in the sequence as it was presented, with as much repetition as was necessary. This instructional unit was improved after tryout with groups of patients.[43]

Motion pictures and television

If motion is necessary, as it may be for teaching procedures, motion pictures and television are available. In many health agencies, the most available piece of the more complex audiovisual equipment is the 16-mm. motion picture projector, because it is used for personnel training. Films are available from university film centers, state health departments, and private companies and may be borrowed on a rental or a free basis. These agencies have listings of their films, with descriptions of the length, content covered, use of color or black and white, and the basis on which they can be borrowed. Health agencies may buy the films they intend to use frequently, as in a prenatal teaching program. Single-concept films in the form of 8-

mm. cartridge loops have been prepared for patient teaching. The programs are short (about 4 minutes) and, with a small portable projection system, the equipment can be taken to patients' rooms, clinic examining rooms, or patients' homes.[40]

Television requires more complex equipment than do motion pictures. There must be monitors or receivers on which learners can view the television. The program may be videotaped and played back or may be presented live, the former requiring a machine to play the tape and the latter considerably more equipment. Sometimes the nurse-teacher will do the program live, as in a hospital in Salem, Massachusetts. Here the nurses give a baby bath demonstration twice a week in a studio, with the maternity patients watching on the television monitors in their rooms.[46] Teaching by television requires many of the same skills as doing an in-person demonstration but involves additional concern for getting camera shots that show what the teacher wants the viewer to see. It has the advantage over regular demonstrations of being able to show a close-up or an over-the-shoulder view to many people at the same time. This enlarging feature can be used to show labels on packaged foods and to show classes various amounts and combinations of foods that could have been adequately seen by only a few individuals. Videotapes can be used as "triggers," providing an instructional stimulus to be followed up by discussion groups. Since color television is not usually available in hospitals and clinics, it cannot be used to teach such things as color coding on insulin bottles, subtle color changes in skin with inflammation or with applications of heat and cold, or alterations in the color of normal body discharges.

Most motion pictures and television presentations combine audio and visual communication. Although these media are unique in their ability to store visual images of motion, the audio portion also teaches. The way in which it explains and enhances the visual may be more or less well done. Strictly audio presentations, in the form of phonograph records or tapes, are generally less useful for the content nurses teach, since so much of what nurses do is visual. They do have special pertinence in the teaching of speech patterns.

Since films and television can be so real, a viewer can rehearse changes in his own behavior by identifying with a film character. Perhaps what expectant parents are asking for or need when they request a film on labor and delivery is to have the experience of birth made "real" to them so that they can better understand the feelings before labor. For this reason, it is believed that prospective parents need an adequate background of knowledge with which to interpret what they will see and time and a comfortable atmosphere in which to discuss their feelings and reactions.[27]

Videotaped feedback was found in one study to improve the degree of motor learning and ambulation performances of amputee patients, in comparison with a group of like patients who were videotaped but did not see a playback of their performances until the last session. Videotaping seems to have several advantages over the use of a mirror. When a patient is asked to walk while observing himself in the mirror, he must divide his attention between two tasks. Patients reported that when viewing was separated from doing, they were able to pay full attention to either activity. In addition, videotaping allows the patient to observe his gait from different perspectives as often as he wants.[1]

Audiotapes and closed-circuit television

The technology for making and distributing audiotapes is now very simple. Audiotapes are infrequently used in patient education, perhaps because without video they seem to lack motivation. However, in some instructional situations audiotape is the best technique to use. For example, it provides an accurate portrayal of one's verbal behavior without the distraction of

pictures of the accompanying nonverbal behavior that is a part of communication. The audiotape was used well by a nurse whose patient had to learn to do long-term (16 months) parenteral hyperalimentation at home. The nurse, in addition to supervision, dictated the entire procedure onto a casette audiotape to assist the patient in managing the numerous complicated steps. The tape allowed time to perform each step; when the patient became more adept and the tape moved too slowly for him, it was redictated at a faster pace. After several weeks, he was able to proceed confidently without the tape.[5]

Both dial access (audiotape) systems[7] and a closed-circuit television (CCTV) system within a hospital have been used for patient education.[6] The dial access, sponsored by the San Bernardino County Medical Society, received more than 150 inquiries per day. Evaluation was done by the number of calls for each tape and by interview by staff members at the end of a message to determine if the caller's needs were met and what areas of ambiguity existed n the tape.[19] Fairview General Hospital in Cleveland made tapes at a local television station and tied into the TV distribution system already in use at the hospital, thus avoiding need for more than minimal equipment. Nurses coordinated the scripts, and no new personnel were hired. The first tape made was "Orientation to the Hospital" and the second, "Bathing Baby." This hospital believes that CCTV takes the place of repetitive teaching so that nurses can now do follow-up teaching and assessment of learning.[6]

Screening and preparing audiovisual materials

All audiovisual materials must be viewed and evaluated before they are used for teaching. If they are procured from outside sources, as is a rented motion picture film, preview is necessary because film catalogs usually do not comment on the quality of the presentation and do not

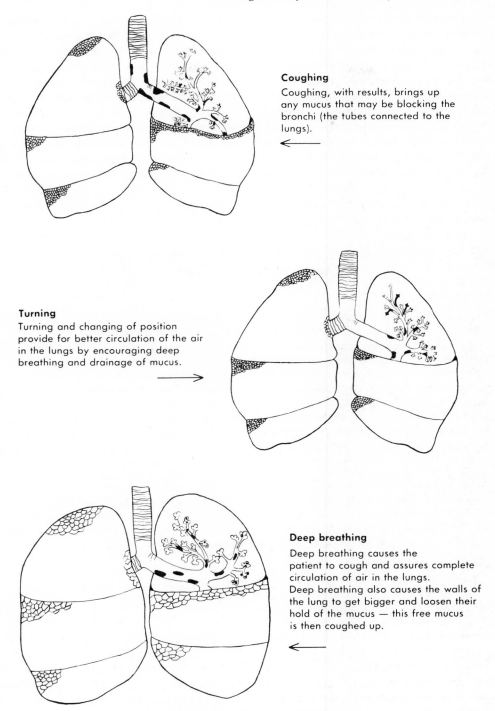

Coughing

Coughing, with results, brings up any mucus that may be blocking the bronchi (the tubes connected to the lungs).

Turning

Turning and changing of position provide for better circulation of the air in the lungs by encouraging deep breathing and drainage of mucus.

Deep breathing

Deep breathing causes the patient to cough and assures complete circulation of air in the lungs. Deep breathing also causes the walls of the lung to get bigger and loosen their hold of the mucus — this free mucus is then coughed up.

Fig. 10. Sample poster with limitations.

provide sufficient description of the content so that a teacher knows, before viewing, if a particular film supports the objectives of a lesson. If the teacher is concerned that children know the kinds of agents with which they can cleanse their teeth, he or she needs to know ahead of the class whether or not the film on toothbrushing presents this information adequately. If it does not, the teacher needs time to find other means to present it. This kind of detail is necessary for planning the rest of the class. Previewing is also done to identify material that the teacher believes is incorrect or is contradictory to other sources being used. If the children have been taught that both nylon and natural bristles on toothbrushes are acceptable and the movie strongly recommends only natural bristles, there is confusion on the part of the learner as to which is correct. The reason for the contradiction may be explained, but, depending on how many errors and contradictions occur and how major they are, it may be better to omit the film

---

IMPORTANT! PLEASE READ THIS NOW AND READ IT AGAIN WHEN YOU GET HOME*

Dear patient:

One of your prescriptions is for a medicine called **ampicillin.** There are certain things you should know about this medicine which will help you get well and stay feeling well.

Your doctor wants you to take ampicillin because you may have an infection. There are many kinds of infections, and everybody gets an infection at one time or another.

Infections are caused by germs growing in your body. These germs grow very fast and make more germs just like themselves. Naturally, the way to get rid of the infection is to kill the germs which cause the infection.

When you take your ampicillin medicine it will kill these germs, but it will kill the weakest ones first. After a few days you may begin to feel better, event though the ampicillin has not killed all the strong germs yet. If you stop taking your ampicillin before it kills all of these germs, they will grow fast again and make more strong germs again. **And you may get sick again.**

That is why it is important for you to take **every** capsule of this medicine at the time of day when you are supposed to take it, and why you must keep taking the ampicillin until it is all gone.

Remember, **take every capsule of the ampicillin at the time you are supposed to take it.** If you are going to be away from home for part of the day, take the medicine with you so you won't miss taking the ampicillin during the day.

Remember also, take the ampicillin **until all the capsules are gone.**

Take your ampicillin like this:
Take one capsule **when you get up** in the morning.
Take one capsule **a half hour before lunchtime,** even if you don't eat.
Take one capsule **a half hour before suppertime,** even if you don't eat.
Take one capsule **before you go to bed** at night.
Keep taking the medicine until all of it is gone.

Please save this and refer to it again when you get home.

---

and substitute another film or a teacher presentation. It also is possible, of course, that the error may have been in the teacher's presentation, which underscores the need for careful preparation. Other causes for rejecting an audiovisual aid are that it may be beyond the level of understanding of the learners or that it may be too peripheral to the objectives. A film that explains the chemical and microbiologic formation of calculus may only detract if the main objective is to learn the motions for brushing the teeth.

Fig. 10 is a visual aid that was made by a nursing student and used in the form of a poster. It was originally done with white lettering and pink lungs on a black poster, a good combination for catching attention. The size was 28 by 22 inches, sufficiently large to be seen by several viewers at once. The objective of this poster seems to have been to increase comprehension of coughing, turning, and deep breathing for health of the lungs. Probably, drawing the lungs inside the chest and using motion or a series of pictures to show the process of coughing, turning, and deep breathing and their effect on secretions in the lung would better explain the differences and similarities of their functions. In this poster all three drawings look alike. The error in drawing three lobes for each lung is not so serious in the attainment of this objective. Extension of the alveoli and bronchioles to the entire lung surface could clutter the drawing, but it should be made clear that other areas of the lung can become involved. These errors could have been anticipated by a knowledgeable teacher, particularly if he or she asked a colleague to check the materials. Other errors resulting in learner misconceptions do not become evident until the materials are used, since it is difficult for even an experienced teacher to view the materials as many learners from different backgrounds will. Thus, evaluation of the audiovisual aid goes on constantly, as does evaluation of other teaching techniques, to determine whether or not it contributes to learning.

Nurses design and approve visual and written materials for both class and take-home use, and, once these materials have been tried out with a number of patients, they can be revised to the point that they present a minimum of difficulty. Good design, particularly for home use, is important. Those most confident in taking their medications often have a schedule describing each medication, number of pills to be used, and time they were to be taken posted on the wall at home. Directions for taking medications were written on prescription blanks that these patients turned in to the pharmacy rather than on the container of medicines they received,[42] which shows the need for carefully planned visual aids.

The Office of Cancer Communications of the National Cancer Institute has gained experience in pretesting of cancer communications and offers a health message testing service. Pretesting is useful in early steps of development of the message or material and provides information to be used in judgment about improvement.[38]

STUDY QUESTIONS

1. Consider the pamphlet in Fig. 4 on pp. 146 and 147. What objectives could be met or partially met by use of this pamphlet?
2. The following terms were used in the index of a catalog of community nurse services. Each of these words or phrases was found by some patients to be difficult to understand. Indicate an alternative for each term, and then turn to the suggested answers in the Appendix for a list of the alternatives suggested by the users of this index.[48]

Maternity care
a. Menstruation
b. Father's role
c. Adjustment to parenthood
d. Uterus
e. Episiotomy care
f. Signs of illness in pregnancy
g. Fetal growth
h. Conception
i. Antepartum
j. Postpartum

k. Mood swing

l. Anesthesia

Infant care

a. Layette

b. Genitals

c. Weaning

d. Immunizations

e. Growth and
development

Child care

a. Sibling rivalry

b. Enuresis

c. Communicable dis-
ease

d. Peer relation-
ships

e. Socialization

Family planning

a. Birth control

b. How to control
pregnancy

c. IUD

d. Condom

e. Anatomy and physiology

3. Provide a critique of the information sheet on p. 166 used with adults who received a prescription of ampicillin.

4. Read the article by Judith McFarlane and Carolyn C. Hames, ''Children with Diabetes Learning Self-Care in Camp'' (*American Journal of Nursing* 73:1362-1365, August 1973).
   a. List the different instructional techniques used.
   b. Given the evaluation information from the questionnaires, what judgment would you make about the teaching effectiveness of the camp?

5. Patients with gout were tested for knowledge based on having read a particular booklet on gout, half having used an unillustrated booklet and half a booklet with the same text but illustrated with 89 cartoons. No significant difference was observed in either the overall test scores between the two groups or between individual question scores. The author suggests that possible reasons for these findings include a strong interest factor of patients reading about their own disease and technical factors such as page layout and picture-text imbalance.[36] What other possible reasons for these findings can you think of?

REFERENCES

1. Alexander, J., and Goodrich, R.: Videotape immediate playback; a tool in rehabilitation of persons with amputations, Arch. Phys. Med. Rehabil. **59:**141-144, 1978.

2. American Lung Association: Chronic coughs; the facts about your lungs, New York, 1973, The Association.

3. Anderson, M. C.: Basic patient care, Philadelphia, 1965, W. B. Saunders Co.

4. Aradine, C. R.: Books for children about death, Pediatrics **57:**372-378, 1976.

5. Baker, D. I.: Hyperalimentation at home, Am. J. Nurs. **74:**1826-1829, 1974.

6. Ballantyne, D. J.: CCTV for patients, Am. J. Nurs. **74:**263-264, 1974.

7. Bartlett, M., and others: Dial access library patient information service; an experiment in health education, N. Engl. J. Med. **288:**994-998, 1973.

8. Caron, H. S.: An evaluation of the booklet, Planning low sodium meals, Washington, D.C., 1955, Behavioral Studies Section, U.S. Public Health Service (unpublished manuscript). Cited in Knutson, A. L.: The individual, society and health behavior, New York, 1965, Russell Sage Foundation, pp. 189-190.

9. Carroll, J. B.: The potentials and limitations of print as a medium of instruction, National Society for the Study of Education Yearbook, part I, Chicago, 1974, The Society.

10. Clark, C. M., and Bayley, E. W.: Evaluation of the use of programmed instruction for patients maintained on warfarin therapy, Am. J. Public Health **62:**1135-1139, 1972.

11. Collen, F. B., and Soghikian, K.: A health education library for patients, Health Serv. Rep. **89:**236-243, 1974.

12. Coultas, R. N.: Patients use props to plan diabetic menus, Am. J. Nurs. **63:**104, Aug. 1963.

13. Crow, M. M., and others: True to life; a relevant approach to patient education, Am. J. Public Health **62:**1328-1330, 1972.

14. Dwyer, L. S., and Fralin, F. G.: Simplified meal planning for hard-to-teach patients, Am. J. Nurs. **74:**664-665, 1974.

15. Fellows, B. J.: The role of the nurse in a chronic dialysis unit, Nurs. Clin. North Am. **1:**577-586, 1966.

16. Fry, E.: A readability formula that saves time, J. Reading **11:**513-516, 575-577, 1968.

17. Fulton, M., and others: Helping diabetics adapt to failing vision, Am. J. Nurs. **74:**54-57, 1974.

18. Gursslin, O. R., and others: Social class and the mental health movement. In Riessman, F., and others, editors: Mental health of the poor, New York, 1964, The Macmillan Co.

19. Harer, W. B., Jr.: Tel-med; a public medical information service by phone, Calif. Med. **117:**68-70, Aug. 1972.

20. Iepson, L.: A study of the comparison of the education level of patients to the readability level of the patient's bill of rights (unpublished plan B paper), University of Minnesota School of Nursing, 1974.

21. Isquith, R. N.: Health-related audiovisual aids for Spanish-speaking audiences, Health Serv. Rep. **89:** 188-202, 1974.
22. Kersh, B. Y.: Programming classroom instruction. In Glaser, R., editor: Teaching machines and programed learning. II. Data and directions, Washington, D.C., 1965, National Education Association.
23. Klare, G. R.: Assessing readability, Reading Res. Q. **10:**62-102, 1974-75.
24. Klausmeier, H. J., and Ripple, R. D.: Learning and human abilities; educational psychology, ed. 4, New York, 1975, Harper & Row, Publisher.
25. Lanese, R. R., and Thrush, R. S.: Measuring readability of health education literature, J. Am. Diet. Assoc. **42:**215-217, 1963.
26. Lenahan, M. J.: Looking for teaching aids? Nurs. Outlook **16:**48-49, Oct. 1968.
27. Leppert, P., and Williams, B.: Birth films may miscarry, Am. J. Nurs. **68:**2181-2183, Oct. 1968.
28. Levie, W. H.: Pictorial research; an overview, Viewpoints **49:**37-45, 1973.
29. McDonald, G.W.: A new dimension in health education, Nurs. Outlook **12:**46-48, June 1964.
30. McFarlane, J., and Hames, C. C.: Children with diabetes; learning self-care in camp. Am. J. Nurs. **73:** 1362-1365, 1973.
31. Mager, R. S.: Preparing instructional objectives, ed. 2, Palo Alto, Calif., 1975, Fearon Publishers.
32. Maternity Center Association: Prelude to action, New York, 1969, The Association.
33. Mattar, M. E., and others: Pharmaceutic factors affecting pediatric compliance, Pediatrics **55:**101-108, 1975.
34. Mayberger, H. W., and Bell, B.: Patient package inserts and oral contraceptives, J. Legal Med. **5:**14-17, Sept. 1977.
35. Mohammed, M. F. B.: Patients' understanding of written health information, Nurs. Res. **13:**100-108, 1964.
36. Moll, J. M. H., and others: The cartoon in doctor-patient communication; further study of the Arthritis and Rheumatism Council handbook on gout, Ann. Rheum. Dis. **36:**225-231, 1977.
37. Morris, L. A.: Patient package inserts, a new tool for patient education, Public Health Rep. **92:**421-424, 1977.
38. National Cancer Institute: Pretesting in cancer communications, Bethesda, Md., 1978, U.S. Department of Health, Education and Welfare, publication no. (NIH)78-1493.
39. Pyrczak, F., and Roth, D. H.: The readability of directions on non-prescription drugs, J. Am. Pharm. Assoc. **16:**242-267, 1976.
40. Remillet, J. G.: The 8-mm film in student and patient education, J. Nurs. Ed. **7:**27-35, April 1968.
41. Scanlon, J. W.: Do parents need to know more about innocent murmurs? Clin. Pediatr. **10:**23-26, 1971.
42. Schwartz, D.: Medication errors made by aged patients, Am. J. Nurs. **62:**51-53, 1962.
43. Self-instruction for stroke victims, Bull. Clearinghouse Self-Instruc. Mater. Health Care Facil. **3:**1-3, April 1969.
44. Sharpe, T. R., and Mikeal, R. L.: Patient compliance with antibiotic regimens, Am. J. Hosp. Pharm. **31:** 479-484, 1974.
45. Skiff, A. W.: Programmed instruction and patient teaching, Am. J. Public Health **55:**409-415, 1965.
46. Spiegel, A. D.: Every patient has a front row seat, Am. J. Nurs. **64:**86-88, Oct. 1964.
47. Thrush, R. S., and Lanese, R. R.: The use of printed material in diabetes education, Diabetes **11:**132-137, 1962.
48. Tiede, J., and others: Report of the evaluation of A community nurse's catalogue, Minneapolis, 1970, Combined Nursing Service.
49. Tosti, D. T., and Ball, J. R.: A behavioral approach to instructional design and media selection, AudioVis. Commun. Rev. **17:**5-25, 1969.
50. Twyford, L.: Educational communications media. In Ebel, R. L., editor: Encyclopedia of educational research, ed. 4, New York, 1969, The Macmillan Co.
51. Valentine, L. R.: Self-care through group learning, Am. J. Nurs. **70:**2140-2142, 1970.
52. VanVechten, D., and others: Health education literature for parents of physically handicapped children; an update, Am. J. Dis. Child. **131:**311-315, 1977.
53. Whitten, C. F., and Fischoff, J.: Psychosocial effects of sickle cell disease, Arch. Intern. Med. **133:**681-689, 1974.
54. Wingert, W. A., and others: Why Johnny's parents don't read; an analysis of indigent parents' comprehension of health education materials, Clin. Pediatr. **8:** 655-660, 1969.
55. Wood, M.: 300 valuable booklets to give to patients and their families; a source guide, parts I and II, Nurs. '74 **4:**45-50, April 1974; **4:**60-66, May 1974.

CHAPTER 8

Teaching: planning and implementing

GENERAL CONSIDERATIONS ABOUT PLANNING

All the items necessary for constructing a teaching plan have now been at least introduced. Evaluation, which is also part of the plan, is considered in more depth in Chapter 9. Since the purpose of a teaching plan is to force the teacher to examine the relationships among learner receptivity, objectives, content, teaching methods, tools, and evaluation, a plan should be written for all but incidental teaching.

The mastery concept of instruction

The mastery concept of learning and instruction, developed primarily with schoolchildren, has profound implications for both the potency of teaching and for planning. In essence, the mastery concept is that an individual's ability to learn the criterion is dependent on the amount of time and the quality of instruction he is given. Some data suggest that learners differ by a ratio of about 5:1 in their learning rates: that is, the slowest 5% of the learners take about five times as much time to reach the criterion as do the fastest 5% of the learners. General intelligence test scores correlated with this finding in the magnitude of .5 to .7.[7] Particular modes of instruction require particular aptitudes, and so the use of a single mode hampers the learning of subjects who are weak in the aptitude required

to learn in that mode. The quality of instruction seems best defined by the clarity and appropriateness of the instructional cues for each learner, the amount of participation and practice of the learning by each student, and the amount and types of reinforcements given to each. Extremely high quality instruction operates to help most learners to achieve the same high quality levels.[6]

The translation of this research to patient education is more complicated because diversity of groups with which we deal is assumed to be greater than that in schools. However, a plan should include amount of time a patient requires for learning. One chooses instructional materials that can be evaluated according to the above criteria and provided in multiple modes and constructs feedback and correction procedures. In general, people who have high ability to understand and profit from instruction are little affected by variations in the quality of teaching, whereas individuals with low ability to understand instruction are much more affected by variation in quality.[6]

A study has been done comparing mastery (emphasis on mastering of task increments) and nonmastery learning approaches in training patients to do hemodialysis. The mastery learning approach patients completed training 10 days earlier, indicated greater feelings of confidence in their ability to handle minor problems and emergencies, and unanimously reported positive feelings about receiving ongoing documented feedback regarding task mastery.[19] Although the study needs to be replicated, the results are encouraging.

Planning decisions and dilemmas
A suitable approach

A common dilemma occurs when one is faced with a number of possible teaching approaches, but none has been adequately evaluated, and a clear choice is difficult to make. It is suggested that drug education is in such a situation. The techniques commonly used include conferences, symposia or workshops, lectures, journals or other printed materials, rap sessions, confrontation or sensitivity sessions, inculcation of values, and tapes, films, and records. Programmatic approaches are: (1) appeal to authority—for medical or ex-drug users, (2) negative reinforcement through recall or bad consequences, (3) logical argumentation or exhortation, (4) new cognitive structures (factual approach), (5) self-examination and attitude confrontation, (6) role or status enhancement, including that with peers, (7) role playing and simulation, and (8) simulation through novelty, humor, drama, and art. None of these foci has predictable outcomes for either drug abstinence or any other drug-prevention goals, and few individual programs have been evaluated. It is known that drug education can lead to increasing drug abuse.[13] What does one do in such a planning situation? One's choice is based on availability of approach and its suitability to learner readiness. Perhaps it is best to use multiple techniques or at least have them available in the event that one begins to fail. Teachers with a new program usually go through a period of finding and honing a "good" approach (effective for their situation and group) and then may become wedded to it.

If one is planning education for a community, one should be aware that members can be quite different from each other in many characteristics—behaviors for which they are ready, needs for instruction based on health problems in their life styles, and so forth. For example, one study of where citizens go for information, including health information, found one community with a heavy dependence on printed media, telephone, and television; another very dependent on family and friends—the interpersonal communication network; and a third on institutions and agencies. The choice of communication sources was far more predictable on the basis of community than by the particular kind of information desired.[29]

Sequence

Planning almost always includes a decision about sequence, unless one decides to allow the learner to move from section to section within the teaching plan in the order he chooses. Sequence can be a trap, because it is easy to assume that the sequence one chooses is the only "right" one. Subject matters do vary in their structures: in vertical learning, each task depends on having learned the previous one; in horizontal, any element can be learned in any order; and pyramidal learning is a combination of the vertical and horizontal.[9] Of the academic subject matters, the structure of math has been most thoroughly studied. There are, to my knowledge, no such studies in topics that would be taught to patients. The best word of advice is to question, try to analyze logically, and finally try teaching in different sequences for a particular subject area. The maximum amount of flexibility is sometimes needed in this area in order to make programs available to people and less expensive and to avoid unnecessarily "turning off" a patient who wants to learn in a different sequence.

TEACHING PLANS

There are many formats in which teaching plans can be written. The major criterion in judging the format is whether it facilitates the

SAMPLE TEACHING PLAN

Learner's readiness: Interested male adult with 2-year college education has been in a hospital once before but had only blood tests. Does not seem to know much about upper GI tract but (through conversation) says physician has told him a duodenal ulcer is suspected. Does not seem anxious.

Main objective: To participate in an upper GI test.

Subobjectives:

1. To explain the reason that patient is to have the test.
2. To list the sequence of events before, during, and after the test, particularly those steps that the patient controls.
3. To fulfill his role in taking the test with confidence.

Content	Teaching action
	General approach: sit at patient's bedside. Encourage questions and discussion. Watch for clues that indicate patient's confidence in fulfilling his role. Follow up, if patient seems to lack much confidence, with discussion of fears.
Test—a means of getting information about how the body is functioning.	Discuss how he feels about having the test; then give information he needs.
Digestive system—includes esophagus and stomach, small intestine, large intestine or bowel. These organs made of muscle, something like those in your arm. Function is in swallowing and digesting food. Upper part of this system, for purposes of this test, ends with upper part of small intestine.	Show picture of upper GI tract in Johnson, *Common X-ray Examinations,* p. 79, and point out parts.
X-ray—records shadows on film. Records best those things opaque to the x-ray film, such as bone. Because muscles are not opaque, tract is filled with something that is is called barium. In this way the x-ray film records the position of these organs and shows the condition of the lining, including the place where the physician thinks the ulcer is. This is called an upper GI test.	Show x-ray film of upper GI tract with an ulcer visible.
Procedure—nothing by mouth after midnight so nothing in stomach to take up space. Barium should fill stomach and outline walls and cannot do so if you have eaten or drunk anything. The nurse will take your water away at midnight, and you will receive no breakfast. These are the only restrictions on you.	Give him ''Directions to the patient who is to have an upper GI test'' (see end of lessson plan for copy) and point out section on preparation.
You will be taken to x-ray department by wheelchair when they are ready for you. In x-ray room it will be dark, so that films can be taken. A radiologist will be there behind	

SAMPLE TEACHING PLAN—cont'd

the machinery, with goggles on, to watch the x-ray of your swallowing and the filming of your stomach and intestine.

You will be asked to drink barium, and x-ray films will be taken, some with the table tilted so that the barium will flow into the intestinal loops. There will be periodic checks as films are taken by the machine. This will take about 15 minutes.

Show patient barium and have him taste it.

Point to intestine in picture of GI tract.

Back to your room. More films will be taken in the x-ray department in 6 hours to check progress of barium. You can eat when the nurse tells you.

Point to picture. Point out this information on ''Directions'' sheet.

You will be given a laxative because barium can be constipating. Your stool will be white—this is normal after having barium.

''Have you had much experience with taking laxatives?''

Your physician will get a report of the test from the x-ray specialist. There will be a technician in the x-ray department to help.

Stress this.
  If you have not had attitude response by this time, ask how he feels about having the test.

EVALUATION

Objectives 1 and 2: At the end of lesson ask patient to explain the reason he is having the test and the sequence of steps in it.

Essential point for Objective 1: To visualize stomach and duodenum with barium, which is opaque to the x-ray film. The objective is to outline any ulcer that might be on the lining of the duodenum.

Essential points for Objective 2:
  1. Nothing by mouth after midnight.
  2. To dark x-ray room.
  3. Drink barium.
  4. X-ray films taken with table tilt and time lapse of 6 hours.
  5. Stool white. Cathartic necessary.

Objective 3: Observe patient and consider observations by others. Did he maintain NPO? Seemed afraid morning of test (listen to conversation)? Did he drink barium with no surprise? Not alarmed at white in stools? More than mild anxiety while taking the test?

DIRECTIONS TO THE PATIENT WHO IS TO
HAVE AN UPPER GI TEST

1. Take nothing by mouth after midnight.
2. No breakfast.
3. You will be taken to the x-ray department when they are ready for you.
4. Since it may be necessary for you to return to the x-ray department for another picture, do not take anything by mouth until notified by a nurse that the test has been completed.
5. You may receive a laxative after test is completed.

relationships between its parts. One possible format is shown on pp. 172 and 173. Note that the sequence of topics is that frequently used in teaching: objectives are dependent on learner receptivity, and content and teaching actions are dependent on objectives.

Consideration of this sample teaching plan will indicate those points that are essential and those that may or may not be included, as the teacher sees fit. The information given about the learner's readiness is important but not sufficient. One would hope for more information about readiness for specific objectives, such as how much the patient knows about the meaning of his symptoms, about the specific test, about anatomy and physiology of the gastrointestinal tract, and about x-ray techniques in general. This information would allow the teacher to relate material the patient is to learn to that he already knows. Since content is derived from objectives, it is necessary to compare the two. If there is content present that does not relate to any objective, the content may be superfluous and should be eliminated; it may, on the other hand, be important and point up the need for another objective. If there is no content in the teaching plan relating to a particular objective, the teacher has to consider whether the content has been left out by error or whether the objective is really necessary. (Such was the case for the sample teaching plan on pp. 172 and 173, which originally contained material about why ulcers occur. This content was not relevant to the objective.) If the patient indicates an interest in knowing more than the plan includes, an objective can be added.

Content and teaching actions are determined from the behaviors to be learned. The content can be written in sentences that will actually be spoken or in outlined phrases. The sample on pp. 172 and 173 tends to contain verbatim the material that will be given the patient, which is often helpful for beginning teachers. With experience, paticularly in teaching the same material repeatedly, teachers may use outlines in words or phrases to bring entire ideas to mind. Note that some entries of content have a notation in the "Teaching action" column, which means that a specific teaching action should be taken with that particular content in addition to the general approach. These actions may include the use of audiovisual aids, learner experiences, demonstrations, or particular questions. It is a good idea to write actual questions that should elicit the desired response, such as "How do you feel about having this test?" Having several such questions in written form will help the teacher to keep the lesson on the right tract, particularly if the patient is nervous and unable to think well on his feet. Examples of nurses's statements designed to elicit thinking behaviors such as describing, analyzing, and formulating have been suggested by Peplau.[22]

As can be seen from the sample plan, it is easiest to indicate actions that are teacher controlled; it is much more difficult to plan precisely when there is more freedom for the learner to control the direction of the class, as in discussion. When this lesson is carried out, it is best if the content can be presented in an easy give-and-take manner, with at least some of the sequence being determined by the learner's questions. This allows the class to be directed by the learner's readiness, not the teacher's, and should help provide satisfaction in learning. Writing the content and teaching actions in side-by-side columnar format enables the teacher to note whether there are large blocks of verbal content that would be enhanced by visual aids or too many aids for a small block of material. It also allows the teacher to reflect on whether or not the objectives can be met by the methods indicated. If the objective is for a mother to learn to dress a child's wound at home and all the teaching actions center on discussion, one would wonder how she can learn to do this skill.

The evaluation is directly related to desired learning outcomes and should be listed by objective, as on p. 172. An effort is made to check learning at the end of the lesson; if the material to be learned is complex or the time between the lesson and the x-ray filming is more than a day, the learner's retention of knowledge is checked shortly before the GI examination. Essential learnings are those that the teacher has identified as crucial to a successful performance, and every individual should reach this level of learning. If not, reteaching is necessary. There is also built into the evaluation an assessment of teaching. If after undergoing the lesson several learners are unable to attain the desired level of performance, the methods of teaching, objectives, or teacher effectiveness in carrying them out must be examined.

Note that an effort has been made to follow principles of learning, some of which have been indicated in the preceding discussion. The lesson is organized around concepts, which are developed from the level at which the teacher thinks they exist in the patient to a level satisfactory for meeting the objectives. Much of the presentation is verbal, which is consistent with this patient's educational level, but studying visuals and tasting the barium are included because descriptions would be less effective. The concepts begin with the most general—description of a test—which might be viewed as an advance organizer. This kind of organization, rather than just listing the steps of the procedure, is meant to increase transfer to future times when the learner will want to know about tests, x-ray films, and the digestive system. There is also acknowledgment in the plan that learning about the test (cognitive) may help to achieve confidence (affective) but is not sufficient in itself.

Usually teachers are not expected to remember the entire plan they have constructed; rather, they use the written plan to guide them while they are teaching. They should have the material well enough in mind that they do not read the lesson to the learner, but they should follow it sufficiently to see that content is not omitted and to remind themselves of the objectives if the discussion rambles. This use of the lesson plan is most acceptable in the cognitive and psychomotor areas. When teacher and learner are discussing feelings, rapport can be damaged by diversion of attention to notes. Therefore, a very inconspicuous plan written on a 3-by-5-inch card or no written plan at all is likely to be best. Since discussions about feelings are considered confidential, it is usually preferable for the teacher not to jot down notes about objectives, readiness, and other parts of the plan, as might be done during discussions about self-care when anticoagulants are used.

Other means of communication that may be included in the teaching plan are story-telling for children and adults alike and pantomine for those who cannot understand speech or the English language. These methods as well as varying the terminology in an explanation and using visuals are based on the knowledge that all learners may not understand one mode of expression.

INSTITUTIONAL PLANNING AIDS

Some health agencies have developed teaching guides for lessons that are commonly taught by nurses in that agency.[2,28] For example, for tuberculosis patients at a particular hospital, teaching outlines were set up for seven lessons; after each lesson the nurse recorded the date, the patient's response to teaching, questions asked, answers given, and suggestions for further visits.[28] These teaching outlines may have been produced by nurses who act as patient education coordinators for the health agency and often do considerable patient teaching themselves.

The patient education coordinator or various departments or committees may produce a wide range of teaching aids specific to the procedures of that agency. These may represent small projects, such as single sheets explaining procedures for tests and orientation booklets given to the patient and family on admission, or be on a larger scale, as in the case of a patient guide explaining many of the experiences that the patient will undergo during a long-term hospitalization. An example of the latter is the patient's guide developed to be used in conjunction with the teaching outlines in the tuberculosis hospital previously cited. The patient's guide describes the physical plan of the hospital, services available, the disease of tuberculosis, the more commonly used diagnostic and treatment methods, and definitions of medical terms frequently used—abdomen, aerosol, bronchogram, cavity, culture, inhalation, mediastinum, pleura, sputum, trachea. The book is so designed that supplemental pages can be added dealing with ex-aminations or surgery that not all patients will undergo.[28]

Teaching outlines and aids save teachers' time in constructing their own materials and provide some common understanding among staff as to what basic behaviors clients should learn. Using these guides does not absolve the nurse from the responsibility of comprehending the material in some depth and being a skilled teacher. Reading to the patient information one does not understand, without knowing whether he needs the information, is not teaching. It is best to operate under the maxim, "If you [the teacher] don't understand it, neither will they [the learners]."

Text continued on p. 186.

UNITED HOSPITALS, INC.
RESPIRATORY REHABILITATION/EDUCATION*

Working diagnosis: _____

If you wish to have your patient participate in the Respiratory Rehabilitation/Education Program, please *date* the following:

The patient needs to know about:
Date _____ nature of his disease and preventive practices
Date _____ breathing and relaxation techniques
Date _____ postural drainage (education)
Date _____ oxygen therapy and pulmonary equipment
Date _____ medications
Date _____ nutrition
Date _____ (Referral coordinator) evaluation of discharge plans
Date _____ (P.T.) adjust physical tolerance to optimum level; develop home exercise program
Date _____ (O.T., daily) work simplification and energy saving techniques
Date _____ (O.T., 2 sessions) home-making
Date _____ May return to hospital for educational purposes as an outpatient if necessary

If you do not wish to have your patient participate in the Respiratory Rehabilitation/Education Program, check here: □

Anticipated further length of stay: _____

Sign: _____

*From United Hospitals, Inc., Miller Division, St. Paul, Minn. Reprinted with permission.

UNITED HOSPITALS, INC.

MR - 103

CHART COPY

DIABETIC EDUCATION

If you wish to have your patient participate in the Diabetes Education Program please check (✓) the following:

☐ is a newly diagnosed diabetic

The patient needs to know about:

☐ insulin administration   ☐ good health practices

☐ oral hypoglycemic drugs   ☐ diet

☐ urine testing   ☐ exercise

☐ is to maintain physical tolerance while hospitalized (energy-expanding activities equal to those at home).

    Has exercise restrictions: ☐ minimal activity, ☐ light, ☐ moderate

☐ may return to Hospital for educational purposes as an outpatient if necessary.

If you do not wish to have your patient participate in the Diabetes Education Program, check here: ( )

Anticipated further length of stay: _____.

Date: Sign:

CARDIAC EDUCATION

If you wish to have your patient participate in the Cardiac Education Program please check (✓) the following:

Diagnosis: ☐ Angina ☐ Myocardial Infarct ☐ Congestive Heart Failure

The patient needs to know about:

☐ symptom recognition and prevention

☐ medications to be given after discharge

☐ diet

☐ need to quit smoking

☐ principles of physical activity

☐ is to participate in the PHYSICAL RECONDITIONING PROGRAM

    (if so, indicate activity level on Reconditioning Order Sheet)

☐ May return to Hospital for educational purposes as an outpatient, if necessary.

If you do not wish to have your patient participate in the Cardiac Education program, check here: ( )

Anticipated further length of stay: _____.

Date: Sign:

Diabetic and Cardiac Education

From United Hospitals, Inc., Miller Division, St. Paul, Minn. Reprinted with permission.

United Hospital, Miller Division Inc.
Diabetes Education

PLANNING SHEET

A.   PRESENT LEVEL OF CONTROL OF HIS DIABETES

*PHYSIOLOGICALLY:

Please check (√) and date
when completed:

☐ _____ Patient Interview
☐ _____ Questionnaire
☐ _____ Dietary Assessment
☐ _____ Knowledge Quiz
☐ _____ Educational Planning
Conference

*KNOWLEDGE AND SKILLS:

1. DEFINITION

   Cause
   Why ℞ daily
   Fears

2. HYPOGLYCEMIC TABLETS

   Prescription
   Drug action
   Fears
   When sick
   Safety

3. INSULIN

   Prescription
   Technique
   Drug action
   When sick
   Fears
   Safety

4. URINE TESTING

   Prescription
   Why test
   Technique
   Fears
   Safety

5. EXERCISE

   Prescription
   Restrictions?
   Why
   When more
   When less
   Buerger-Allen

6. HYPOGLYCEMIC REACTIONS

   What it is
   How to recognize
   Treatment
   Fears
   Identification

7. ACIDOSIS OR COMA

   What it is
   How to recognize
   Treatment
   Fears

8. DIET

   Prescription
   Understanding
   Motivation
   Obese
   Food for sick days
   Exchanges
   Preparing foods

9. GOOD HEALTH PRACTICES

   FOOT CARE
     Why
     How
     Problems
   DENTAL HYGIENE
   EYE CARE
   SKIN CARE

10. GENERAL

   Economic problems
   Psychological adjustment
   Family relationships
   Self-care

11. OTHER: Secondary
            subjects

*PSYCHOLOGICAL/SOCIAL ADJUSTMENT

*ECONOMICS

CHEC 2 R-5/70

DIABETES EDUCATION

From United Hospitals, Inc., Miller Division, St. Paul, Minn. Reprinted with permission.

*ADDITIONAL FACTORS TO CONSIDER: Religion:

                                                    Age:

*BARRIERS TO LEARNING:

  Physical
    patient's diagnosis:
    physical handicaps:
    degree of illness:

  Psychological
    degree of acceptance:
    IQ: educational level:
    language problem?
    resistance to change:
    family problems?
    other:

*THINGS WHICH WOULD HELP IN HIS LEARNING PROCESS:

*OTHERS TO BE TAUGHT:

B. WHAT IS HOPED TO BE ACCOMPLISHED WITH THIS PATIENT:

C. METHODS TO BE USED: approaches, priorities, sequence, who is to do the teaching, when, where?

DIABETES EDUCATION

From United Hospitals, Inc., Miller Division, St. Paul, Minn. Reprinted with permission.

UNITED HOSPITALS, INC.
MILLER DIVISION

C A R D I A C   E D U C A T I O N

Please date when completed:

Planning Sheet

——————— Patient Interview
——————— Educational Planning
Conference

1. WHAT IS HOPED TO BE ACCOMPLISHED WITH THIS PATIENT? (Use list of objectives in the Education folder as a guideline.)

2. WHAT WILL BE TAUGHT?

**INSTRUCTORS
AND SCHEDULE**

SUBJECTS

3. OTHERS TO BE TAUGHT:

CHEC 8

C A R D I A C   E D U C A T I O N

From United Hospitals, Inc., Miller Division, St. Paul, Minn. Reprinted with permission.

4. DIAGNOSIS AND MEDICAL HISTORY:

5. SYMPTOMS LEADING TO ADMISSION:

6. HT._____WT._____ WEIGH DAILY?
7. SMOKING HABITS:
8. SLEEPING HABITS:
9. USUAL EMOTIONAL STATE:
10. MEDICATION HISTORY:

11. IN HOSPITAL MEDICATIONS:

12. FRIENDS OR FAMILY WITH HEART DISEASE:

13. TYPE OF RESIDENCE: STAIRS:
14. DAILY LIVING PATTERN:

15. SPORTS PARTICIPATION:
16. OTHERS WHO MIGHT HELP DURING RECOVERY:
17. HARDEST THING ABOUT CONDITION:

18. INTEREST IN MORE EDUCATION:

19. EMPLOYER:
20. OCCUPATION:
21. JOB SECURITY:

22. LIVES AT HOME WITH:
23. PATIENT'S PERCEPTION OF HIS ILLNESS:

24. INFLUENCES ON LEARNING: (Fears, Emotional State, Physical Handicaps, Language Problems,
                            Family Problems)

25. THINGS WHICH WOULD HELP IN HIS LEARNING PROCESS:

CARDIAC EDUCATION

From United Hospitals, Inc., Miller Division, St. Paul, Minn. Reprinted with permission.

United Hospital, Miller Division Inc.

PROGRESS SHEET

CHEC 1 R-5 70

DATE	DEP'T. and NAME	NEEDS and PROBLEMS	PROGRESS OF PATIENT AND/OR FAMILY

EDUCATION

From United Hospitals, Inc., Miller Division, St. Paul, Minn. Reprinted with permission.

FAMILY–STAFF INTERACTION GUIDE

SPECIAL CARE NURSERY

MARTIN LUTHER KING, JR. GENERAL HOSPITAL
County of Los Angeles • Department of Health Services

DATE	CALLED	VIEWED	TOUCHED	HELD	BOTTLE FED	BREAST FED	DIAPERED	WRAPPED	BATHED		INIT

RECORD ALL PARENT VISITS. USE CODES & INITIALS

Ⓜ – MOTHER Ⓕ – FATHER Ⓟ – PARENT

Ⓞ – OTHER (GIVE NAME)

	ADMISSION DATE	BIRTH WEIGHT	

	NURSE	M.D.	LIAISON NURSE	CHW MSW
INFORMATION DISCUSSED				
VISITING & PHONING				
ENCOURAGED TO VISIT AFTER DISCHARGE				
SCRUBBING TECHNIQUE				
FACTORS PREDISPOSING TO PREMATURITY				
MEDICAL PROBLEMS				
EXPLANATION OF & NEED FOR				
INCUBATOR				
MONITOR				
IV EQUIPMENT				
OXYGEN EQUIPMENT				
RESPIRATOR				
BILI LITES				
DISCHARGE TEACHING				
BATH DEMONSTRATION				
CORD CARE				
CIRC CARE				
FORMULA PREPARATION				
SIBLING RIVALRY				
INFANT CARE, ROUTINE WHEN TO BATHE, FEED, ETC.				
ACTIVITIES OF THE MOTHER				
ENCOURAGED TO TREAT AS NORMAL INFANT				
DISCHARGED MEDICATION				
FOLLOW-UP APPOINTMENTS				
OTHER TEACHING				

PATIENT IDENTIFICATION

NAME

MLK NO.

MLK-793 (9-73)

Fig. 11. Family-staff interaction guide, special care nursery. (From Cropley, C., and Bloom, R. S.: An interaction guide for a neonatal special-care unit, Pediatrics **55:**287-290, 1975.)

GUIDELINES FOR TEACHING PATIENTS ABOUT NITROGLYCERIN*

Goal: To prepare the patient for the self-administration of nitroglycerin in a safe, therapeutic manner, and to assist him to use good clinical judgment in managing his symptoms.

Before beginning to teach, assess the person's knowledge about his disease and medication. Explore the impact the illness has had on the patient and his family. Determine any fears and questions they may have. Discuss the following material.

Pathophysiology of angina pectoris:

Myocardial oxygen supply-and-demand deficit as it relates to pain.

Patient's subjective symptoms.

Precipitating circumstances (physical and emotional).

Use of rest, in conjunction with medication, to terminate the attack.

Nitroglycerin:

Pharmacological action to relieve symptoms.

Drug to be taken when discomfort is not relieved by rest, but patient should not wait for pain to worsen before taking nitroglycerin.

Route of administration: Sublingual only, *not* effective if swallowed.

Onset of action, 1-3 minutes; duration of action, 10-30 minutes.

If no relief, take 1-2 tablets at 5 minute intervals, but no more than 3 tablets per attack.

If no relief after 15 minutes, call physician immediately.

Nitroglycerin tablets to be carried by patient at all times.

There is no limit to the number of nitroglycerin tablets which may be taken in a 24-hour period.

Nitroglycerin is not addicting; does not lose its effectiveness in relieving pain even after years of use.

Prophylactic use: Take a tablet 3-5 minutes before engaging in activities known to precipitate angina.

Side effects: Headache, often pounding in nature; flushing of the skin; dizziness; occasional syncope. Usually subside after drug is taken for an extended period. Avoid standing after taking nitroglycerin.

Store nitroglycerin in a tightly closed, dark, glass container; avoid heat, air, light, and moisture.

The drug is potent for up to six months only. Fresh tablets produce a burning sensation in the sublingual mucosa. Nitroglycerin may be kept in the refrigerator to ensure potency.

*From Allendorf, E. E., and Keegan, M. H.: Teaching patients about nitroglycerin, Am. J. Nurs. **75:**1168-1170, copyright 1975, The American Journal of Nursing Co.

EXAMPLES OF AMBIGUOUS AND CLEAR
STATEMENTS CONCERNING GOALS*

Ambiguous goal	Clear goal
Improve patient attitude toward staff.	Patient and staff agree on self-care goals.
Assist patient in adjusting to hospital routine.	Patient keeps appointments without being reminded.
Help patient better his communication skills.	Patient explains his problem to staff so that they comprehend.
Better family relationships.	Patient handles her own self-care to family's satisfaction.
Patient accepts his disability.	Patient follows his diet and takes his medications on time.

*From Abrams, K. S., and others: Problem-oriented recording of psychosocial problems, Arch. Phys. Med. Rehabil. **54:**316-319, July 1973.

EXAMPLE OF A MANAGEMENT PLAN*

Problem 1: Patient cries and says she is going to die when subject of going home is mentioned by staff.

Cause:

1. Patient says she is worried that she will have another stroke if her blood pressure goes too high.
2. Patient is taking hypertensive medication and is having her blood pressure monitored daily; her physician wants this routine continued at home.
3. Patient is physically unable to do so and states that her husband is too nervous and upset to check her blood pressure; she knows of no other resources to do this at home.

Goal: Patient to have a way at home of controlling and monitoring blood pressure that is satisfactory to her and to medical standards.

Patient education: Instruct patient about what blood pressure is, what her medication does, and what and acceptable range of blood pressure readings is for her.

Plan:

1. Determine if husband, other family member, or friend is willing and capable of taking and recording blood pressure accurately.
2. If yes, provide instruction and practice sessions prior to discharge.
3. If no, find home health aide to stop in daily at home to take and record blood pressure.

_____
(Signature)

*From Abrams, K. S., and others: Problem-oriented recording of psychosocial problems, Arch. Phys. Med. Rehabil. **54:**316-319, July 1973.

PROGRESS NOTE ON MANAGEMENT PLAN*

Problem 1

Subjective: Patient says that she is no longer worried about going home since her husband is learning how to watch her blood pressure.

Objective:

1. In a meeting with patient and husband, physician and nurse instructed them about blood pressure, her medication, and acceptable range of blood pressure readings for her. They were informed that home health aide or family or friends could monitor her blood pressure. Husband volunteered to do it. The names of two other people were also solicited from him, as fill-ins, if he is not available to do it at home.
2. Several appointments were made for him to receive instruction and practice in how to determine blood pressure. He agreed to contact the other two people to determine whether they in fact would do it when he is not available.

Impression: Husband is willing to learn how to monitor blood pressure at home, and patient is no longer worried about going home.

Plan:

1. Proceed with instruction sessions as scheduled.
2. After husband has contacted other two people willing to take blood pressure, arrange for instruction and practice for them.

_____

(Signature)

---

*From Abrams, K. S., and others: Problem-oriented recording of psychosocial problems, Arch. Phys. Med. Rehabil. **54:**316-319, July 1973.

Charts specific to education have sometimes been developed to aid communication among health team members about teaching. Samples from the Education Program at the United Hospitals, Inc., Miller Division, St. Paul, Minnesota are shown on pp. 176 to 182, including a physician's order sheet, an education progress sheet on which all health team members record their impressions so that they are available in one place, a planning sheet on which the patient's education needs are summarized and recorded and goals are set, and a teaching plan formulated that spells out priorities, sequences, approaches, and time schedules.[27] Fig. 11 is a Family-Staff Interaction Guide used at the Martin Luther King, Jr. General Hospital in Los Angeles. It is used with a separate "progress note" sheet by all disciplines. The list of topics guides teaching and provides quick review to see that objectives are being accomplished.[12]

Institutionally developed guidelines for teaching particular groups of patients are becoming common (see box on p. 184). They standardize content and assist nurses in remembering it.

The problem-oriented format has obvious advantages: It gathers all data about teaching problems in one area and probably increases the possibility that patient education will be identified and worked on by a number of disciplines. The need for specific unambiguous wording that allows for cooperative work on a problem perhaps becomes more evident when a problem-oriented system is used. Suggestions for improving wording and examples of use of such a system are on pp. 185 and 186. Other samples of patient education notes in the problem-oriented format can be found in the literature—for example, in community child health care.[5]

ADAPTING TEACHING STRATEGIES TO CHILDREN

For the teaching of children, the basic tactics described in preceding sections are adapted to the growth and development levels of children. Many possibilities for teaching of young children center around play, which is a primary way in which they learn.[23] Petrillo has written an excellent book on this topic for hospitalized children.[24] Collins suggests that a coloring book be used as a tool to prepare children for surgery and hospitalization. The purpose is to help the children visualize what they and other patients will look like, including their dressings, and to provide a means for parents to describe and explain procedures involved.[11] For children 4½ to 7 years old, use of patient dolls, into which the children place tubes and appliances, and discussion (postoperatively) of what happened to them are aimed at the children's gaining some mastery of the situation and clarification of the difference between fantasy and reality.[23]

Use of puppet play therapy for children ages 3 to 11 years undergoing cardiac catheterization has been studied. In work done by Cassell and Paul, the goal of the play therapy was to help the children understand a fearsome situation by imparting information about the procedure in such a way that they could use it, to facilitate release of the child's emotions by providing opportunity for direct expression of hostility and fear in a warm, accepting relationship, and to help the children realize that the medical staff empathized with them and understood their fears. There was random assignment of 40 children into a control group and an experimental group, the latter participating in two 30-minute periods of puppet therapy, one before the catheterization and one afterward. In both sessions the child and the therapist acted out the procedure, first with the therapist playing the role of physician and giving explanation to the child puppet about what the child would see or feel and then with the roles reversed and the therapist crying and complaining during any potentially frightening experience. In the postcatheterization session, there was only the latter role assignment. The experimental group showed less emotional disturbance during the procedure than did the control group and expressed more willingness to return to the hospital. No differences were found between the groups in emotional disturbance after the catheterization and later at home.[10]

Books and games are also tools for teaching children. In an article on the therapeutic value of literature, Murphy lists books for children of different ages that can be incorporated into nursing care. Books can be used not only for direct instruction but for establishing rapport between patient and nurse, helping to ease the patient's confinement, and for asking and answering questions children may be afraid to ask.[20] Some stories depict children with whom the child can identify; others emphasize the humanity of medical personnel; some stories dealing with mothers and children can help keep ties at home alive and bridge the gap between mother and nurse; others help to deal with the child's feelings openly. Blake has also made lists of these kinds of books available.[5] All have the potential of facilitating discussion and dramatization of expected but unfamiliar experiences such as hospitalization. Games can be used as a tool to promote communication between nurse and school-age children; the mechanics of the game give the children something to talk about, and they can size up the situation to see if the nurse is someone to whom they can relate.[5]

Just as play, which is a natural developmental tool, is useful with children, so identification with a group of peers, a major developmental tool of the adolescent, is useful in teaching them. Sheridan has reported successful use of groups with children of a mixture of ages to focus on the concerns of hospitalization. She reports that the younger ones often act out for the group; older ones are able to act as interpreters for them. The session, called Talk Time, is open to what the children want to talk about within the general focus of the hospital experience. Three to twelve or fourteen children come at a time. The groups remains in the beginning phase since its membership is not stable. An example of a topic they choose is why a blood sample is taken or what is done with it, because most of them have little understanding of this common procedure.[26]

Abbott and others used preventive teaching for children who were so anxious about hospitalization that they could not be reached in an in-hospital teaching program. Since 4- to 5-year-olds seemed particularly vulnerable, a teaching program was taken into the kindergartens. Three nurses went in medical garb, had play clothes and medical equipment for the children to play with, and had a drama. They also showed slides about a child in hospital for surgery. The authors thought those children subsequently admitted were less anxious, but little evaluation was done.[1]

Teaching of a mentally retarded individual follows basic learning principles and depends on the child's developmental level, or readiness. The younger and more severely retarded the individual is, the shorter his attention span will be, the less his ability to learn from verbal instructions, and the greater the necessity for demonstration and imitation that make use of the real situations and objects. For example, manners are taught by games and acting out of situations rather than by verbal instruction. It is important for the teacher to make learning successful by breaking down behaviors into components to be learned, working on only two or three behaviors in a 30-minute period, and by starting near the end of the learning sequences and teaching the last step first so that the person feels success. Perhaps the biggest teaching problem is trying to elicit desired behavior from many of the severely retarded, since they are not responsive to verbal direction. However, quite specific directions on how to teach many individual skills are available.[4] Programs for development of motor skills, such as walking, use exercises to develop necessary component skills before attempting to get the child on his feet. Stevie, a retarded child described by Barnard, learned through a series of exercises carried out with a parent: swaying in the sitting position and catching himself by putting his arm out to the side to develop equilibrium responses, following the same schedule in the kneeling posture, rolling on a partially inflated beach ball to learn how to balance himself with feet and hands, coming from a bent kneeling position to upright kneeling to establish trunk support, riding a tricycle, and coming from a supine position to sitting and from kneeling to standing to develop control of the lower truncal area and extremities.[3]

IMPLEMENTATION

The actual implementation of teaching is difficult to describe in a book and perhaps better left to an audiovisual medium.[21,25] In purposeful, planned teaching, one carries out the plan. It will not work perfectly, but one can use it as a guide unless or until feedback from the patient indicates clearly that it is inappropriate or not working. One then redoes the planning process with new data. Experienced teachers can do that on the spot and move ahead. Others will need to break the teaching session and, if possible, replan and implement again. The kinds of questions that come up during implementation include substitution of learning experiences. The patient may request the substitution, what is planned may become unavailable, or something much better comes on the scene. The decision to be made is whether the substitution is good.

One obviously does not memorize a lesson, but the teacher's behavior should be sufficiently under control that his or her intent is generally carried out. The following interactions probably represent instances in which teaching was not planned, so there was no planned intention. Notice how nonpurposeful these conversations are. Such conversations seem to have a harmful effect on parents.

Conversation 1*

MOTHER: (about four-month-old child) He has a real temper!

NURSE: We'll hope he'll outgrow it. Has he been well?

(Later)

NURSE: Any problems?

MOTHER: No, not really. He's just a monster.

NURSE: Is he? Can he roll over now?

(Later)

NURSE: You can get him dressed now.

MOTHER: If he'll let me. . . .

(No response. Nurse leaves the room.)

Conversation 2*

MOTHER: She beats me on the chest with her fists and throws herself backwards. You can't quiet her when she's like that.

NURSE: Wait until she gets to be two, right?

MOTHER: Ohh!

NURSE: Then you'll have a little fanny to paddle.

MOTHER: You're right. What do you do when they're this young?

NURSE: Did she have any reaction from her first DPT?

Conversation 3*

MOTHER: . . . then for the last two days he's been vomiting, and this morning he started . . .

DOCTOR: (interrupting) When did the diarrhea start?

MOTHER: This morning. About four times he vomited.

DOCTOR: OK. How long has he had the runny nose? . . . any fever?

MOTHER: Oh, just a little bit, and he is unable to keep anything on his stomach.

DOCTOR: Hmmm . . .

MOTHER: Even plain water comes back!

DOCTOR: All right. Has he been urinating today?

Conversation 4*

MOTHER AND FATHER: Uh . . . what kind of pneumonia is that, would you say? What was it he had before this?

DOCTOR: H-hm.

MOTHER AND FATHER: Bronchial? . . . Broncular? . . . Lobar or what? . . .

DOCTOR: M-hm. OK?

MOTHER: Uh . . . what kind of pneumonia is that, would you say? What was it he had before this?

DOCTOR: M-hm.

FATHER: Bronchial? . . .

MOTHER: Bronchial? . . .

FATHER: Broncular? . . .

MOTHER: Lobar or what? . . .

DOCTOR: Bronchial . . . it's the same thing.

MOTHER: Is that what it is, bronchial now?

DOCTOR: M-hm. OK?

Teaching on a broader scale may be essentially planned, or implementation may be planned and carried out by many individuals with no one tending to the overall plan. For example, Brazelton complains that too much is written for the new mother. Most of it is aimed at giving her advice, and very little offers her support for her own individual reactions and intuition. The different advice she receives may

---

*From Freemon, B. L., and others: How do nurses expand their roles in well child care? Am. J. Nurs. **72:**1866-1871, 1972.

---

*From Korsch, B. M., and others: Practical implications of doctor-patient interaction analysis for pediatric practice, Am. J. Dis. Child. **121:**110-114, Feb. 1971. Copyright 1971, American Medical Association.

conflict so thoroughly that she is left in a serious quandary—overwhelming her baby with love on the one hand and giving him independence from her on the other. When she cannot follow all this advice, she becomes even more confused and guilty. She finds that many of her instinctual reactions to her baby are frowned upon by one authority or another. The literature that was designed to support her becomes an undermining influence.[8] If Brazelton is right, this is an example of a field of patient education planned in individual programs but unplanned as an overall field.

The decision to move to U100 insulin is an example of an overall coordinated plan that was based at least in part on the simplicity it would bring in administration. Whether patient understanding will also increase is another question. The concept of ''units'' as opposed to ''volume'' seems to cause a great deal of confusion. Patients have said they will get the new insulin but use the old syringe![18]

SUMMARY

Teaching involves providing conditions under which learning will occur. This is accomplished first by a relationship that motivates. The teacher is also skilled in deciding what experiences are likely to be profitable for a particular individual to reach certain objectives and in helping him to carry them out.

STUDY QUESTIONS

1. You are a clinic nurse. It has become evident that Mrs. Paganelli is not taking her digitalis and her diuretic. She is 80 years old, with arteriosclerotic heart disease, congestive heart failure, and cataracts in both eyes. She says she cannot see well enough to read the directions on the bottle or to clearly see the shape and color of the pills as she removes them from the bottles. She seems to be discouraged. What can you do?
2. Following are descriptions of general teaching situations. Indicate ways in which you might alter teaching activities for patients with various levels of readiness to learn.
   a. The patient has had a hysterectomy and has been told that some blood flow will occur until the tissue heals; that if the odor becomes noticeable or if the flow increases or turns bright red, she should report this at once to her physician; and that unless specifically ordered, she should not douche.
   b. The patient with a permanently implanted pacemaker is taught to check his pulse daily and to notify his physician immediately if any vertigo, syncope, pulse rate variation, visual change, or chest pain occurs. He is told that an increase in pulse rate may indicate that the batteries are weakening.
   c. It often is valuable to ask patients in whom the diagnosis of congestive heart failure has been established to identify the earliest symptom or combination of symptoms they remember noticing when the disease first appeared. This same pattern remains consistent for most patients, and they can be taught to identify trouble early and notify their physician or nurse when it arises.[16]
   d. Assimilation of a disability includes shift to an asset value system as opposed to comparison by the patient with what he used to be able to do.[14]
   e. A goal of patient education for labor and delivery is to feel satisfaction with one's own behavior.
3. A mother comments to you, ''My baby has clumsy fingers.'' You determine that the child's growth and development are normal for his age but that he could profit from environmental stimulation to develop his eye-hand coordination and prehension. What kinds of general teaching approaches might be used?
4. The following problem situations from the Diabetes Education Center in Minneapolis were used for discussion with groups of patients and their families. Suggest ways in which they might be used as teaching tools.
   a. Patty is 6 years old and has had diabetes for 6 months. At 7:30 A.M. today she received 2 units regular and 10 units NPH insulin. At 3:00 P.M. Patty came home from playing in the park and complained of being shaky and hungry. Patty has always been high-strung, but her mother immediately took a urine specimen. It showed 2+ for sugar. Patty routinely has a snack at 3:30 P.M. of milk and crackers. What should her mother do now, and what should she do tomorrow?
   b. Jerry is 13 years old and has just come to a new school. He has had diabetes for several months. At school he does not want to feel ''different'' taking a snack before gym in the morning, and he does not want to carry his lunch for this same reason, even though the school lunch menu is not suitable to his exchange diet. He has not told anyone at school about his diabetes and just recently went into a reaction at gym time, which was very embarrassing. What do you think Jerry and his parents should do to help the situation?

c. Mrs. Elliot is 56 years old and has had diabetes for 10 years. She has always been able to control her diabetes by the oral medication Orinase. Lately, however, she has not been adhering to her diet, is beginning to gain weight, and has been showing 3+ and 4+ urine sugar tests much of the time. She is afraid to go to the doctor because he might put her on insulin. What risks is she taking and what suggestions might you make to Mrs. Elliott?

d. Mr. Hanson is 65 years old and has been diabetic for 3 years. He has not been testing his urine because he says it always tests negative. He has not been following his meal plan and refuses to see the doctor. Mrs. Hanson has noticed that the last 3 months her husband has been tired and weak and occasionally experiences blurred vision. Otherwise he says he feels fine and really doesn't have diabetes at all anymore. What advice would you give to Mr. Hanson? Explain.

5. Provide a critique of the following problem-oriented record*:

Problem: Obesity.

Subjective: Has been overweight since young adulthood. Many members of the family share obesity problem. Has been impressed by relation of obesity to problems in postoperative recovery.

Objective: Weight, 214 pounds; height, 5 feet 2 inches. Dietary habits discussed: carbohydrates predominate; economics also a serious consideration.

Assessment: Believe patient desires to alter diet patterns by her initiating the request for aid. Believe she has been convinced of effects of obesity on her health. Believe she is motivated to change in order to improve outlook for her children who have already adopted poor habits of nutrition.

Plan: Begin instruction in basic nutrition; work with meal planning considering life-long patterns and low-income status. Discuss with nursing staff to encourage and reinforce teaching. Will follow up during hospital stay and on return visit to gynecology clinic.

Registered dietician

REFERENCES

1. Abbott, N. C., and others: Dress rehearsal for the hospital, Am. J. Nurs. **70:**2360-2362, 1970.
2. Amend, E. L.: A parent education program in a children's hospital, Nurs. Outlook **14:**53-56, April 1966.

*From Cadmus, M. G.: Problem-oriented gynecology; a nursing renewal, J. Obstet. Gynecol. Neonatal Nurs. **1:**45-48, June 1972.

3. Barnard, K.: Teaching the retarded child is a family affair, Am. J. Nurs. **68:**305-311, Feb. 1968.
4. Bensberg, G. J.: Teaching the mentally retarded, Atlanta, 1965, Southern Regional Education Board.
5. Blake, F. G., and others: Nursing care of children, ed. 8, Philadelphia, 1970, J. B. Lippincott Co.
6. Block, J. H., editor: Mastery learning; theory and practice, New York, 1971, Holt, Rinehart and Winston, Inc.
7. Bloom, B. S.: Time and learning, Am. Psychol. **29:**682-688, 1974.
8. Brazelton, T. B.: Infants and mothers; differences in development, New York, 1969, Delacorte Press.
9. Briggs, L. J.: Sequencing of instruction in relation to hierarchies of competence, Pittsburgh, 1968, American Institutes for Research.
10. Cassell, S., and Paul, M. H.: The role of puppet therapy on the emotional responses of children hospitalized for cardiac catheterization, J. Pediatr. **71:**233-239, 1967.
11. Collins, R. D.: Problem solving a tool for patients too, Am. J. Nurs. **68:**1483-1485, 1968.
12. Cropley, C., and Bloom, R. S.: An interaction guide for a neonatal special-care unit, Pediatrics **55:**287-290, 1975.
13. Einstein, S.: Drug-abuse prevention education; scope, problems, and prospective, Prevent. Med. **2:**569-581, 1973.
14. Fordyce, W. E.: Psychology and rehabilitation. In Licht, S., editor: Rehabilitation and medicine, Baltimore, 1968, Waverly Press.
15. Freemon, B. L., and others: How do nurses expand their roles in well child care? Am. J. Nurs. **72:**1866-1871, 1972.
16. Hanchett, E. S., and Johnson, R. A.: Early signs of congestive heart failure, Am. J. Nurs. **68:**1456-1461, 1968.
17. Korsch, B. M., and others: Practical implications of doctor-patient interaction analysis for pediatric practice, Am. J. Dis. Child. **121:**110-114, 1971.
18. Lawrence, P. A.: U-100 insulin; let's make the transition trouble free, Am. J. Nurs. **73:**1539, 1973.
19. Lira, F. T., and Mlott, S. R.: A behavioral approach to hemodialysis training, J. Am. Assoc. Neph. Nurses Techs. **3:**180-188, 1976.
20. Murphy, D. C.: The therapeutic value of children's literature, Nurs. Forum **11:**141-164, 1972.
21. Olson, F., and others: Self-analysis of patient teaching behavior (videotapes and study guide), Lincoln, Nebraska, n.d., Nebraska Television Council for Nursing Education, Inc.
22. Peplau, H. E.: Process and concept of learning. In Burd, S. F., and Marshall, M. A., editors: Some clin-

ical approaches to psychiatric nursing, New York, 1963, The Macmillan Co.

23. Petrillo, M.: Preventing hospital trauma in pediatric patients, Am. J. Nurs. **68:**1469-1473, 1968.

24. Petrillo, M., and Sanger, S.: Emotional care of hospitalized children; an environmental approach, Philadelphia, 1972, J. B. Lippincott Co.

25. Redman, B.: Patient teaching; a guide for analysis (videotapes and study guide), Lincoln, Nebraska, 1970, Nebraska Television Council for Nursing Education, Inc.

26. Sheridan, M. S.: Talk time for hospitalized children, Soc. Work **20:**40-44, 1975.

27. Ulrich, M.: Introducing an educational program for hospitalized diabetics, St. Paul, Minn., United Hospitals, Inc., Miller Division.

28. Weaver, B., and Williams, E. L.: Teaching the tuberculosis patient, Am. J. Nurs. **63:**80-82, Dec. 1963.

29. Williams, F., and others: Where citizens go for information, J. Commun. **27:**95-99, 1977.

CHAPTER 9

Evaluation of health teaching

■ Evaluation is a process by which the value of something is judged. Most commonly in patient education that "something" is teaching and learning with a particular client. Evaluation reinforces correct behavior on the part of the learner, helps him to realize how he should change incorrect behavior, and helps teachers to determine the adequacy of their teaching.[7] Evaluation involves measuring behavior and interpreting the results in terms of desired behavior change—which is complicated by the fact that all such measurement contains error. Program evaluation is also necessary and, although based on the same principles as evaluation of an individual's learning, does involve different ways of thinking, problems of aggregating data, and different standards for judging the value of the activity. Program evaluation is discussed later in this chapter.

The goals of this chapter are for the reader to (1) identify appropriate measurement techniques for objectives from cognitive, psychomotor, and affective domains; (2) identify major sources of error; and (3) comprehend the process of interpretation and subsequent replanning in order to evaluate both individual learning and the overall program.

OBTAINING MEASURES OF BEHAVIOR

All measurement may be said to involve observation of behavior. These observations are more or less direct—more direct if the method of measurement involves viewing of actual behavior as it occurs and less direct if it involves the subject's responding to substitute situations that may be largely verbal. Each method contains certain weaknesses that can produce error in measurement.

Since the purpose of measurement and evaluation activities is the prediction of how the individual will behave in the future, it would seem most accurate to base this prediction on observation of actual behavior (direct measurement). The basis for this position is well known. Response to a situation is very complex, involving conscious and subconscious levels of mental activity, varying with how the individual feels, what has just happened to him, what previous experience he has had with similar situations, and so forth. Thus, what people say they would do and what they actually do may be different. It is known that people often respond in ways that are the most socially acceptable, which may or may not involve conscious alteration of response. Perhaps the most difficult measurement of behavior occurs with behavior in the affective domain, for the individual can easily control the expression of feelings. The best opportunity for accurate assessment here seems to be by direct observation of behavior in a situation in which the individual is unaware that he is being observed for this purpose.

Although indirect measurements have their perils, they also have advantages that can con-

193

tribute greatly to accurate assessment. Natural behavior is often inaccessible in that it occurs in private, as in family interactions. It may occur infrequently and in various places, for example, in response to emergencies that require resuscitation measures, in response to insulin shock or diabetic coma, or in response to ingestion of poisons by a child. It may also occur relatively infrequently, as when a parent provides sex education for a child. Thus, the observer cannot be present or it is inconvenient for him or her to be present when the actual natural behavior occurs. The strategy behind most tests used in indirect measurement is to control the situation in such a way that the desired behavior can be stimulated at will,[13] in the form of written, oral, or performance response to a mock situation. Especially for behaviors that are complex, the test can be much more accurate if the learner responds to situations on video tape or motion picture film than merely to written test situations.[8]

Thus far in this chapter several major sources of error in measurement have been identified: One source is the constant possibility that indirect measures may present a false picture of how the individual might really behave. A second source of error is the complexity of behavior, which accounts for the frequent inability to identify what causes it, or the inability to measure thought patterns and attitudes even by direct observation. A third source is the bias of human observers, who are limited by the amount of stimulus to which they can attend and which they can record and who tend to assign meanings according to their own views of a situation. A fourth source of error is sampling. It is often not feasible in terms of time and effort expended to observe an individual's or a group's behavior repeatedly in order to take into account the variation in performance from day to day and from situation to situation. Neither is it possible to inventory in great detail an individual's knowledge about all aspects of a subject. Rather, it is necessary to get enough

samples over a period of time and in general areas of subject matter to decrease error to an acceptable level.

The degree of error allowable depends on the predictions—and decisions—that need to be made and on the precision of the best tool for measurement that is available. One would be more concerned with being sure that a learner knew what to do about a blood pressure drop or a blood leak during home hemodialysis than with whether or not a mother knew how to fold diapers with extra thickness for her baby boy. In both cases, observation of the learner doing the behavior would be appropriate for evaluation, but for hemodialysis the teacher would want to observe many times, measuring the learner's behavior against objective criteria agreed on by experts. In order to be sure of the learner's understanding, the nurse would supplement the observation with oral or written questioning of what constitutes a blood pressure drop, what can cause it, and how it can be corrected. Without the learner's knowledge, the nurse might add some blood to the dialysate to see if he detects it and how he responds. Since all methods of measurement are prone to particular errors, the best information on which to base a decision can often be gained by using a combination of methods.

Measurement involves obtaining a record of pertinent behavior. Not only is it quite difficult to record all that occurs, but also this mass of information is not useful. The guideline for the pertinence of behavior to be recorded is the objective, and, if its statement has met all the specifications for preciseness and clarity that were outlined in Chapter 4, it becomes much easier to decide what information is useful to record. Envision the difference in trying to evaluate these two objectives: "To know injection sites," and "To draw on his own skin five areas suitable for injection of insulin." In regard to the former objective, not only is it difficult to know what content and behavior to measure, but also the teaching may have been haphazard because of this lack of specificity. Note also that there is no time stipulation on this objective. Tests in which the time is limited are appropriate only if the behavior to be learned requires speed.

In considering methods of measurement to be used, the taxonomy of educational objectives in Chapter 4, which provides a general classification of behaviors, may again be used as a guide.

USING MEASUREMENT TECHNIQUES

There are a number of units in which behavior can be measured: the most common are speed, accuracy, probability of occurrence, originality, persistence, amount, and correctness. Of these, measurement of persistence is often neglected, thus leaving us with little knowledge about retention of health teaching. These measures are made through a variety of techniques, which are described in subsequent sections.

Direct observation of behavior

As in much of nursing practice, observation skills are used considerably in teaching, but they are more effective in evaluating learning in some areas than in others. In the absence of many well-developed, readily available tests for the measurement of attitudes, the best course is to become skilled in examining behavior that expresses feelings and values. Cognitive skills are more difficult to observe, since thinking is an internal act that may or may not be expressed in actions. This includes cognitive skills underlying motor acts, such as the basis on which one decides that the irrigated catheter is patent, and behavior more completely cognitive, such as a mother's reasoning for bringing her child to the physician. Thought processes are most often measured by verbal means: through oral questioning or written tests.

The recording of observations, necessary when observation is being used in the evaluation of learned behavior, varies with the type of learning that is being evaluated. Since attitudes often change slowly and are expressed in many different ways, the form for recording observations might best be relatively unstructured and adaptable to long-term use. Motor skills, on the other hand, are much more uniform in their expression, so that the recording form for observation of them can describe specific steps that every learner will do. The products and processes of learned behavior also can be described—the way the diaper looks after it has been secured and the process of putting it on. Indeed, some products are difficult to evaluate without seeing the process, as in the case of a paraplegic patient learning to irrigate his catheter.

Rating scales and checklists

The most complete recording of behavior would be obtained by film or video tape. These tools have the advantage of replay of the performance, which aids in obtaining an accurate description of what happened and in pointing out relevant behavior to learners. However, these tools are expensive and rarely available and, by themselves, do not summarize the kind of behavior seen or identify its meaning in relation to objectives. To fill this need, a rating scale, which describes pertinent behavior in words, may be constructed. In order to reduce error in measurement, the words must be precise so that misinterpretation is avoided. For example, the rating scale on p. 196 should be refined to the point that several nurse-teachers who would look at a learner's behavior could independently classify it at one of the three points with little variation. For those points on which the raters could not agree, the wording probably needs to be clarified. After the scale is refined, individual nurses can use it alone, although as a prerequisite they should know the subject matter well enough to be able to make quickly the observations of behavior required by the rating scale.

It is, of course, possible for an individual to be displaying behavior from two different levels

SAMPLE RATING SCALE

Subobjective: To obtain 1 ml. of aqueous fluid for injection from a 2-ml. vial with a 2-ml. syringe, 22-gauge needle, using sterile technique.

●	●	●
Consistently uses contaminated syringe, needle, or top of vial. Cannot push needle diaphragm. Is rarely aware that she is erring and if so usually does not know how to correct the error.	Occasionally contaminates. Can push needle through diaphragm. Has difficulty withdrawing all the fluid and obtaining accurate measurement (within 0.1 ml.). Can usually diagnose her errors while doing the procedure and correct them.	Rarely contaminates. Can obtain last few drops out of vial without damaging needle. Can measure within 0.1 ml. even if bubbles present. Can change needle or syringe if defective or contaminated. If makes error corrects it by herself.

(Other scales would be developed for other subobjectives of the skill of giving an injection.)

of functioning (see descriptions of behavior in sample rating scale): for example, he may contaminate the syringe and needle fairly often (lowest level) but be quite skilled at removing bubbles from the syringe and measuring accurately (highest level). Usually, the behaviors will at least be at adjacent levels on the rating scale, since these skills involve comparable levels of coordination. The difference may be that the learner is careless about contaminating. Checks can be made beside individual statements at various levels of the description, so that the teacher does not lose information about the learner's performance by just checking one of the categories on the line. Another alternative is construction of several scales for this particular subobjective, each dealing with one set of behaviors—maintenance of sterility, obtaining and measuring of fluid, handling of errors. Space is usually left below each rating scale for comments, but a well-developed scale will include all pertinent points and will rarely require extra written comments. In fact, this kind of form is developed to prevent having to record behavior by writing it out in great length.

There are other factors in the construction of a rating scale, besides preciseness of the descriptions, that contribute to its quality as a measuring instrument. The number of levels of achievement represented in the behavior descriptions is one of them. In the sample scale above, three steps have been used since it is difficult for an observer to discriminate between any more than five levels of achievement. Four or five steps could have been used. Note that the kinds of behaviors described in the scale are those that are crucial to the success of the skill as described in the objective—asepsis, accuracy of measurement, ability to perceive and correct one's own errors. Concerns such as whether the needle goes precisely through the center of the rubber stopper or the particular manner in which the syringe is grasped are not considered to be crucial.

The rating scale is designed to summarize a series of trials, for instance, trials in practice sessions in learning to obtain fluid for injection. It also has the advantage of describing levels of attainment of the goal so that the teacher and learner know what improvements need to be made.

An instrument closely related to the rating scale is the checklist. Crucial steps are chosen; in the example given, remember that other sub-objectives would deal with other behaviors crucial to giving an injection. Directions for using a checklist should indicate that a check or a letter means that the step was either done or not done and, if done, was satisfactory or unsatisfactory. The following is an example of a checklist that could be used in lieu of the sample rating scale given on the opposite page:

☐ Scrubbed top of vial with disinfectant sponge.
☐ Punctured rubber vial with needle, without contaminating.
☐ Withdrew all of fluid from vial.
☐ Expelled excess air from syringe without losing fluid.
☐ Measured fluid to within 0.1 ml. of the correct dose.

To determine progress in learning the skill, checking may be done periodically. Since the checking is done as the skill is performed, there is less likelihood of error in trying to summarize several trials. Learner and teacher can see in which steps errors occur, particularly if successive ratings show which errors are consistent.

With either a rating scale or a checklist, some decision has to be made about what is an acceptable level of performance. In order to give an injection by himself, the learner should have reached the top performance level, whereas the second level is sufficient if he will have supervision. In terms of the checklist, the individual should consistently be performing all steps satisfactorily in order to function independently and perhaps fewer of the steps if competent supervision will be given.

Anecdotal notes

Other behaviors do not lend themselves as easily to the kind of preset description found in the rating scale, particularly behaviors expressing attitudes, in which the context is often important to interpretation. A more useful form for recording such behaviors is, perhaps, the anecdotal note.

This technique consists of recording pertinent behavior described in objective terms and comparing anecdotes over a period of time, noting change or lack of it. Again, far too much time and effort are needed to record all kinds of behavior; what is considered pertinent behavior is that which is related to the objective. For the objective in the sample anecdotal notes on p. 198, notes about what the patient knew about toothbrushing or what he told his roommate about the time that breakfast is served are not likely to be pertinent. His explanation to the roommate as to why he was in the hospital may have relevance if it expressed feelings regarding his illness, his treatment, or his physician. It can be seen that the third anecdote contains material that is not objective. The expressions "cocky," "like a banty rooster," "bragged," are definitely colored with the nurse's feelings toward this patient, preventing others who read the reports from drawing their own conclusions. In addition, the wife's response during this situation, which is most important to an assessment of what may be contributing to the behavior, is omitted.

The only interpretation that might be made on the basis of these three notes in the sample is that Mr. Jones is not accepting activity and smoking restrictions and that in particular circumstances his feelings seem to have been stronger than in others. These notes and others may serve as a baseline against which to compare behavior as teaching is occurring. Anecdotes like those in the sample anecdotal notes do appear on patients' charts, but not consistently, particularly if the learning objective is not clearly defined. They also tend to be scattered among the daily notes and thus are difficult to find. It would seem wise to collect notes specific to teaching-learning on a special form

SAMPLE ANECDOTAL NOTES

Subobjective: To accept the restrictions on activity and smoking.

January 19, 1965, 1:30 P.M. Patient: James Jones
    Diagnosis: Myocardial infarction
    Recorded by: S. Smith, L.P.N.
    Found Mr. Jones in his room leaning over the bed to get urinal out of bedside stand. I asked him
      why he was doing that since he was supposed to be on absolute bedrest. He stated, ''Dr. won't
      let me have cigarettes, so I didn't see why I should lie still for him.'' I said, ''But you're
      making such good progress and rest is essential for that.'' Pt. turned head and looked at wall.
      He did not answer when I called his name three times. I left the room.
January 21, A.M. Patient: James Jones
    Recorded by: M. Jones, R.N.
    When I was giving bath, patient said he hoped Dr. would come in soon so he could discuss with
      him why he could not smoke.
January 21, 4 P.M. Patient: James Jones
    Recorded by: M. Jones, R.N.
    Pt.'s wife came to visit. He seemed very cocky with her—like a banty rooster.
      Bragged that he was going to tell the Dr. off because he wasn't going to be confined to bed and
      be told he couldn't smoke.

---

that would outline the entire teacher-learning plan. In order to obtain more valid measurement of learning, an effort must be made to collect notes regularly and to write them within an hour or so after the events occur. The records may be reviewed periodically to determine progress and plan teaching tactics. As with other evaluation techniques, measurements are continued until the goal is reached or until it appears that the behavior is static over a period of several observations. Then a reassessment of the goal should take place.

It is fortunate that the nurse usually deals with individuals or with small groups of learners, for observation procedures using the rating scale, checklist, or anecdotal notes are expensive in time. Full attention is usually required to observe one learner at a time, and the opportunities for observing cannot always be made to occur at the nurse's convenience. For example, whereas a patient can be asked to demonstrate a motor skill almost any time, interaction with his family can be seen only when they are present.

As these methods of observation are used to collect data, interpretation of the data begins.

Evidence of behavior change

It is very easy for nurses to err in their thinking about what evidence is necessary to indicate that a behavior change (learning) has occurred. For example, in teaching coughing, turning, and deep breathing to a surgical patient, the nurse may have as a criterion absence of complications, which is too all encompassing. There are many other factors that contribute to development of atelectasis besides the patient's failure to do the prescribed exercises. Similarly, an objective for a patient to follow an ulcer diet cannot be evaluated by whether or not he has a recurrence of the ulcers. If a decreased absentee rate is used as a criterion of successful health teaching in an industrial nursing situation, evidence must be present that the decreased rate was due to the teaching and not to other factors, such as change in administrative policy about absences. Too many other factors affect these criteria to make them the sole measures of the effectiveness of teaching and learning unless elaborate measures are taken to control or account for other factors that could be causing the behavior change. Evaluations of learning with such controls could become experimental studies. However, practicing nurses are usually not equipped to do such studies; therefore, they gather together as many clues as possible and proceed. In the example previously given, the practicing nurse would note that the atelectasis had occurred, review the available medical evidence about what had caused it, and on this basis perhaps decide to review with the nursing staff and patient how the coughing, turning, deep breathing, and patient teaching for it had been carried out.

The evidence is most supportive of teaching effect when the behavior occurs close in time to the teaching action or when the intervention seems to be the major change in the situation. For example, nurses caring for patients with cardiac disease noticed rises of as much as 20 points in both systolic and diastolic blood pressures whenever the patients' wives showed unhappiness or apprehension during visits. The nurses began to ask the wives to stop to see them before they visited their husbands. Then, within the limits set by the physician, the nurse discussed with the wife the patient's condition, his progress, his diet, his medications, and so forth. In some cases the nurses believed that the wife's apprehension was so obvious that they asked the physician to talk with her before she saw her husband. The nurses supported the success of his teaching intervention with the observation that there were fewer sudden rises in blood pressure during wives' visits, fewer phone calls from family members trying to contact the physician to check on a patient's condition, and less uneasiness on the part of the patients' wives when they came to visit.[36]

Even more lax than the nurse who errs in determining the criteria of learning is the one who uses a pamphlet as the major means of teaching and evaluates the learning only by asking the patient whether or not he has read the pamphlet. Similar comments can be made about the criterion of the number of patients attending teaching sessions. This kind of criterion is often cited as evaluative of teaching programs, and, although it may indicate valuable interest in the program, it may not be an accurate indicator of the learning that is occurring. Superficiality of evaluation became evident during a study of ambulatory elderly patients.[29] Nurses or physicians were found to be asking patients whether or not they understood explanations. It appeared that some patients were saying they understood in order to avoid hurting the physician's or nurse's feelings. The patients then departed in ignorance, having learned almost nothing.[29]

Not only do patients sometimes give false information, but health practitioners are unable to judge whether a private behavior is occurring even as they gain familiarity with the patient. In one study, which generally reflects the results from others, the relationship between stated (by the patient) medication intake and actual intake was 0.42, and the relationship between the physicians' judgments and actual intake was 0.48. The degree of error both in patients' reports and in physicians' judgments about their patients can be large.[26]

The nurse must also be wary of statements that imply that considerable behavior change has taken place, with no supporting evidence presented. The following quotations are examples. In one situation, sex education classes were said to be successful because "gone were the giggly innuendoes and street-corner terms. Instead, there was a new respectfulness and frankness. . . ."[28] A report on teaching preparation for open heart surgery stated that:

. . . our patients had a better understanding of what was about to happen to them. They felt closer to their physician and were therefore less fearful and anxious about the actions of hospital personnel. Because the patients and their families were encouraged to partic-ipate in the nursing care, they cooperated well and seemed to feel personal satisfaction in the patient's achievements leading to recovery. . . . The patients felt more like individuals and felt that the nursing staff was highly interested in them. . . . There were fewer postoperative complications. The nurses, in turn, showed more interest in, and empathy for, these patients.*

These reports indicate a lack of evidence to support the conclusions made. Sometimes such statements are made because either the absence of learning objectives or the presence of unreal-istic ones leads to confusion about what out-comes should occur. The resulting lack of di-rection greatly handicaps whatever efforts are made toward evaluation.

Other examples from the nursing literature do show more relevance in the relationship be-tween the learning goal and the criteria of be-havior change. Criteria for learning to be a patient with cardiac disease are that the patient does fewer things for himself during the acute phase of his illness and that he makes fewer expressions of inadequacy. Although a little more difficult to measure, the goal of under-standing of the physiologic process of the cause of pain after a myocardial infarction is that the patient show less apprehension when he has pain.[22]

A study was made of a preoperative teaching program for children who were to have eye, nose, or throat surgery. The criterion used to evaluate the teaching was how relaxed the chil-dren were as they entered the operating room. This study showed that before the teaching pro-gram, an estimated 25% to 34% of them were in unsatisfactory condition; after the teaching pro-gram 96.6% were either asleep or well relaxed.[2] Results such as these are exciting, but they

would become even more useful if the other factors that could have caused the change had been considered. In this particular study, these could have included differences in the timing or kinds of medications given preoperatively and differences in the way that the staff interacted with patients, possibly brought on by the staff's knowing that the study was occurring. It also would be necessary to know on what basis de-gree of relaxation and degree of anxiety were determined and whether or not the observers making these judgments knew of the teaching program. Also, more than three or four patients should have been studied. All these factors can present bias and taken together can greatly limit the certainty that it was the teaching program that really made the difference.

Oral questioning

Oral questioning is a very flexible form of measurement and often is used in combination with other techniques, such as observation. It attempts to get at those behaviors that cannot be easily observed, such as whether or not the pa-tient understands the bases for his action in per-forming a psychomotor skill. It also allows construction of hypothetic situations that are not present in the actual teaching environment. Examples of these practices include asking a person learning to irrigate his colostomy stoma why he is preparing the equipment as he is or asking a mother what she would do if her baby turned blue, which may include a demonstra-tion of resuscitation techniques.

The method of oral questioning can be ex-pensive in time, particularly if done in a one-to-one teacher-student relationship, but its strength over written testing is that the teacher knows immediately whether or not the learner under-stands the question and can let the learner know immediately whether or not he gave the right answer. In a group teaching situation, this kind of direct interchange is limited, although the reaction of one learner to another's answer can be very educational. In large groups the ad-

---

*Varvaro, F. F.: Teaching the patient about open heart surgery, Am. J. Nurs. **65:**111-115, Oct. 1965.

vantages of oral questioning are somewhat lost since not every individual is able to respond to an oral question unless he does so in writing.

The verbal nature of both oral and written questioning may handicap those individuals who have difficulty expressing themselves, although it is more likely that people will find it easier to express themselves orally than in writing; or the individual who is verbally quite facile may seem to know more than he actually does. For these reasons combinations of methods such as observation of behavior and oral questioning can often provide a truer picture than can a single method.

It is a common misconception that oral questioning is a method that does not require much preparation on the part of the teacher. This is not true. Questions must be very carefully phrased so that the learner can understand them and so that they test the objective. With knowledge of the individual's prior exposure to an idea, questions can be phrased to stimulate thinking at any level of the cognitive domain. On p. 202 are sample objectives taken from Chapter 4 and questions that should test various levels of thinking.

A series of questions is often needed to encourage the learner to do the entire evaluation task (see boxed material on p. 202). An example of this is the question on safety (testing application). At other times the learner may not remember the entire question or may just need the continued interest of the teacher to complete the answer. If the patient who designed an ileostomy bag talked only about how he had designed the appliance so that it had a better seal, the nurse might prompt him to suggest its characteristics with regard to cost, odor control, and strength of the bag, all of which are important to an adequate ileostomy appliance. Additional questioning may also serve the purpose of determining the extent of an individual's knowledge. After the mother has correctly answered the question about the effect of worry on breast milk, she might then be asked, "Does

this mean that this mother should not allow herself to become angry?" Such a question requires a higher level of thinking than the level of knowledge.

Any question, whether written or oral, can be stated in such a vague manner that the learner does not know what the teacher wants and becomes frustrated trying to guess. An example of a vague question is "How do you take care of Jimmy?" It is not clear whether this question refers to who takes care of Jimmy, how his mother manages to care for him, or what theories of child rearing she believes are useful. A clearly stated, broad question, such as "What do you think is the most important thing to do in caring for a child?" does serve the purpose of obtaining general attitudes and values. Some less-educated or less-motivated people would find it difficult to answer this broad and abstract a question. They respond best to specific questions about concrete items: "What do you do when Jimmy uses words you don't like?" It is only the more mentally facile individual who can assess his thoughts about the many areas of child care, summarize them, and state them.

Tact must be used in presenting questions. People do not like to feel that they are being grilled, and there is likely to be a lack of acceptance of the traditional teacher-in-authority role that may be acceptable in formal classroom situations in a school. This does not mean that evaluation should not be done with patients who seem resistant and somewhat forbidding to a young nurse. It can be done in subtle ways, such as by noticing questions or comments that arise naturally during a discussion or by observing a motor skill when it is practiced. For example, a woman discussing a booklet she was to have read on breast self-examination may say to other learners or to the nurse, "I don't see why it's necessary to look at the breasts besides feeling them." Such a comment may indicate an emotional rejection of observing the breasts; it may mean that this point was not explained in the booklet; or it may be that it was explained

SAMPLE OBJECTIVES AND ORAL QUESTIONS FOR EVALUATION

Objectives	Questions
To state what effect worry in the mother may have on her breast milk (level of knowledge).	"What effect can worry have on a mother's breast milk?" (This question presumes that the learner has read or been told of this relationship.)
To translate instructions for time and route on a medicine bottle into appropriate action (level of comprehension).	Present to the learner several medicine bottles with directions for time and route different from those on his own bottles. "How and when does the physician want these taken?"
Given general knowledge of safety, to plan how to rid a house of safety hazards (level of application).	"How would you make your kitchen safer?" Repeat the question for bathroom and other rooms, being certain that areas covered include fire safety, electrical hazards, safety from poisons, safety from falling.
To distinguish how a quack's argument differs from scientific reasoning (level of analysis).	This can be analysis only if the individual has not been told or has not discussed the difference. If he has, he will probably be repeating thoughts that are not the product of his own mind and would be at the level of knowledge or comprehension. Several examples of quack and scientific reasoning may be given to him and the learner asked to state differences based on those samples.
To design an ileostomy bag that suits one's needs better than do available commercial ones (level of synthesis).	"For what reasons did you design the bag this way?" This would be combined with observation of the bag.
To assess the health care one is receiving in terms of its completeness, one's satisfaction with it, and the results obtained (level of evaluation).	"What quality of care would you say you have received? Consider its completeness, your satisfaction with it, and the results that have occurred."

and forgotten or not clearly understood. The nurse-teacher should know what was stated in the book and should do further observing and questioning.

In addition, questions need to be carefully phrased to avoid cluing the patient to the socially desirable answer or "the answer" the nurse wants, which may be an inappropriate reiteration of what the nurse has told them.

There are times when drill on those facts that

an individual is learning helps him to learn and remember them. However, one should beware of pat answers on the patient's exact replication of words he has heard, since this may indicate lack of sufficient comprehension to express the idea in alternative ways. It is difficult to know when a learner is responding with a socially desirable answer to which he has no commitment; the following question attempts to reduce this possibility: "Some mothers like to prop the bottle up on a pillow and feed the baby that

---

ISOLATION CARE*

Your doctor has requested that you be cared for in isolation. The main principles of isolation are to avoid introducing any new micro-organisms to you and to prevent the spread of that micro-organism which caused you to be ill.

Isolation care is carried out for several reasons, some of which are:

1. Your doctor may be evaluating your illness with several possible diagnoses in mind. Until he positively determines the cause of your illness he may request that special precautions be taken in your care.
2. When ill you are significantly more susceptible to other illnesses because your resistance is low. For this reason, those who take care of you will assume additional precautions to avoid subjecting you to unnecessary exposure.
3. Your illness may be transmitted to others. Isolation can avoid this possibility.
4. Depending upon your diagnosis, certain city and state public health regulations can make it necessary to place you in isolation.

We know that various micro-organisms, such as bacteria and viruses, can cause different types of illnesses. We also know that various types of micro-organisms enter and leave the body in various ways. Therefore, the precautions taken for isolated persons vary. In some instances the nurse will wear both mask and gown while coming in close contact with you. Some suspected or confirmed communicable diseases require the nurse to use the gown only.

It may be necessary to use precautions in handling the dishes and equipment used in your care. Your nurse will explain this to you on the basis of your diagnosis.

We want to protect your visitors from possible exposure, too. They will wear a gown and/or mask just as your nurse does. Your visitors should refrain from handling things in your room and from kissing you.

Your nurse will further explain your care in isolation. Thank you for your cooperation.

---

*University Hospital: Information to patients (isolation care), University of Washington, Seattle.

way, and others like to hold them when they feed them. Which do you find works best for you?''[30]

Written measurement

Written measurement is indirect and demands at least some reading skill and knowledge of how to take tests on the part of the learner. It offers a marvelous opportunity to measure learning at all levels of the cognitive domain with considerable efficiency of teacher time, after the items are once constructed by the teacher. Written tests seem most appropriate in teaching situations in which the learners are well, since solitary concentration for a certain length of time is required.

General considerations

Tests are prepared by individuals or groups of teachers in a particular institution and used within that institution, or they may be developed by test experts and sold. Those sold commercially should provide a manual with information about the purposes for which the test was designed and evidence that it accurately measures the goals that it claims to measure. This evidence includes information about how well the test covers the subject matter; for example, if it is meant to test knowledge of nutrition, does it include items on all the major concepts in nutrition today? This quality of a test is called content validity. There also should be information about how well the test score is related to actual patient behavior in the present (concurrent validity) or the future (predictive validity). For example, if a diabetic patient scores high on the test, how likely is he to be giving good self-care now and in the future? A similar kind of statement about future self-care would be needed for those doing less well on the test. If a test contains a high degree of validity, its value for decision making is greater than if validity were present to a lesser degree.

It is very rare that tests developed locally by teachers are this adequately studied. The teachers who use their own tests gain, if they have continuing contact with the same patients, a feeling for how closely the test relates to their patients' actual behavior, but they very rarely perform studies that provide them with accurate information of this kind. Standardized tests must be general in order to sell in sufficient numbers; therefore, they are not likely to fulfill all the needs for evaluation. Those tests commercially available in the health area at present primarily test comprehension of general health and hygiene topics.[5,6] As the availability of commercially produced tests increases, nurse-teachers will need to scrutinize particular tests to see whether or not they are of good quality and then to fit them into evaluation programs, continuing to design their own tools when others are not available or adequate. This may only require nurse-teachers to supplement commercial tests with a few questions of their own dealing with local practices or other special content.

Nationally distributed tests can have a very beneficial effect in decreasing unnecessary parochialism. It is easier to teach a patient how something is done in the institution where he receives care than it is to teach him by broad principles that will help him to transfer knowledge to other institutions and situations. Examining the content of a national test can help the nurse see limitations in the nurse's own objectives through review of what others expect their learners to be able to do.

Both so-called objective questions—multiple-choice, true-false, and matching items—and essay questions have their place in measuring health learning. Essay writing requires considerable skill in organizing and expressing ideas, which is more appropriate in a school situation than with most patients. Thus, such questions to patients are usually shortened and made more specific; they can then be asked in either oral or written form. An example is "What should be done if your child eats poison, and why should it be done?" Note that this question, whether oral or written, requires recall of information. This is a different behavior from discrimination between answers that are already present, as in multiple-choice, true-false, and matching items. Ability to recall is desirable for information used frequently and essential for emergency situations, such as what to do in case of child poisoning or how to recognize and deal with diabetic coma or seizures. Since the objective is for the person to act on the information, he must be able to produce it from his memory, not just recognize it from among several alternatives. Periodic self-testing of memory for specific information will strengthen retention of infrequently used material. The strength of the recognition item is that it can require the learner to discriminate between ideas, some of which he might not otherwise consider, thus helping to test his depth of understanding.

As in the box above, items can be written to test all levels of cognitive behavior. Since the

Test items on various levels of the cognitive domain

Knowledge   T F The hospital is required by law to use isolation with certain diagnoses.

Comprehension T F A patient will not be retained in isolation after a diagnosis is made.

Application   Isolation is a means of containing the spread of microorganisms. How can these methods be used with a person at home who has a cold?

Analysis   The basic principle(s) of our society that relate(s) to the reason isolation is used is (are):
a. Certain institutions have the right to carry out certain functions for the society.
b. An individual has certain rights.
c. The majority rules.
d. *a* and *b*.
e. *a, b, c*.

Synthesis   Suggest a set of rules for isolation that will maximize the well-being of staff, visitors, and patients.

Evaluation   It seems necessary to isolate persons with communicable disease to varying extents in order to protect others from the disease. Which one of the following policies would best achieve protection of the public and the welfare of the ill individual?
a. After diagnosis allow the individual and family a choice between hospital care and being restricted to home.
b. Have a team of health personnel to enforce the proper degree of isolation in a hospital and the reporting of communicable disease.
c. Allow individual physicians and health agencies considerable latitude in establishing such policies.
(NOTE: The answer must not be in terms of opinion but must show evidence of judgment in terms of particular criteria, such as safety and psychologic and sociologic well-being.)

level measured by a particular question depends on what information the learner has received, written material on which the questions are based is first given. It can easily be seen in the boxed material that the information in the pamphlet about isolation care is aimed only at knowledge and comprehension. From the level of application up, the questions require increasingly more information than was given in the explanation. These questions are presented in the illustration only as examples of questions that might be given to test learning on higher levels. It is not necessary for the patient to reach these higher levels of thinking for subjects such as isolation, in which the patient does not function independently. However, some patients may function at this level because their general level of knowledge and thinking is this high, but these objectives are not common. For home hemodialysis, in which the patient and his family function much more independently, objectives requiring more complex levels of thinking are more common.

The true-false item form is most adaptable

for testing knowledge or comprehension. The multiple-choice form is more flexible and can be used at all levels. Since synthesis requires independent thought, it is more likely to be tested by methods in which no suggested answers are given. At all levels, visual materials can be incorporated into written questions, for example, showing a mother four photos of umbilical cords and asking her to indicate which need(s) to be called to the attention of the physician or which will likely drop off soonest.

Item construction

There are numerous errors in the construction of single items and groups of items that can prevent a true assessment of an individual's knowledge. The skills required to construct written tests are complex. Without additional training, many nurse-teachers will not become accomplished in construction, but they should learn to avoid at least obvious errors. The points considered for making oral questions specific and understandable by learners hold as well for written questions. A good way to test whether these criteria have been attained with written (essay) and oral questions is to outline a suggested answer. Frequently, ambiguities that are not otherwise evident will be uncovered. For all items the final test is trying them out on learners to discover how they interpret the items.

An error to avoid is the testing of trivia or of irrelevant material. Consider the nurse who shows a film in conjunction with baby care classes. The following questions are irrelevant to the objectives of most baby care classes:

1. The name of the movie you saw about your baby's bath was
   a. "Your Baby's Bath"
   b. "Bathing Baby"
   c. "Morning Adventure"
   d. "Mother Loves Baby"
2. The company that sponsored the movie you saw was
   a. Pet Milk Company
   b. Carnation Milk Company
   c. Curity Diapers
   d. Foremost Milk Company

Examples of trivia would be asking the size of the room in which the bath was given or whether the nurse held the washcloth in the right hand or left hand during the demonstration. Notice that triviality and irrelevance are so defined in terms of the learning objectives.

Clues in the language of the item give away the correct answer to someone who is test wise. The following example, based on the pamphlet explaining isolation care, suffers from one clue—the exact same terminology as that used in the teaching presentation:

T F   Your illness may be transmitted to others.

In such a case the individual learns to recognize the words without necessarily knowing what they mean. A similar clue occurs in the previously stated question 1, in which the correct answer occurs in the lead-in phrase before the choices (the "stem"). There are also grammatical clues, as when a singular verb is used in the stem, making several of the choices in a multiple-choice question grammatically incorrect. Following is an example using a plural verb:

3. Areas under the scalp where bone has not yet filled are known as
   a. Meconium
   b. An umbilicus
   c. Fontanels
   d. All of the above

The following matching item illustrates several problems with clues, ambiguity, and vocabulary level:

Directions: Match the body part with the action that best describes how to wash it.

Body part	Washing action
____ 4. Vulva	a. With a pointed object
____ 5. Neck	b. With a soft washcloth
____ 6. Soft spot	c. Vigorously but gently
____ 7. Ear	d. With a twisted piece of cotton

Mothers may not know the term *vulva* unless it has been specifically introduced to them. Some learners would eliminate choice *a* since they would know that one never washes the body with pointed objects. The fact that choice *a* is so much easier an item than the others makes it less plausible—a clue. This does not mean that the idea is not important to test, but it probably should be made into a separate item. The directions indicate that a single choice is better than any other; however, more than one of the washing actions given are equally good for several of the body parts. If the correct answer is not clear-cut to the teacher, the question will probably be ambiguous and frustrating to the learners; therefore, the teacher should try to clarify it. This is true with any item form. Such ambiguity is particularly difficult to avoid when the difference of opinion as to what is correct is cultural:

T F   Meat should be eaten once a day.

True-false items are notorious for having clues and may also be ambiguous. Statements containing absolute terms such as *all, always, certainly,* and *entirely* are much more likely to be false than true. Statements with words that qualify, such as *generally, sometimes, as a rule,* or *may,* are much more likely to be true than false.[7] An example of a qualified statement is as follows:

8. T F   Cords generally become detached from the body between the fifth and eighth days after birth.

Some qualifier must be used in order to make this item clearly true or false; in this case another kind of item, such as a multiple-choice question, might be better to use. Question 8 can be stated to foil attempts at taking advantage of clues; "tenth and fourteenth days" can be substituted for "fifth and eighth days." Uncertainty about the correct answer ensues when part of a question is true and part of it false, as in the following example:

9. T F   The umbilical cord may be swabbed with alcohol in order to dry it and sterilize it.

Direction should be clear that, if any part of the item is false, the item should be marked false.

For all kinds of items, the best distractors (incorrect choices) are misconceptions that are common among learners. It is easy to get an idea of what these misconceptions are by listening to patients talk among themselves, with visitors, or with nurses or by watching them perform certain skills. Following is an example:

10. T F   The soft spot should not be touched when giving the baby a bath.

Remember that because of the differences in training and sometimes in cultural background, learners' incorrect ideas are not the same as nurses' would be.

In construction of a test, the goal is to produce items that will provide true information about what the learner knows. Clues and implausible distractors help the learner to get the correct answer by guessing; this makes the individual appear to know more than he does. On the other hand, ambiguity makes it difficult for the learner to demonstrate the knowledge that he actually has. Testing of trivia may be reliable in providing information, but it is about unimportant learning. Thus, these errors are to be avoided.

For adequate testing of a set of objectives, a number of items are grouped, and various kinds of measurements are used. A plan for the kinds of items and tools needed is made before their selection or construction. A major objective for instruction about a baby bath might be as follows: to cleanse the baby safely. First of all, much of the evaluation of learning in this situation should be done by observation of the mother's motor skills. For cognitive skills a group of written items may be collected. Consider the previously stated items 1 through 10 as a test of the basic cognitive aspects necessary for meeting this major objective. There are large areas of content that are left untested, such as correct temperature of the water, reasons for

TOOL FOR MEASURING MOTHERS' INTENDED
ACTIONS FOR CHILDHOOD SYMPTOMS*

Vignettes of symptoms and situations "What would you do if?"

1. Your child has had signs of a cold during the day but now is breathing very rapidly and with difficulty?
2. Your child ate some rat poison?
3. Your child fell off the steps onto his (her) head and began vomiting about an hour later?
4. Your child begins to cough?
5. You were polishing a table and your child took the bottle of polish and drank part of it?
6. Your baby ate two cigarette stubs from an ash tray?
7. Your child played outdoors all afternoon and now he complains of a pain in his foot?
8. Your child cries every time he (or she) passes urine?
9. Your child is having a convulsion (fit) that has lasted more than 5 minutes?
10. Both of your child's eyes are watery and red and his (or her) nose is running with thin mucus?
11. Your 2-month old baby has been crying steadily between 6:00 P.M. and 10 P.M.?
12. Your baby just lies flat; he (or she) seems too weak to lift his head?
13. Your child had a convulsion (fit) that lasted 5 minutes?
14. Your child who is not old enough to go to school has a hoarse voice and a cough?
15. At suppertime, when your baby is usually wide-awake, you notice that he (or she) is very tired and drowsy?
16. Your child has sneezed several times during the afternoon; at bedtime he sneezed again?
17. Your child has a cough and also complains of pains in chest?
18. Your child fell on the playground and came home with a bump on his forehead (1 inch across)?
19. Your child swallows a nickel?
20. Your child vomits her (or his) breakfast before going to school?
21. Your baby eats half of a bottle of baby aspirin?
22. Your baby has been crying more than usual and has begun to wet its diaper several times every hour?
23. Your child is stung by a bee?
24. Your baby has dirtied 8 diapers with bowel movements between breakfast time and suppertime?
25. Your baby has not wanted to play all during the day?
26. Your baby, who usually spits up a little bit, vomited most of his evening feeding with great force?
27. The urine that your child has just passed in the toilet bowl is quite red?
28. Your child's eye is red and the eyelid is swollen?
29. Your child has hot dry skin (if you take its temperature, the thermometer reads 101.5)?
30. Your school child tells you that it hurt when he moved his bowels and that there was blood and phlegm on the toilet paper when he wiped himself?
31. At bedtime you realize that your baby has not had a bowel movement since yesterday morning?
32. For no apparent reason your baby does not seem hungry for solid food or for his evening bottle?
33. Your child's knee has become red, swollen, and so painful that he (or she) does not want to walk?
34. Your child has a rash (that you have never seen before) on her face and chest?

*From Stine, O. C., and Chuaqui, C.: Mothers' intended actions for childhood symptoms, Am. J. Public Health **59:**2035-2045, 1969.

TOOL FOR MEASURING MOTHERS' INTENDED
ACTIONS FOR CHILDHOOD SYMPTOMS*—cont'd

35. Your boy is crying because he wants to void (pee) but the urine won't come out?
36. Your child plays at the playground until suppertime when he complains of feeling tired and hot (if you take his temperature, [the thermometer] reads 103)?
37. After eating only part of his supper, your child complains of pains in his stomach?
38. Your child has been crying, held his (or her) breath, and then "fell out"?

Precoded answers to "What would you do if?"

1. Take the child to the doctor as quickly as possible.
2. Call the doctor to see the child at home.
3. Telephone the doctor to ask his advice.
4. Take the child to the doctor the next day.
5. Ask a neighbor or relative for advice.
6. Ask the druggist for medicine.
7. Try aspirin or another medicine that you have in the house.
8. Put the child to bed until he or she is better.
9. Keep the child in the house.
10. Do nothing.

---

care of the eyes and the genitals, and many more. All the questions test at the level of knowledge or comprehension. Subobjectives would be defined in the learning plan and would indicate more specific behaviors, but it is quite likely that testing at the levels of knowledge and comprehension would be sufficient to evaluate learning. Again, careful definition of goals is essential to teaching but must be supplemented with other skills.

Measurement of attitudes by written test differs from measurement of cognitive skills in that there are no right answers, only desired attitudes. Usually measurement is taken through a series of statements designed to elicit expression of the degree of acceptance of the attitude. This may be on a scale from "strongly agree" to "strongly disagree" or on a scale of how many people are characterized by particular behaviors or thoughts. Following is an example of an item that might be answered on the former scale:

Illness isolates a person.

•   •   •   •   •

Strongly   Disagree   Uncertain   Agree   Strongly
disagree   agree

A number of such items would be used in an attempt to elicit expression of feeling about dependence, for example, or about a group of attitudes common to illness. The person who develops such a tool and interprets results must know a considerable amount about attitudes and how they are exhibited. This is particularly true since attitude scales are easily faked, and persons with the same attitudes will manifest different behaviors. Because of the skill needed and the limitations of this method, usually only standardized tests are used and then combined with other behavior observations. Because of the recent concern about the level of relationship between attitudes and behavior, perhaps direct measurement of behavior is a more useful approach when behavior change is the goal.

Sample test

Instruments for assessing patient knowledge and evaluating their learning after an instructional program are rarely reported in the literature. This is unfortunate because it is through such tools that one probably obtains the clearest notion of objectives and standards of outcome in patient education. Moreover, without tools, it is probably reasonable to assume that needed evaluation will not be done. The box on pp. 208 and 209 contains an example of what seems to be a useful tool, even though its measurement characteristics were not reported as being highly developed. The subject matter of the tool is, of course, important as one component, although not always the decisive one, of successful health care.

EVALUATING THE TEACHING-LEARNING PROCESS

Measurement is carried out so that evaluation of the teaching-learning process can be done more accurately than it would be by using general impressions. Evaluation must go beyond measurement in that it involves making a value judgment about learning and teaching. This involves summarizing the evidence and determining to what degree the objectives are being met.

Measurement and evaluation occur continuously as teaching is done, thus serving to redirect activities of the teacher and learner. Information about how learners are progressing is gathered by having them respond to questions or perform periodically or both. The expressions on learners' faces—of boredom or interest, confusion or enlightenment—are clues to whether they understand what is being taught. For example, a class of parents may look confused after the inheritance patterns of mongolism have been explained, or Mrs. Smith may be unable to fold her baby's diapers after a demonstration. Some individuals can tell the teacher what they do not understand; others cannot identify or express their uncertainty. Retracing of the explanation or skill demonstra-

tion, interspersed with questions or performance of the skill by the students, will help to identify what is not clear. This technique may point up terms used by the teacher that the learners did not understand. It may also suggest that Mrs. Smith was so confused with being taught three different methods of folding diapers that she could not distinguish one from the other. Trying to reteach without determining the nature of the learning problem prevents the nurse from knowing how to avoid making the same error again. It is unwise to teach for a very long period of time (even one lesson period) without requiring the learner to respond so that errors can be corrected.

There comes a time when adequacy of learning must be evaluated in terms of meeting the final objectives. Of course, if satisfactory evaluation was done as the teaching was going on, the degree of attainment of final objectives or the time needed to meet them can be quite accurately predicted. Too often what happens when nurses are teaching hospital patients is that there is not much leeway in the time available for teaching, and the entire teaching-learning process, particularly evaluation, gets short shrift. Having only a short time for teaching does impose restrictions, but many nurses seem to assume that because an individual has been taught, he has learned. Do not take this for granted!

Key decisions regarding the patient, such as whether or not he can live alone, revolve around the degree to which the objectives of learning have been attained. The identification of the minimum performance necessary in order for the individual to function is most important. Certain basic knowledge and skills must be learned because they are crucial to performance of a particular task; others may also be crucial, depending on how independently the individual will be functioning. Therefore, what may be an adequate level of performance for one individual may not be sufficient for another.

In measuring, teachers focus on what they

have identified as crucial. In a test the learner should probably be able to answer or perform nearly 94% of all crucial behaviors. This figure allows for some error in the measurement tool. The patient ought to be followed up with questioning and reteaching of those crucial items for which he cannot give a correct response. In giving a written test, the teacher may easily lose sight of the difference between essential learnings and other items. The score may be added up, and, if the learner has passed half the items, he may be considered to have learned adequately. But the question may never be asked: what exactly is it that he knows? Observers of motor skills are more likely to intuitively realize that, if the individual is not placing his crutches in the proper position to his body, he will have difficulty learning to walk with them.

Special plans need to be made to be sure that the series of items that is constructed measures an individual's ability to transfer knowledge and skills beyond the context of the instructional situation to other situations that the objectives describe or suggest. The reason that thorough testing of transfer is necessary is that there is insufficient knowledge about how to produce transfer and to be certain that it has occurred, without careful measurement. Problem areas include how to make sure that initial learning is well enough established to allow for transfer, how to make sure that there is sufficient stimulus variation (a variety of situations and tasks) in the initial learning to produce transfer, and how to determine rapidity with which instruction and difficulty of tasks should move at various stages in the progression of learning.[9]

Suppose that related objectives are as follows: To take diuretic in the prescribed dosage and at the prescribed time. To recognize desired and undesired effects of the medication. To contact the physician when undesired effects occur. Instruction for such objectives would no doubt include information about the purpose of the medication, how to take it and why, pictures and descriptions of desired and undesired effects, and descriptions of situations related to taking the medication correctly. It is not possible and should not be necessary to give instruction about all possible situations an individual will encounter, since, if representative situations are used for teaching, most individuals can transfer information to similar ones. For checking the amount of transfer the patient actually can make, questions should be constructed that deal with those variations from or combinations of themes already presented that represent situations he might encounter. It is possible by a series of such questions to map the areas he does and does not know. Questions that should require transfer (if they have not been used in original instruction) might be as follows:

1. Suppose you have intestinal flu with vomiting and diarrhea for several days. How would this affect the taking of your diuretic?

2. If over a period of 3 days the belts on your clothes feel tighter, what should you do?

3. You are visiting friends for a few days and find that they do not have any citrus fruits. What should you do?

The interpretation of evaluation by teacher and learner is of utmost importance. Learners will have varying degrees of insight into their progress. Rather, allowing for teacher bias, teachers and learners will agree to varying degrees on the amount of progress that has been made. The learner should be asked for his assessment of the progress, and differences and similarities with regard to the teacher's assessment should be discussed. This kind of interchange is likely to help each party, but when differences of opinion persist, the nurse must maintain responsibility. For example, a public health nurse may be teaching a daughter to give bed care to her elderly mother. After several sessions, the daughter believes that she is performing adequately; however, the public health nurse observes that the daughter is careless about keeping side rails up on the hospital bed, provisions for washing the mother's genitals are lacking, regular turning is not being carried out, and the footboard is not being used—all of which have been taught. Whatever the reason, emotional or otherwise, for the daughter's not giving essential care, the nurse is faced with a choice. One alternative is to find the basis for lack of learning and to reteach, weighing the learner's likelihood of changing against the relative adequacy of the care. The other is to suggest that some other arrangements for care be made, since the nurse is responsible for supervision of this care. The learner may become hostile to the nurse, sometimes as a way of expressing a desire to get out of the situation. In contrast, Auerbach speaks of the rewards to the participants in parent education when they find themselves thinking and acting differently and experiencing a new sense of power.[3] Evidence of positive change in the learners is tremendously rewarding for teachers.

Entangled in evaluation is the relationship between learner competence and teacher competence. To some extent this relationship depends on who in it is regarded as more responsible for learning. Sometimes it is obvious that a teacher cannot communicate or does not understand the subject matter, in which case the teacher needs to be helped to develop teaching skill. It must be remembered that teaching has the potential for being harmful as well as ineffective and that there is such a thing as professional incompetence in this area of nursing as in any other. Possible harmful effects include leaving the patient with incapacitating confusion, a loss of self-confidence, and an inability to accomplish necessary reintegration into a family or other social group.

Evaluation of teaching and learning must also be viewed within a perspective of the known limitations of teaching today—particularly in the area of motivation of individuals. At present, knowledge of the determinants of behavior is both limited and fragmented, and a practical means of assessing the relative influence of

each factor is virtually nonexistent. Therefore, in a particular situation it is difficult to estimate the degree to which each factor already present is influencing particular behavior and how new factors might affect it. In many of the complex situations that require learning, reality factors such as poverty, health, and family crisis limit the effect that teaching can have. In such situations, small and not-too-decisive effects are characteristic of even the "good" programs. One solution has been to use several complementary kinds of interventions, of which teaching may be one, in order to maximize the effect. Sometimes nothing seems to have an effect, and the individual or family does not recover from illness or achieve high-level wellness. Explanation may be sought through inquiry into the patient's perceptions, motives, values, intelligence, and grasp of relevant knowledge, or it has been suggested that his situation might reflect a condition such as powerlessness, in which his ability to learn is only one of the behaviors affected. Powerlessness reflects an expectancy that one's own behavior cannot determine the outcomes one seeks. There is presently no baseline, or norm, beyond which one can say with reasonable certainty that powerlessness is a significant factor in determining behavior in a given patient situation, but the concept is intriguing.[20] There may be other such behavioral syndromes, and since learning is a central means by which individuals and groups adapt, it would be likely to commonly be affected. Limitations in our knowledge of factors that affect learning, description of their effects, and predictions that can be made about learning influence the effect teaching programs can have. Although the educational approach involves freedom for participants to accept, adopt, or reject, this approach may allow too much freedom for some objectives that are important to society. Institutional controls, although more difficult to establish, can be more effective in controlling behavior.

Thus evaluation both during and at the conclusion of a segment of teaching-learning is a summation and interpretation of the results of measurement. It serves to reinforce successful behaviors of both learners and teachers. It also provides a time for analysis of lack of progress and for redirection of activities.

Since many teaching programs are aimed at long-term behavior change, it is necessary to do some evaluation at varying time periods after instruction. Although such assessments are necessary, their meaning for the teaching program is clouded by intervening factors in the patient's life that have affected his behavior and memory. An example of such a study was done by a general hospital with patients on its cancer registry who had had colostomies from 6 months to 8 years previously. Some general areas in which patients felt they had been adequately taught did emerge and included preoperative preparation and the technique of irrigations. Other areas—such as what to do about problems of fecal impaction and of delay in return flow and information about services of the American Cancer Society—were believed to have been not so adequately taught.[19]

How is such a study useful to present practice in that hospital? It is one piece of information that is limited because it represents patients' perceptions, which may not correlate highly with their actual performance, and because it represents teaching done at a previous time. It should be checked against studies of the effectiveness of present teaching programs. A similar evaluative survey of the patient teaching program was done in a hospital in suburban Boston. Over a period of 8 months, patients were interviewed about questions they had when leaving the hospital. They commonly requested time to talk with the physician in privacy and at times other than rounds, simple answers with less medical terminology, explanation of what had been done to them and why, explanation of what to expect postoperatively or after treatment (65% of patients said they had not received this), and better communication

between physician and family. A committee of this hospital utilized the information from this evaluative survey by recommending a checklist for discharge instructions, with each topic to be marked by the physician when instruction was given, establishing a discharge office for patient and families to ensure adequate education, developing a list of common patient questions and answers that all physicians agreed to as suitable for distribution, and providing a library of audiovisual and printed materials on health for patient use.[18]

Inevitably, if teaching fails, one faces the same question asked before entering the process of teaching: is the behavior change necessary? The answer is not always clear. Such uncertainty arises, for example, when one asks whether teaching could or should reverse abortion recidivism. In one center, 2 weeks after an abortion the patient was offered contraceptives and an intensive counseling program in abortion and family planning. Generally it was found that the counseling program did not significantly decrease abortions, whereas insertion of an IUD immediately after abortion was well accepted by patients and showed no increase in abortion morbidity. The author presents no evidence about the impact the program had on altering sexual behavior. It is very likely that the immediate insertion was better and that no educational program could alter sexual behavior to a great extent. However, one pertinent question is, are repeat abortions truly a health problem?[27]

Perhaps this question of what is the proper patient behavior is nowhere more unclear than in the affective domain. For parents of disabled children, there is said to be a widespread common-sense ideology of "acceptance" used by both medical personnel and parents. "Gratefulness" and "self-help" are noted to be common themes in the journals, and there seems to be a lack of support for public disagreements with the official morality.[33] One wonders if the cost of "bucking the system" on this implied educational objective is not very high.

PROGRAM EVALUATION

Whether a program is more diffuse or structured, each activity within the program has to be judged for its merit. A program is diffuse when it is part of the service offered and is periodically "pulled out" and looked at. Other more structured programs are carried out as the sole assignment of individuals who have a definite time plan for offering services and a fairly small, identified clientele.

Audit procedures include a look at patient education activity, as do instruments that measure quality of care, allowing an evaluative look at that portion of the care for a particular group of patients, over a whole institution.

The experience of one committee when auditing records of cholecystectomy patients does not seem uncommon. They found the highest deficiency rate in documentation of patient knowledge on discharge. Subsequently, the following criteria for this group of patients were written:

Outcomes—cholecystectomy*

1. Knowledge
   a. Patient verbalizes knowledge of discharge diet as ordered by physician.
   b. Patient verbalizes knowledge about returning to normal activities in 4-6 weeks.
2. Physical status
   a. Ambulates
   b. Afebrile
   c. Wound clean and dry

Both outcome and process criteria are probably needed in evaluation of patient education. In other areas of care, it has been found that outcome and process studies on the same patients do not correlate highly.[4] Sometimes health status at the end of the study period is most dependent on the initial status, with process measure playing little role. The importance of process of care apparently varies for sub-

---

*From Rinaldi, L. A., and Kelly, B.: What to do after the audit is done, Am. J. Nurs. **77:**268-269, 1977.

groups of patients.[25] Because we know so little about what kinds of outcomes are attainable with patient education, process audit can provide some control to the quality of service, even though process can become an end in itself.

Various standards can be used to make the judgment involved in evaluation. There are historical standards, normative standards, absolute, theoretical, negotiated, arbitrary, and perhaps other bases for standards. Health education usually has used historical or normative standards,[14] although there are significant areas of the practice of patient education in which measurement seems to have been so lacking or so primitive that the level of effect historically or across programs is not really known. As the field accumulates more of a body of literature, theoretical standards should be possible.[14] The translation of the mastery concept to patient education could provide one theoretical standard. Green's best estimate of the average success rates of serious health education programs is 50%. This is an impression based on the literature in family planning, nutrition, immunization, cancer screening, dental health, smoking cessation, and primary care utilization studies. Possible reasons for such a level include the fact that community health education is aimed at common motives of the largest number of people and thereby misses the unique motives of many, unless a special effort is made to reach them. Also, studies show that health professionals are more supportive and giving of information to those clients who need it least.[14]

Most new improvements in teaching (as opposed to providing the service where it has not previously been available) have had small effects; it is difficult to obtain large, dramatic effects. There is some evidence, however, that the accumulation of these effects over years can make an impact on a problem if the knowledge can be disseminated to enough people.[34]

Formal evaluation of educational programs is a relatively recent activity. Methodology and conceptual frameworks are still being developed and often have to be individually designed for a project because generalized evaluation designs are lacking. The serious student of program evaluation in education should consult Worthen and Sanders's book, *Educational Evaluation: Theory and Practice.* Actual techniques by which empirical evidence is collected and judged are similar to those used in research. This includes use of experimental design.[20] An additional design, useful when one cannot afford two new programs for comparison groups and when one is concerned about the ethical implications of withholding patient education, is the midcycle switch design.

Experimental group	O	X O		O
Control group	O		O X	O

O = observation, X = treatment.

With random assignment, the design is strengthened.[1]

Times of measurement and interpretation in light of other possible reasons for the effects obtained are important. Fig. 12 provides some examples. Curve A illustrates the error that would be made in underestimating the impact of an educational program if the effect were measured as the difference between O_1 and O_2. This pattern can occur when the audience must go through an attitude change between the educational exposure and the actual change in behavior. Curve B illustrates the overestimation of impact if observations at time 3 were taken as permanent. This backsliding effect is not uncommon with behavioral changes that are complex, such as smoking cessation, diet changes, and complicated medication regimens. Some

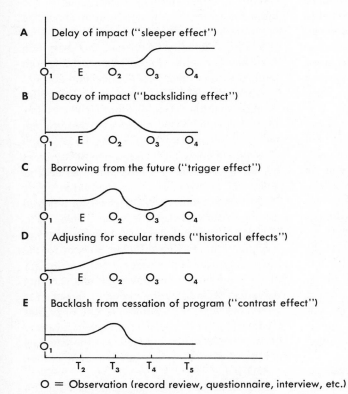

Fig. 12. Points of observation relative to different educational inputs. (From Green, L. W.: Evaluation and measurement; some dilemmas for health education, Am. J. Public Health **67:**155-161, 1977.)

O = Observation (record review, questionnaire, interview, etc.)

E = Educational intervention

educational effects are really only triggers to behavior that would have changed eventually anyhow (curve C). The gains at O_2 may be offset at O_3, so the net long-term gain is zero. This phenomenon is most notable in some mass media campaigns designed to recruit new patients to a screening clinic or a family planning clinic. The gains immediately after the broadcasts turn out to be patients who would have appeared within a few months anyway. Curve D shows why control groups are important: apparent gains or losses may have been occurring anyway, as part of general trends or extraneous events. Finally, curve E shows a relapse that can occur from premature termination of the educational treatment, as in self-care, smoking, or diet programs.[15]

It does not seem likely that formal evaluation will be common in patient education programs for some time; there are few people trained to do such evaluation, and the field of patient education is not well established. What appears to be essential are some standards for evaluation that are adequate enough to support the practice of a particular program—and are always done in a more or less formal, nonbiased way. The administration usually makes decisions about programs, and so do accrediting teams, but these decisions are based on professional judgment, which can often be strengthened with an empirical evidence base. The following points, though in an extremely formulative stage, are standards, or guidelines, for evaluation of a patient education program:

1. There must be a combination of goal-attainment and goal-free evaluation, which means that the teacher has to look at unintended as well as intended effects and at the quality of the objectives in light of the overall goals patient education shares with all of medicine—intelligent compliance and rehabilitation to optimal social functioning.

2. The evaluation should summarize all instances of the service so that its quality can be known and hopefully controlled.

3. There must be comparison with some empirically based standards: at this time these will mostly be historical (what the program was previously able to attain). Normative standards should accrue as programs report their results and have instruments that are of good enough quality to allow for valid comparison.

4. The program should meet absolute standards in terms of what is medically safe. That is, the learning goals must represent at least minimal knowledge and skills for safe self-treatment, and there should be evidence that every patient meets at least those minimal goals on exit from the program. If it is determined that patients cannot meet the minimal standards, a noneducational therapy must be substituted.

5. Multiple evaluation methods and measurements should be used, since each is too limited to allow for generalization about the program.

6. There should be an operational description of behavioral units to be attained, for both minimal and optimal patient education goals.

Although not mandatory, most programs should use formative evaluation (feedback) during the developmental phase after the program has been set up and is operating for a while. This should allow for conservation of resources by rapidly molding the program to an acceptable level of effectiveness, as opposed to letting it function at reduced effectiveness for a period of time because evidence is not available. Also, it is a far better strategy to develop a strong teaching program with sufficient potency for the job and to evaluate the necessity for an element of the program by withdrawing it and studying the effect.[16] In a strong program the teacher intervenes when the readiness is high or creates readiness; practice is always involved; a variety of learning modalities and levels of materials are provided; and teachers and environment are persuasive.

Special norms, especially guidelines 3 and 4 on this page, should probably be kept for differ-

---

CLASSES OF PATIENTS FOR PATIENT EDUCATION BASED ON READINESS AND ON BEHAVIORAL-DISTANCE-TO-TASK CAPACITY*

Profound difficulty: Judged not to be amenable to educational therapy.

Maximal difficulty:

Months or years of continual training required. Cannot profit from highly verbal, mass methods or massed instruction.

In the meantime, cannot be counted on to do the task well enough to be self-sufficient.

Intermediate difficulty:

Learning distance is considerable, but patient learns well in several modes, although often requires help with synthesis of the ideas and application to reality.

Learning distance may be intermediate, but patient able to learn well in only two modalities; motivation may be moderate.

Minimal difficulty:

Behavioral distance small, and patient successful at self-instruction.

Can be given as normal part of care or requires less than one-half hour nursing time.

Delayed:

Motivation not up to learning now—may be ready in the future.

Also includes periodic reeducation of patients with chronic illnesses.

---

*Readiness = motivation, skills already possessed, and learning skills.

ent categories of patients, as shown in the box above.

EVIDENCE OF THE STATUS OF KNOWLEDGE IN GROUPS AND POPULATIONS

With large groups, the evidence for evaluation comes in different forms than with individuals: it comes in statistics that indicate prevalence of health problems, use of health resources, and number of individuals who can answer questions of health knowledge. Such studies are expensive to carry out and often suffer from incomplete data, with resulting difficulties in interpretation. It is necessary for nurses to have some knowledge of how to interpret these data for at least three reasons: First, those who work primarily with individual patients and families in institutional or community settings will find from statistics a perspective within which to view the readiness their patients bring. Second, all nurses have a professional stake in the health of the community and a commitment to utilize their influence toward its health and well-being. Third, nurses whose work involves responsibility for groups and communities should interpret the statistics as part of an assessment of need for health care and as a base for planning intervention.

Statistics also serve as a form of evaluation. For example, suppose that data about perinatal mortality and morbidity indicate need for a goal of comprehensive and early medical care for expectant mothers. Various means of intervention, including patient education, are utilized to try to meet this goal. Indications of the success might be the increased proportion of expectant mothers registering for care in the first trimester or the large percentage of those mothers under nursing supervision receiving specified tests and services. An additional approach would be to ask a number of prenatal patients their reasons for seeking medical care at the point they did. These indicators not only provide an evalu-

---

POSSIBLE ERRORS IN TEACHING-LEARNING PROCESS IF GOALS ARE NOT BEING MET

Readiness-goals:

1. Did the learner ever accept the goals, or were you teaching about what only *you* believed to be important?
2. What evidence do you have that the goals were appropriate?
3. Were goals clearly written and understood by teacher and learner?
4. Were goals broken into sufficient intermediate steps to provide guidance?

Teaching-learning:

1. Had teaching materials previously been tried with persons of ability similar to your patient and found successful?
2. If previous experience with the materials was not available, in what ways did their characteristics match the patient's readiness?
3. Were evaluative data gathered often during teaching, to give evidence of areas of success and lack of success?
4. Was teaching continued for sufficient time for learning to be thorough?
5. Were the data gathered for evaluation sufficiently valid and reliable to form an adequate basis for the evaluative decision?
6. Were baseline data obtained for measuring change? People rarely start with no knowledge.

---

ation of the program that has been implemented but also serve as a basis for replanning and reteaching or monitoring of the need on a continuous or intermittent basis. For nurses who are used to obtaining from individual patients frequent feedback and evaluation as to how the teaching process is proceeding, the feedback offered by results of infrequent surveys and prevalence data may seem inadequate: the feedback may be affected by a great many variables besides the program the nurse wishes to evaluate; the data may not be immediately available as a guide for proceeding with teaching; the data may not be as specific to the goals of the teaching program as would be desirable; and the data may seem impersonal and detached from the meaning of the learning to the patients. However, nursing has too long enjoyed the luxury of individual patient contact without exploring to the limit less expensive ways of creating behavior change.

SUMMARY

Although evaluation is the end step in the process of teaching-learning, it is forward looking in that its message redirects activity. (See box above.) The information necessary to the evaluation of how well objectives have been met is gathered by various measurement techniques. A concerted effort is made to gather reliable information by perfecting measuring tools and by using combinations of them. This method provides a sounder basis for decisions about competence of the learner to behave in the manner specified in the objectives.

STUDY QUESTIONS

1. You observe a nurse who has been teaching a patient how to give himself an injection. The nurse asks the patient the following questions as he goes through the procedure:

   Is it all right to give the injection with the syringe and needle you used yesterday without changing it?

   Review why you are wiping the skin that way.

Table 9. Interview schedule for patients being discharged on a regimen of diuretics, pretest and posttest*

1. What is a diuretic? (or "fluid pill"? or "water pill"?) An agent used to reduce excess fluid in the body, by means of increasing the urine.
2. Do you know what a "side effect" to a drug is? An effect which is not desired, but which sometimes occurs in certain individuals.
3. Do you know what one of the side effects is which occurs with some diuretics? Hypokalemia (decreased potassium from the body).
4. Do you know that there are other causes of loss of potassium from the body besides a diuretic? Yes (or) no.
5. Can you name any of these other causes?
   a. Vomiting.
   b. Nasogastric suctioning (stomach-pumping).
   c. Diarrhea.
   d. Intestinal drainage.
   e. Starvation.
   f. Dietary deficiency.
   g. Infusions without potassium additives.
6. Do you know some of the signs and symptoms (ways of detecting) that your body is losing too much potassium?
   a. Malaise.
   b. Weakness of muscle.
   c. Constipation.
   d. Increased gas pains.
   e. Decreased ability to void.
   f. Leg cramps.
   g. Apathy: drowsiness and/or irritability.
   h. Dizziness on rising from sitting or lying position.
   i. Very slow heart beat.
   j. Anorexia.
   k. Excessive thirst.
   l. Nausea.
   m. Progressive weakness, leading to flaccid paralysis.
   n. Weakened voice.
   o. Shallow breathing.
7. Do you know what digitalis is?
8. Did you know that a heart patient who is also on digitalis therapy must be very careful to avoid having "digitalis toxicity" (overworking of the digitalis) when he is also on certain diuretics? Yes (or) no.

9. Do you know some of the bad effects of digitalis—that is, when the digitalis is "overworking"?
   a. Anorexia (loss of appetite).
   b. Increased salivation.
   c. Nausea and vomiting.
   d. Diarrhea.
   e. Lethargy, with or without mental confusion.
   f. Visual problems:
      (1) "Halo" vision.
      (2) Decreased or dimmed vision.
      (3) Visual "blind spots."
      (4) Double-vision.
   g. "Thumping" or palpitations in the chest.
   h. *Very* slow pulse or irregular rhythm.
10. Do you know any ways of preventing or making up for this loss of potassium from the body?
    a. Potassium supplements—if prescribed by the doctor.
    b. High-potassium foods.
11. Can you name any of the high-potassium foods?
    a. Bananas.
    b. Peaches.
    c. Apricots.
    d. Raisins.
    e. Prunes.
    f. Raw carrots.
    g. Raw tomatoes.
    h. Orange juice and other fresh, frozen, and canned juices (except apple and cranberry).
    i. Potatoes.
    j. Meats.
    k. Fish.
    l. Nonstarchy vegetables.
    m. Nuts.
    n. Milk solids.
    o. Cereal grains.
    p. Tea.
    q. Sanka coffee.
    Note: The patients were allowed to answer No. 11 before No. 10a if they did this spontaneously after answering No. 10b.
12. What should you do if you begin to recognize of the signs and symptoms of potassium loss in your body? Or if you become too nauseated to eat the foods high in potassium? Or if you have prolonged diarrhea? Call the doctor, or go to see him.

*From Fournet, Sr. K. M.: Patients discharged on diuretics; prime candidates for individualized teaching by the nurse, Heart Lung **3:**108-116, Jan.-Feb. 1974.

What would you do if the tip of the needle touched the table as you were picking up the syringe?

What would you do if you touched the skin now? (After it has been cleansed with the alcohol sponge and before the injection is given.)

State the subobjective that the nurse is evaluating.

2. A public health nurse is teaching a wife and a daughter how to care for a bedfast elderly father and husband. The patient moves little but has not been incontinent. He has had no skin breakdown to present but according to the wife has been allowed to lie in one position for 4 hours. The main objective, which follows, is part of the more-encompassing objective: To avoid harmful consequences of bed rest.

Main objective: To avoid decubitus ulcer formation.
Subobjectives:

A. To recognize any evidence of tissue breakdown by criteria of color, sensation, and response to massage.

B. To reposition the patient at least every 2 hours so that the body is resting on the same surface only every fourth time.

C. To keep all linen wrinkle free.

D. To massage vigorously at every turning the skin that has been receiving pressure from body weight.

E. To report to the public health nurse or physician evidence of incontinence or skin breakdown within a day after it is observed.

Answer the following questions concerning this situation:

a. What methods of measurement might be used to evaluate the learning in such subobjective?

b. During a subsequent visit the nurse found that both mother and daughter could identify evidence of skin breakdown in all five photographs shown. They could not identify areas reddened by sheet wrinkles on the patient's back as potential sites of breakdown. They reported that the patient had not been incontinent and that they usually turned him every 2 hours except when he put up a big fuss. What should the nurse do?

3. How is the notion of transfer utilized in evaluation?

4. You are trying to teach a mentally retarded youngster self-dressing skills, and he is inattentive and rebellious. It is obvious that he is showing lack of readiness to learn. List three possible factors that might be producing this behavior, and indicate what action a nurse-teacher might take in response to each.

5. You are the teacher in a class for diabetic patients, some of whom make the following comments. What evidence does each question or comment give about the individual's understanding?

a. "Would blood sugar be the same for man, woman, or child?"

b. "I don't feel I'm really a diabetic because I don't have to take insulin." (Patient is a 19-year-old girl in whom pregnancy precipitated signs and symptoms of diabetes. The physician has ordered that she be controlled by diet.)

c. Father whose 8-year-old son has newly been diagnosed as having diabetes, talking to a college student who has been insulin dependent for 2 years, "Are you able to hunt?"

6. Read Sister Michael Joyce's article, "Assignment: East Harlem" (*American Journal of Nursing* **69:**1497-1502, July 1969). Analyze the article in terms of the entire teaching process, especially the adequacy of the evaluation.

7. How adequate is the interview schedule shown in Table 9 as a pretest and a posttest for patients being discharged on a regimen of diuretics?

8. Read the article by Edward N. Peters and Robert A. Hoekelman, "A Measure of Maternal Competence" (*Health Services Reports* **88:**523-516, 1973), and write a critique of the tool development for maternal competence.

REFERENCES

1. Alkin, M. C., and Fitz-Gibbon, C. T.: Methods and theories of evaluating programs, J. Res. Devel. in Educ. **8**(3):2-15, 1975.

2. Amend, E. L.: A parent education program in a children's hospital, Nurs. Outlook **14:**53-56, April 1966.

3. Auerbach, A. B.: Parents learn through discussion, New York, 1968, John Wiley & Sons, Inc.

4. Brook, R. H., and Appel, F. A.: Quality-of-care assessment; choosing a method for peer review, N. Engl. J. Med. **288:**1323-1329, 1973.

5. Buros, O. K., editor: The seventh mental measurements yearbook, Highland Park, N.J., 1972, Gryphon Press.

6. Buros, O. K., editor: Tests in print. II. An index to tests, test reviews, and the literature on specific tests, Highland Park, N.J., 1974, Gryphon Press.

7. Cronbach, L. J.: Educational psychology, New York, 1963, Harcourt Brace Jovanovich, Inc.

8. Edling, J. V.: Educational objectives and educational media, Rev. Educ. Res. **38:**117-194, 1968.

9. Ellis, H. C.: Discussant to three conceptual approaches to research. In Gagne, R. M., and Gephart, W. J., editors: Learning research and school subjects, Itasca, Ill., 1968, F. E. Peacock Publishers, Inc.

10. Feldman, J. J.: The dissemination of health information, Chicago, 1966, Aldine Publishing Co.

11. Fournet, Sr. K. M.: Patients discharged on diuretics; prime candidates for individualized teaching by the nurse, Heart Lung **3:**108-116, Jan.-Feb. 1974.

12. Fuchsberg, R. R.: The diabetes supplement of the national health survey. II. Methods and techniques, J. Am. Diet. Assoc. **52:**121-124, 1968.

13. Furst, E. J.: Constructing evaluation instruments, New York, 1958, David McKay Co., Inc.

14. Green, L. W.: Toward cost-benefit evaluations of health education; some concepts, methods, and examples, Health Educ. Monogr. **2**(Suppl):34-64, 1974.

15. Green, L. W.: Evaluation and measurement; some dilemmas for health education, Am. J. Public Health **67:**155-161, 1977.

16. Green, L. W., and Figa-Talamanca, I.: Suggested designs for evaluation of patient education programs, Health Educ. Monogr. **2:**54-71, 1974.

17. Holland, W. M.: The diabetes supplement of the national health survey. III. The patient reports on his diet, J. Am. Diet. Assoc. **52:**387-390, 1968.

18. Hospital patients want their questions answered, Public Health Rep. **82:**224-225, 1967.

19. Hungelmann, J., and Kolba, Sr. M. T.: Bridging the gap between hospital and home, R.N. **9:**26-27, 1969.

20. Johnson, D. E.: Powerlessness; a significant determinant in patient behavior? J. Nurs. Educ. **6:**39-44, April 1967.

21. McDonald, G. W.: The diabetes supplement of the national health survey. I. Introduction and overview, J. Am. Diet. Assoc. **52:**118-120, 1968.

22. Nite, G., and Willis, F. N., Jr.: The coronary patient; hospital care and rehabilitation, New York, 1964, The Macmillan Co.

23. Peters, E. N., and Hoekelman, R. A.: A measure of maternal competence, Health Serv. Rep. **88:**523-526, 1973.

24. Rinaldi, L. A., and Kelly, B.: What to do after the audit is done, Am. J. Nurs. **77:**268-269, 1977.

25. Romm, F. J., and others: Correlates of outcomes in patients with congestive heart failure, Med. Care **14:**765-776, 1976.

26. Roth, H. P., and Caron, H. S.: Accuracy of doctors' estimates and patients' statements on adherence to a drug regimen, Clin. Pharmacol. Ther. **23:**361-370, 1978.

27. Rovinsky, J. J.: Abortion recidivism; a problem in preventive medicine, J. Obstet. Gynecol. **39:**649-659, 1972.

28. Schima, M. E.: Starting sex instruction for sixth-grade boys, Am. J. Nurs. **62:**75-76, Sept. 1962.

29. Schwartz, D.: Medication errors made by aged patients, Am. J. Nurs. **62:**51-53, Aug. 1962.

30. Spaulding, M. R.: The effectiveness of tape recordings with primiparas of the lower socioeconomic group in coping with mothering tasks. In Batey, M. V., editor: Communicating nursing research; problem identification and the research design, Boulder, Colo., 1969, Western Interstate Commission for Higher Education.

31. Stine, O. C., and Chuaqui, C.: Mothers' intended actions for childhood symptoms, Am. J. Public Health **59:**2035-2045, 1969.

32. University Hospital: Information to patients (isolation care), Seattle, University of Washington.

33. Varvaro, F. F.: Teaching the patient about open heart surgery, Am. J. Nurs. **65:**111-115, Oct. 1965.

34. Voysey, M.: Official agents and the legitimation of suffering, Sociol. Rev. **20:**533-551, 1972.

35. Weiss, C. H.: Evaluating action programs; readings in social action and education, Boston, 1972, Allyn & Bacon, Inc.

36. Wollert, W. M.: Achievement through clinical practice—a practical approach to patient care. In American Nurses' Association: Exploring progress in nursing practice, New York, 1965, The Association.

CHAPTER 10

Present delivery of patient education

■ The health education enterprise does seem to be growing, and its deficiencies are painfully obvious. Its goals are fractionated, its outcomes not clear, its organization largely molded to the medical model, and commitment to it tentative.

PRESENT DELIVERY SYSTEM FOR PATIENT EDUCATION

The President's Committee on Health Education, although it did not carry out a comprehensive study, did provide a view of the health education endeavor in this country. The broad strokes of the report and of those who have written about it are clearly damning.[103,134] The whole field of health education is described as fragmented, uneven in effectiveness, and lacking any base of operations. No agency in or outside of government is responsible for or even assists in setting goals, maintaining criteria of performance, or measuring results. The effort is underfinanced: the Department of Health, Education, and Welfare budget for health education is less than ¼ of 1%, and state budgets allot less than ½ of 1% for health education.[103] There is an enormous expenditure for health information but relatively little in the way of effective education (the extra component that would help an individual act on what he has been exposed to). The Committee found only two instances of agencies seeking to evaluate the effectiveness

of their materials; one insurance company was spending $2 million a year for materials and in 20 years had never evaluated them. There are 7,000 hospitals in the United States, but the Committee could find no more than four that were doing an effective job of patient education. School health is in total disarray in the United States.[134] The Committee recommended a national center for health education with divisions for research in the following areas: health education, demonstration programs, communications in health education, community health education centers, and a clearing house for health information and education. Of interest is the concern of one member of the Committee about the apparent lack of commitment to the report from the professional health organizations.[103]

A recent survey deliberately sought out (by means of literature review, consultation with technical experts, and extensive discussions with health education evaluators themselves) and studied those programs in which strong evaluation was believed to exist. The survey found that the ability of consumer health education programs to foster beneficial short-term impact on patient knowledge, attitudes and behavior, and health status had been reasonably demonstrated in a number of different settings, for a number of different health problems, using a number of different techniques. The long-term effects of consumer health education programs have generally not been measured, perhaps in part because few programs themselves exist for a long period of time. A large majority seem to operate over a period of 3 to 4 months; the study staff encountered very few programs that had been in operation continuously for more than 2 years. The kinds of programs that exist can be thought of as self-care programs, system utilization programs, disease control programs, and others. They have been sponsored and funded by hospitals, regional medical programs, public health departments, health maintenance organizations, voluntary associations, and insurance companies. Hypertension, diabetes, and nutrition were found to be highly prevalent as topics in consumer health education programs in almost all settings. Hospitals have inpatient programs, outpatient programs, and community-oriented programs. Public health department involvement in consumer health education is typically multiple-focused, short-term, and nonintensive; most frequent topics were child care and nutrition education for young parents; education on health services and resources available; and common public health problems such as drugs, venereal disease, and lead screening. Insurance companies have been involved primarily in facilitation of program development rather than in front-line delivery of educational services.[69,135]

On a more specific program level, Hart and Frantz found that two thirds of hospitals that had active open heart surgery programs and answered the questionnaire carried out patient education programs to prepare patients for postdischarge.[48] Forty-five percent of the hospitals used a planned instructional sequence. More than half had no continuity in teaching personnel. Forty percent did not include follow-up visits as part of the teaching program. There did appear to be acceleration of the trend for hospitals to implement such programs.

Perhaps such a set of findings was to be ex-pected because of general characteristics of the health care delivery system and its previous lack of support for health education. That system has been described as consisting of thousands of autonomous units, only a few of which at present undergo careful and systematic planning. Hospitals are said to have neglected the distributive processes and use of community-based health indices toward optimal health services.[73] Sidney Garfield's model health care delivery system (Fig. 13) aims to include components that would be most important for patient education.

The American Hospital Association has available a collection of professional accreditation and legal statements that support patient education.[5] Such statements are important in that they form a base for implicit standards of care. It will be important to watch the legal base for patient education practice; there is much potential for activity that could clarify issues.

Within the present delivery system, a number of organizational activities in patient education are reported. One survey, representing 70% of the members of the American Society for Health Manpower and Training (640 responses from the 900 members listed as of December 1971), provided data about trainers in hospitals. Training activities included personnel inservice and orientation as well as patient education. Forty-five percent of these persons were located in the nation's large medical centers, whereas only 19% of the hospitals were in these centers. Separate departments of education were found mostly in large hospitals; in smaller hospitals the training function was frequently located in the department of nursing. Many of the trainers held credentials in nursing, and 65% had been in their current positions for less than 3 years. Trainers in education departments were more likely to have had previous experience in training and education than were trainers in nursing departments, of whom 31% reported having no training experience prior to their current positions. Eighty percent of the trainers said patient

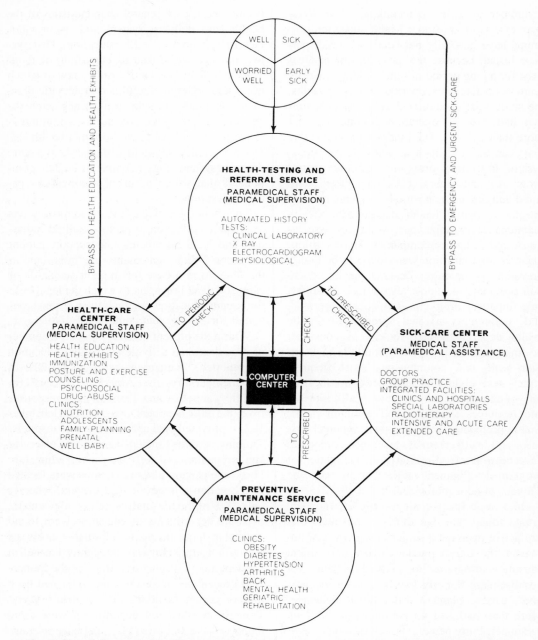

Fig. 13. New delivery system. Separates sick from the well by establishing a new method of entry, the health-testing service. (From Garfield, S. R.: The delivery of medical care, Sci. Am. **222**:15-23, April 1970. Copyright © 1970 by Scientific American, Inc. All rights reserved.)

education needs to be increased in their hospitals, but only 30% reported having planned or conducted patient education. In community health education 68% saw a need for development, but only 23% had had such experiences.[10]

The American Association of Medical Clinics (AAMC) and Core Communications in Health report joint development of a comprehensive patient education program that is being tried in four clinics. The development includes a mixed media curriculum combining slide presentations monitored by a health educator (many of whom are registered nurses) with written questions and answers, lectures, group sessions, family consultations, and take-home materials ranging from books and tape casettes for adults to coloring books for children. Topics are selected by the AAMC Patient Education Advisory Committee from a list of topics suggested by physicians and patients. The only access to the program is physician prescription. Virtually 100% of the patients accepted the program despite the fact that, at the time this report was written, the charge for this service would not be reimbursed by insurance companies.[112]

There are many reports of individual health education programs. A few examples follow:

A storefront that belonged to Lenox Hill Hospital was converted to a health education center and was staffed with the hospital's community relations department and trained volunteers. If the questions are too difficult, they can be referred to the hospital's outpatient department. There are weekly special programs such as those on breast self-examination. There is a VD hotline. The service will be taken to different communities by mobile van, and it presently sees 1,200 persons per month.[2]

The Rogue Valley Memorial Hospital in Oregon established an education department and has become both a regional patient health information center and a provider of educational programs for hospitalized patients via closed-circuit television. Its organization chart can be seen in Fig. 14.[56]

Home care programs organized in hospitals often include a significant patient education component. The Continuing Care Unit of the Lemuel Shattuck Hospital, devoted to chronic disease, is staffed largely by nurses. It was established because a study found large variance in patients' following of advice after discharge, and some poor quality advice being given. These nurses perform such functions as contacting patients after discharge, teaching them, and showing family members what patients can do for themselves.[91] No evaluation of the effectiveness of the unit is reported.

In two sites, demonstration projects with medically indigent populations have shown important outcomes for patient education. At Yale University a study was done of utilization patterns of 31 multiproblem families for 30 months of comprehensive care provided by a family-oriented health care team (physician, public health nurse, health aide, and consultants). The program, aiming to provide continuity, coordination, and constant availability of care, found a change from an illness response in the emergency room to a health-oriented response pattern, with increasing use of nurse counseling, psychosocial guidance, employment assistance, health education, marriage counseling, and rehabilitation and decreasing use of physician services for illness care. The authors suggest that for the urban poverty group, care of acute episodic illness may not be the primary need. Continuing positive experiences with a comprehensive health care system that helps patients cope with their social and emotional problem may be of greater importance in improving health behavior and functioning. The no-show rate for clinic appointments changed from 15% to 2% to 7%.[11]

Los Angeles County University of Southern California Medical Center, serving 600 indigent

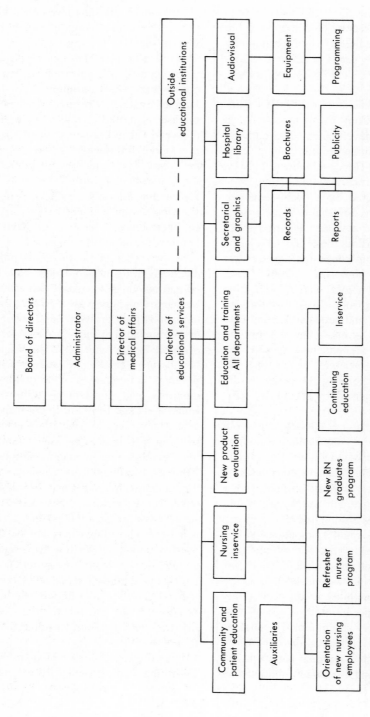

Fig. 14. Functional organization chart of the Department of Educational Services, Rogue Valley Memorial Hospital. (Reprinted with permission from Hospitals, Journal of the American Hospital Association **48**(19):149-153, Oct. 1, 1974.)

diabetic patients, instituted a telephone answering service and implemented a policy for nurse practitioners or residents from the diabetes service to screen all candidates for admission. Emergency room visits by this group were markedly reduced, and such preventable admissions as diabetic coma reduced by two-thirds. The average period in hospital annually is no longer appreciably different from that of a typical nondiabetic population. All of these improvements have resulted in tremendous cost savings.[80]

Both of these studies emphasize coordinated care that is accessible to the patient. The diabetic patient seeking medical advice or adjustment of medication or diet could previously obtain it only through a clinic visit or an inpatient admission. Although the study with diabetic persons did not measure the effect of this new service on patient learning and compliance, it seems that access to timely and appropriate information may have played a role. Indeed, the addition of a follow-up clerk increased the return of emergency room patients for follow-up care in one institution.[33] It is not clear if this was the result of extra attention or of a clarification of the confusion such patients often exhibit about what they are supposed to do. But access to information and education in use of health services cannot be dismissed.

A report from Children's Medical Center in Dallas describes another pattern of delivery of patient education. It employs a pediatric nurse clinician as parent-teacher and counselor. This nurse reports directly to the director of nursing and is not assigned to any particular nursing unit. On physician's written order, he or she provides parents with a series of services: gives parents of children in intensive care units (ICU) progress reports by phone or in person; gives orientation tours of the ICU for patients scheduled to have elective surgery; teaches, often using a family of teaching dolls to reenact a hospital stay; and does discharge preparation.[8]

Another type of organizational pattern for incorporation of health education into an institution can be seen in Fig. 15. A registered nurse heads the Therapeutic Health Education Section, also staffed by a nurse, dietician, pharmacist, and occupational therapist. They do direct teaching and act as resources to hospital staff to prepare them to teach patients.[130]

At one tertiary care institution responsible for the management of 1,800 patients with diabetes mellitus, a computerized information service was developed. It allows much better planning and management for the diabetes teaching service, through listing of diabetic inpatients and outpatients and summarization of previous exposures of patients to specific bedside and classroom education.[17]

A perceived major difficulty with patient education has been financing. In the past, this service has not been recognized as a reimbursable expense by most insurance companies, although many are now reevaluating this policy.[36] The Blue Cross Association has formulated guidelines about kinds of programs that would meet reimbursable standards and how they should be financed: the program should have specified goals and methods and must be a basic component of patient care; educational treatment must be given to specific patients for specific problems; and the effects of such treatment on the cost and quality of care must be a part of the patient's record.[14] Successful attempts to obtain reimbursement have been reported. The request included thorough documentation of the program, including evaluation and follow-up, evidence of cost-effectiveness, qualifications of the patient educators, and functioning of the patient education committee. The request was first made to the local plan of Blue Cross; although national Blue Cross does have a White Paper supporting patient education, the local plans determine reimbursement. Approval of one carrier can be used as precedent with others. Patient education is viewed as an allowable routine service cost under Medicare regulation.[86,87] A critical element seems to be that the education be shown to be integral to care.

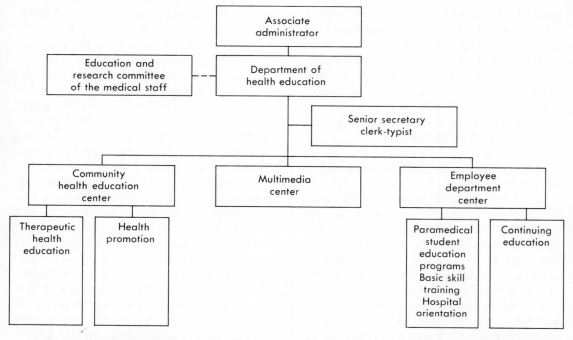

Fig. 15. Organizational pattern of the Department of Health Education. (Reprinted with permission from Hospitals, Journal of the American Hospital Association **46**(8):59-65, April 16, 1972.)

Notions about cost-benefit are not completely developed for patient education. There are reports in the literature of considerable and of more modest savings. For example, for a diabetes education program, a rigorous study would be necessary to separate the effects of education from the effects of other variables, such as concurrent discontinuation of oral agents because of concern about vascular complications from them. Still, decreased admissions from diabetic ketoacidosis may well be traceable to patient education efforts. In mass programs, notions of threshold spending (amount necessary to obtain an effect), saturation spending, point of diminishing returns (more money will not yield more effect), and booster spending (investment to reenliven a program whose effect has waned) must be developed to direct wise use of resources.[42]

Besides third-party payers, patient education has been funded from patient tuition fees, grants, and leftover funds in health care institutions.

There are several long-range system goals for patient and health education. Clearly, cost containment is one. Decrease in malpractice suits is another. The patient should be educated to have reasonable expectations from the medical staff and to be responsible for self-care. These goals are based on meeting requirements of informed consent and perhaps on the hope of improving the relationship with the patient, since there is some evidence that patients are more dissatisfied about the information they receive from their physicians than they are about any other aspect of medical care.[73]

Team or not?

An obvious question in the delivery of patient education is whether to use a team or not. I know of no data that guide such a decision, but in their absence a number of practical matters can be considered. Some patients' learning tasks require the subject matter expertise of different disciplines; rehabilitation of a paraplegic patient is an example. Whether a patient education generalist, such as a nurse with special rehabilitation training, can do as adequate a job as a full team in some situations has not been determined.

Within nursing, there seems to be a continuum of delivery patterns for patient education; some patterns are dependent on the general mode of delivering nursing care in a particular setting. Where team nursing is practiced, patient education may well be delivered as part of that team's duties. It has been suggested that patient education is better accomplished by primary nursing (akin to case method) than by other organizational systems, since the nurse has an opportunity to develop a trusting relationship with a patient, understand and take advantage of his moments of natural readiness to learn, learn which teaching methods are most effective with him, and better evaluate presence or absence of behavioral change. There seem to be no overwhelming data to support this position. The underlying assumption is that all nurses are effective helpers and will be so with the patients to whom they are assigned as primary nurse. It may well be that team nursing saves the patient, for it puts him in contact with a number of nurses, some of whom may be effective teachers with him. On the other hand, one might argue that since learning takes place over a period of time and may be enhanced by more knowledge about and a good relationship with the patient, team nursing can be hampering, especially if coordination and communication within the team are not excellent. It may be that, within general bounds of availability of information about the patient necessary to help him learn, the quality of the professional is most important, not the organizational methods of delivery of care.

Teaching is a special kind of skill that many staff nurses seem not to have. Perhaps even more important than formal classroom teaching skills are habits of general informativeness, which have been studied.[18] It has not been unusual to find that teaching of patients is required for clinician positions, nor is it uncommon for hospitals to hire patient teaching specialists, such as a teaching nurse for diabetic patients. The number of such specialists may gradually increase: the first teaching specialist may work with diabetic patients; often the next to be hired is a cardiovascular teaching nurse; then a parent education teaching nurse and others, as needed, are hired. Such individuals, even if they do group teaching of patients, can rarely provide enough service to meet the patients' needs; they are not available every day. Other health personnel are needed to reinforce the specialist's teaching. Thus, the specialist delivery system can be modified to the advantage of all by the addition of a specific role for other staff members, who must know what was taught and provide follow-up, reinforcement, and supervision of the patient as he practices tasks taught by the specialist. A further modification of the specialist delivery system is to have staff nurses do much of the patient teaching, with the teaching specialist available for referrals when difficult patient education situations arise. Such difficulty often involves a nonmotivated patient, situations of conflicts between health professionals or with families about what a patient is to learn, or patients with limited learning abilities. Often, the specialists provide staff preparation in the subject matter and skills of teaching. The final point on the continuum is for patient education to be delivered by all staff members—all would be skilled in teaching. Perhaps a variation is for nurses on a paticular unit to each specialize in teaching a particular kind of content or dealing with a particular kind of learning problem, but for each to be competent in some area of patient education. They then use each other as consultants.

The choice of a paticular delivery format depends on how well the general mode of delivering nursing care is working and on the competencies of the staff in patient education. In a situation where the team communication system is marginal and most nurses do not see patient education as part of their jobs and are not skillful in it, the employment of specialists may indeed get the job done and be a means of altering the staff's attitudes and abilities about patient education.

The actual functioning of teams, either interdisciplinary or intradisciplinary, in delivery of patient education is relatively unstudied. The presence or absence of a team opinion was studied in three dialysis units, each with a team of about ten members. Each member was asked to describe a good dialysis patient, physically and emotionally, and to rank these characteristics. One team had no opinion; the other two did, one with very high expectations and one very low expectations, especially regarding work and the social life of patients. The study leaves several questions, such as what happens to patients when members of a team expect different things of him; when a team has an opinion, how does it affect the clients, especially when it is "unreasonable" for some.[22]

That patient education is becoming a specialty in nursing is evident with the formation of the American Association of Diabetes Educators. Its goals are to aid in professional development of individuals responsible for educating diabetic patients, to foster communications among these individuals, to serve as a resource center for diabetes education, and to develop guidelines for diabetes education programs.[23] Although other specialties may not be so totally oriented to patient education, groups such as the American Association of Nephrology Nurses and Technicians have long been concerned about the teaching aspect of their areas of practice. This is reasonable since major treatment methods (dialysis and transplantation) involve considerable learning on the part of the patient and family.

The childbirth educator is another example of a specialized patient education clinician who can work relatively autonomously. The incompleteness of currently available health care services and their prominent goal of trying to fit the patient into the medical-hospital structure with the least possible amount of resistance create need for this kind of practice. Sources of information, someone to talk with about personal concerns, and a way to gain skills for childbirth are needed and generally can be only partially gained by reading. The childbearing period should also be used for growth-promoting activities, such as learning to use touch, specifically for childbirth but also transferable to other realms, such as sexual functioning. Childbirth educators may operate in direct cooperation with local medical services or as an optional independent addition to regular medical services.[47]

Teaching roles for related professions

Contributing to the confusion is the ambiguity surrounding the teaching role for various professions. What is it? Is it supported or practiced by the profession? How does it complement the patient education role of other professions? An example of the conflict can be seen in the excerpts from the "Statement of the Clinical Role of the Pharmacist" on p. 231 and the "Statement on Pharmacist-Conducted Patient Counseling" below. These statements indicate the direction of this profession. Pharmacy has been conceptualized by a recent study commission as a knowledge system, the product of which is a service. In the opinion of the Commission, the profession is neither effective nor efficient in delivering its knowledge to those who prescribe, dispense, and consume medications. A particular area in which the pharmacist alone is often involved is self-medication, but patient education is being seen more generally as a responsibility of the pharmacist.[82]

Using suitable verbal, written or audio-visual communication techniques and methods, the pharmacist should inform, educate and counsel patients (or their representative or guardian) about the following

---

EXCERPTS FROM A STATEMENT OF THE
CLINICAL ROLE OF THE PHARMACIST*

The following are reasonable functions for the pharmacist to perform: . . .

2. The pharmacist should have a meeting with the patient for the purposes of reviewing instructions and counseling for home use of medications (a) at time of discharge from the hospital or (b) at time of delivery of medication to him at his community pharmacy. These instructions include modes of administration, conditions of storage, time of renewal, and signs of untoward reactions. The patient is advised in the event of an unanticipated drug reaction to contact the physician or, if the physician is unavailable, the pharmacist. . . .

The pharmacist should be capable of performing the following functions: . . .

3. Provide patient education in personal health matters, i.e., smoking, drug abuse, need for annual health checkup, and other preventive measures.
4. Provide patient education and referral when patients are continually using laxatives, antacids, analgesics, etc., or when patients describe symptoms such as one of the cardinal signs of cancer. . . .
6. Provide instructions for home use of medications: how and when to take, how to store, cautions in use, when to reorder, expiration date, when to see the physician.
7. Provide instructions in the use of appliances such as inhalers, colostomy bags, and trusses. Anatomical models and other demonstration equipment are useful. Special facilities to insure privacy are desirable.
8. Interpret physician's instructions as they relate to drug therapy as well as to the total treatment regimen.
9. Conduct rounds in the hospital and develop a system in the community for following a patient's progress when under drug treatment. The monitoring of patients should determine if patients are taking their medicines.

*From Report of task force on the pharmacist's clinical role, J. Am. Pharm. Assoc. **11:**482-485, 1971.

items for each medication in the patient's drug regimen:

1. Name (trademark, generic, common synonym or other descriptive name(s);
2. Intended use and expected action;
3. Route, dosage form, dosage and administration schedule;
4. Special directions for preparation;
5. Special directions for administration;
6. Precautions to be observed during administration;
7. Common side effects that may be encountered, including their avoidance and action required if they occur;
8. Techniques for self-monitoring of drug therapy;
9. Proper storage;
10. Potential drug-drug or drug-food interactions or other therapeutic contraindications;
11. Prescription refill information;
12. Action to be taken in the event of a missed dose; and
13. Any other information peculiar to the specific patient or drug.

These thirteen points are applicable to nonprescription drugs as well as those ordered by a physician or other prescriber. In addition, pharmacists must counsel patients in the proper selection of nonprescription drugs as well as when and if they should be used.*

---

*From Statement on pharmacist-conducted patient counseling, Am. J. Hosp. Pharm. **33:**644-645, July 1976.

It is easy to see overlaps between the pharmacist's position and that of other professions. There appears not to have been an overall interprofessional look at these roles, and the legal scope of practice as defined in state practice acts usually provides no further clarity. The exception is the physician's scope of practice, which is unlimited in the area of health. Perhaps the key question concerns the degree to which health professionals are actually practicing patient education.

It is no surprise that selected lay persons with short-term training have functioned well in teaching-counseling roles. Families of chronically ill children need many forms of assistance, including explanations about the nature of the child's illness, coordination of services, and help with behavioral and educational services. Because of their needs, a 30-hour course was offered to lay persons; it included principles of health education, use of health literature, chronic disease and its effect on families, counseling techniques, advocacy, community resources, and learning theory. Although evaluation was not rigorous, performance of the lay counselors with these families was judged successful.[92]

Still of considerable concern to nurses and, in my opinion, largely unresolved is the legal base for their patient education activities. Only very sketchy answers are available, and in large areas of the practice of patient education none at all.

What discussion there has been seems to focus on informed consent, probably because laws regarding it have recently received so much attention. The court cases involving this issue have been clear and consistent in placing the responsibility on the physician. The extent, or "scope," of disclosure required varies from state to state: some laws demand "full and complete disclosure" and others require "reasonable" disclosure.[38] It is believed that the nurse generally does not have the necessary information regarding a medical procedure, nor does he or she know what alternative procedures are available for the patient. If the patient indicates to the nurse that he has not had an explanation of procedure, the nurse is obligated to notify the appropriate parties so the patient can be given the opportunity to give an informed consent.[51]

Of considerable interest is application of underlying considerations regarding the physician's duty to inform the patient to the nurse's duty to inform patients about nursing procedures. There are few authoritative cases or laws addressing this issue at present. The nurse has a general obligation to the patient to do what is best for him; in the belief of some, remedying deficiencies in the patient's understanding of nursing procedures, which would allow him to decide whether to undergo the procedure, and not concealing information about it would constitute good practice.[38]

One case is reported that centered around the nature of instructions a nurse gave to a patient and whether the patient clearly understood them. It is suggested that nurses have an obligation to make certain that the patient appears to understand the nature of the instructions and appears to have the mental and physical capacities to carry them out as given. It is also suggested that the chart indicate the nature of the instructions and the fact that the patient appeared to understand and appeared willing to cooperate.

Summary

Some description of the delivery of patient education is available, although in no way comprehensive. Patient education has been part of some innovative demonstration projects that have produced considerable improvement in patient use of health care services. Commitment to patient education is still tentative on the part of third-party payers and perhaps on the part of health care professionals, some of whom are interested because of its cost containment potential and improvement in relationships with patients. Most health institutions appear not to hold their practitioners accountable for patient education; therefore, one is likely to see considerable variation in practice based on what an individual practitioner feels is important. Organizational patterns for delivery of patient education are legion, varying in their degree of interdisciplinary participation and, within nursing, in their focus on the use of specialists or "regular" health care workers.

DEVELOPING A PATIENT EDUCATION PROGRAM

Increasingly, nurses are involved in or responsible for developing a patient education program. Some excellent resources are available to assist in this work, besides the real support usually gained from discussions with colleagues who are trying to accomplish the same task. The Maryland Hospital Education Institute publishes a booklet, *Organizing and Im-* *plementing an Inpatient Education Program.*[89] Materials recently collected by the American Hospital Association from many institutions focus on patient education programming at the hospital level and at the specific patient population level. Examples and worksheets are available on the coordinator's role and qualifications; gaining cooperation and support; use of patient education committees; institutional assessment for patient education; policies, procedures, and job descriptions; and financing patient education activities.[4] Experience in the applicability of these kinds of materials across institutions will be gained.

The boxes below and on p. 234 present two authors' notions of how to proceed; they present essentially the same elements but in different sequences and with more or less elaboration. Problems involved in organizing a teaching

---

STEPS IN DEVELOPING A PATIENT EDUCATION PROGRAM*

1. Assess program need.
   This can be done by questionnaires or interviews with health professionals and clients, the medical records department and various community agencies (VNA's [visiting nursing associations] or associations for the disease such as diabetes). When requesting statistics from the medical records department, ask for the top five or ten admission diagnoses, including both primary and secondary diagnosis.
2. Obtain administrative and professional support.
3. Determine potential clients, sources of referral and subsequent follow-up.
4. Plan program content with an interdisciplinary team (committee).
5. Determine program goals, objectives and evaluative procedures.
6. Select learning strategies.
7. Determine and utilize available resources.
8. Recruit, motivate, train and retrain teaching personnel.
9. Implement the program.
   Delay in implementation because of a small number of patients or other reasons can quickly lead to a decrease in interest and enthusiasm for the program.
10. Document teaching.
11. Do follow-up.
12. Evaluate teaching and program.
13. Revise program.

*From Nemchik, R.: Developing an education program. In Guthrie, D. W., and Guthrie, R. A., editors: Nursing management of diabetes mellitus, St. Louis, 1977, The C. V. Mosby Co.

EXAMPLE OF DEVELOPMENT STEPS USED IN ONE PROGRAM*

1. *Needs analysis.* In this hospital, medical records statistics showed 6½% of all discharges in 1974 had either a primary or secondary diagnosis of chronic obstructive pulmonary disease.
2. *Administrative approval.* Take data to administration. If they give the go-ahead for planning, brief them at intervals throughout the planning, and in the final stages gain approval.
3. *Translating needs into objectives.* Specific needs were determined after discussion with the lung association, outpatient clinics for COPD [chronic obstructive pulmonary disease], government agencies. Two consulting physicians and the director of inservice education were frequently consulted.
4. *Designing the program to meet the objectives, through organized methodologies.* Each objective was broken down into four categories: anticipated time necessary to meet it, teaching method, identification of involvement of the patient/family, and learning system used. The number of patients, their eligibility, space, time of day, parking arrangements, transportation for those who had none, were set.
5. *Gaining support.* The program was introduced to the staff physician meeting. Ninety-five percent of physicians signed their consent to have their patients with documented evidence of COPD attend the program, while five percent wanted to have individual control on whether or not their patients were to attend. The program was next introduced to the department of nursing services and the department of respiratory therapy and classes given to them to enable them to feel comfortable in referring the patients with COPD and to integrate COPD classes into the total process of patient care.
6. *Implementation of the program.* Classes ranged from one to five patients.
7. *Reassessing needs through evaluation.* Both patients and physicians are sent evaluation forms, and meetings with the COPD education committee focus on on-going assessment of the cost and quality of the program.

---

*From Wesenberg, C.: Consumer health education: steps in planning and developing a hospital based program, J. Cont. Educ. Nurs. **8**(5):32-34, 1977.

program are to be expected. In these days of "overbedding" in hospitals, it may be difficult to sell a program that, if successful, will probably further reduce bed utilization. It is suggested that partial support from the administration of your agency can be temporarily adequate, at least until the program is off the ground and success seems probable. If there is no administrative support, one obtains and uses support from an influential physician, clients who are convinced of the value of a teaching program, and others. You will need to be able to answer questions about costs, resources available, and community support and reaction.[85] It might well take a year for the program to be planned, gain support, and become operational.

Both of these models focus more on planning programs for specific patient populations (after assessment of which group should have priority), rather than on patient education programming for an institution, which has multiple programs.

THE DISEASE TREATMENT, SYMPTOM, AND DEVELOPMENTAL TASKS SYSTEM OF DELIVERY OF PATIENT EDUCATION

Programs or efforts in patient education often get started around the needs of a particular

Table 10. Public's awareness and use of cancer detection tests: survey of 1,567, over 18 years of age, January 1974*

Tests for detecting cancer	Aware		Ever had		Had in past year	
	1963	1974	1963	1974	1963	1974
Pap smear	78%	87%	48%	78%	23%	52%
Proctoscopic examination	51%	61%	15%	24%	5%	14%
Chest x-rays	83%	88%	56%	72%	20%	36%
Skin examination	63%	63%	13%	22%	6%	13%
Breast examintion	83%	86%	43%	67%	22%	48%
Breast self-examination	70%	83%	49%	66%	14%	23%
	(1970)		(1970)		(1970)	
					(Who report they do monthly)	

*From The public's awareness and use of cancer detection tests; conducted for The American Cancer Society, Princeton, N.J., 1974, The Gallup Organization, Inc.

group of clients for whom learning is seen to be important. This section will review a number of these areas, although they are by no means comprehensive. This kind of organization of effort is useful because it focuses program development efforts on a small enough area that it seems possible to accomplish something. For each area there is specific content to be taught, common goals, and often particular patterns of readiness. The content and objectives are dependent on what is known about how to treat the particular problem, the readiness patterns of patients, general public knowledge about the problem, and the skills that the treatment requires. All areas use common skills in the process of teaching and a wide range of teaching methods, assessment, and evaluation. The disadvantage of such an organization of programs is that those patients with unusual needs (not common statistically) may get no patient education service at all.

Sample areas of program development
Cancer

Everyone is familiar with the danger signals approach to cancer education. There are those who believe that this approach can be too frightening for some individuals and that focus

should be on what can be done about the symptom. This relates to a major focus in cancer education: decreasing the delay time between noticing a symptom and seeing the physician. There is conflicting opinion about whether decreasing delay will significantly affect prognosis. Delay is apparently very widespread.[7] It is known that patients can be fully informed about signs and symptoms and still not respond with promptness.[46] There is also some evidence that there can be longer delay among those who suspect cancer than among those who do not.[1]

A 1974 public opinion poll indicates that awareness and obtaining of examinations for cancer detection have improved. There is a suggestion, however, that some of this improvement may reflect physician initiative. For example, women most often reported having their first Pap test because of a physician's influence rather than their own initiative. This is consistent with the increase between 1963 and 1974 of those who report they have had a complete physical examination within the past year (11% in 1963, 40% in 1974).[97] Further information from this opinion poll appears in Table 10.

Cancer detection requires repeated checkups. Although the Pap test has been known for more than 25 years, only about half of all adult American women have had the test once, and fewer have the test regularly. More than 90% of the women with breast cancer find it themselves. The statement that we could cure 85% of breast cancer but are curing only 40% implies that women do not detect it early enough or, once they detect it, do not seek or obtain adequate care.[52]

Patient education does, of course, play a part in the treatment of cancer as well as in its detection. All patients have to deal with the fear of recurrence and with the social redefinition of themselves that occurs. Means of dealing with school phobia in children with malignant neoplasms is an example of an intervention aimed at maintaining what is believed to be a healthful life pattern.[61] For particular sites of cancer and usual treatment forms, there are educational programs, such as the muscle rehabilitation and prosthesis adaptation after mastectomy and the ostomy care after bowel surgery for cancer.

It is well known that there is tension between the position that patients should be informed about diagnosis and prognosis, even if grim, and the position that such knowledge is not good for them and that they do not want it. Perhaps the most commonly stated position today is that most patients know anyway and should be provided with the information and skills that will help them to cope. What is not clear is what is actually practiced. Older studies describe the kinds of interaction strategies used by health professionals to avoid the issue: speaking in generalities rather than specifics about the extent of cancer involvement and the relative success of surgery or letting the patient take the lead in conversational choices under the guise that this allows him to get the information he wants and needs.[97] Finally, many health professionals, unless they remain current about cancer knowledge, will give very inadequate information to patients: this has been described as often more pessimistic than is warranted.[25]

It has been suggested that since 34% of persons with cancer survive 5 years or more, they might better be served by care organized according to a rehabilitation model. Both the cancer and the therapeutic intervention for it may produce significant long-term or permanent functional loss and psychologic difficulties. Gaps in present services can be filled with the services and philosophy basic to the rehabilitation model.[63]

Cardiovascular area

Reported programs and efforts in the cardiovascular area again follow major diagnostic medical categories or means of treatment for high blood pressure, stroke, pacemaker, myocardial infarction, and hemophilia.

General knowledge about the heart. A 1972 survey done in Calgary, Alberta, described lay perception of heart disease. Some of its findings follow:

Sixty percent knew that cardiovascular diseases in earlier stages could be asymptomatic.

Ninety-two percent could name at least one risk factor.

Although 74% knew that heart disease takes many forms, 40% were unable to name even one type of heart disease. Thirty-three percent equated strokes and heart attacks.

Reported sources for most of the information about heart disease were: 55% print sources, 30% from relatives and friends, 19% from medical personnel. Only 29% indicated they had ever received information about heart disease from a doctor.[74]

High blood pressure. The detection and control of hypertension have become a major public health campaign in the United States. This has resulted in a major report to the National Institutes of Health: the "National High Blood Pressure Education Program," focusing on community and professional education and on resource and impact assessment. Probably the most significant figures summarized in this report are that 15% of adults have high blood pressure. Of those, one half are aware of the condition; of the one half that are aware, only one half are receiving therapy; and of those receiving therapy, only half are under control.[83] Others have tried to tease from various pieces of data possible causes for such a situation: some people do not have their blood pressure checked; some who do are not told what their pressure is or at least in a fashion that would impress them on the implications of their condition; some are not given a prescribed treatment, or they perceive that their physician told them to discontinue therapy.[125] Further potential sources of slippage were described in a public opinion poll:

Between the ages of 17 and 35, 48% of the public and 57% of the hypertensive group saw high blood pressure as serious.

Only 24% knew that hypertension is the same as high blood pressure.

Tension and overweight were seen as the most prevalent likely causes of high blood pressure. That may prevent the public from recognizing that hypertension also exists in the thin and the calm among us and that overt characteristics are not always present.

Forty percent of the general public and 50% of the current hypertensive group said it is likely that one can have high blood pressure with no obvious symptoms.

There appeared to be little doubt in the public's mind that high blood pressure can be controlled. Eighty-three percent understood that treatment must usually continue. There was little appreciation that simply controlling blood pressure is an important way to reduce the possibility of heart trouble or stroke.[96]

Much effort has been aimed at detection of hypertension, recently with the additional focus of long-term control after detection. The position of patient education in detection is secure although often naive about what it can accomplish. Standards for detection programs require an education/counseling component; what happens in actual practice is not known. Innovative means to deliver the educational message have been sought; one suggestion is for the American Heart Association to train volunteers in a certi-

fication program to deliver an educational message about high blood pressure.[84]

More recent efforts have been made to maximize the delivery of care for detection and treatment of hypertension toward the goal of long-term control. Some programs given at the work site, with employer support, have been highly successful. This approach does not involve direct patient cost or time lost from work and perhaps gains strength from a work situation in a cohesive organization, which also be a community, especially in an urban setting.[3] A large, national cooperative study in 14 communities has had high participation at all phases of follow-up, perhaps related to its careful focus on reducing barriers to patient cooperation, with convenient hours of operation, transportation, and location, no cost, and minimum waiting time. Missed appointments were monitored and renewed contact made. The treatment regimen was stepped care, to enable the goal of normalization of blood pressure at the lowest possible medication level. In addition, staff time was used to encourage patients to discuss any therapy problems; this was aimed at minimizing side-effects that could deter patient continuation of needed treatment.[54]

Stroke. Preventive teaching for stroke is similar to that for cardiovascular disease in general but also includes emphasis on how to detect and know the significance of transient ischemic attacks. "Guidelines for the Nursing Care of Stroke Patients" identifies patient teaching actions and teaching materials.[102] Of special concern for stroke patients are special teaching techniques for left or right hemiplegia. Those known to be useful for patients with perceptual deficits, which may have been caused by stroke or other diseases, are minimally available in the nursing literature but used regularly by physical therapists. Another important area of practice is how best to accomplish family teaching. Tasks of families are: (1) to follow an outlined schedule of home treatment, (2) to reorganize the home environment in terms of such problems as visual deficits and hemiplegia, (3) to assist the patient in mastering special devices for communication, such as word boards or special writing aids, and (4) to plan for social carryover of retraining, relating therapy to activities of everyday life, such as vacation, hobbies, and contact with friends.[116]

Pacemaker. A description of a program for pacemaker patients is available in the literature,[59] as is a booklet for patients, published by the American Heart Association. The focus for such a program is to get proper maintenance on the pacemaker, including checking the pulse and adapting one's living activities to the restrictions imposed by the pacemaker. Use of an actual pacemaker is a valuable teaching tool. Pathophysiology can be explained simply: the heart is a pump that delivers nutrition to the body; there are electrical impulses that cause and control its contraction; there are changes in the heart cells that disturb the regular electrical waves an cause uneven or slow heartbeat and pulse. Explanation of the function of the pacemaker can then follow. The teacher must carefully avoid the common misconception that the pacemaker is like a new heart or is a pump itself.

Myocardial infarction. Although instruction in the coronary care unit is important, the educational cycle begins as part of risk factor screening and control. Controversy still exists about the outcome of control of at least certain risk factors; in addition, the changes of behavior required (such as diet alteration and cessation of smoking) are often difficult to accomplish. Such behavioral changes are often attempted after myocardial infarction in an effort to prevent a further infarction; thus, many of the same teaching goals play a part in primary, secondary, and tertiary prevention.

A second source of concern is the number of patients who are lost before they get to a hospital. Mobile cardiac units, training of police and firepersons, and training of the lay public, at least in cardiopulmonary resuscitation, are

attempts toward decreasing this number. Patient delay after symptoms are noted is not understood. It was estimated that as many as one third of the patients delayed longer than 12 hours.[45] Although denial has been hypothesized as a cause, there was evidence that patients, even those with previous myocardial infarctions, were sometimes uncertain of the signs and symptoms.[128] It was reported that a fairly large proportion suffered symptoms of left ventricular failure also (or alone) and did not associate these symptoms with cardiovascular disease, even if they knew they had it. This was especially true of paroxysmal nocturnal dyspnea. Often the role of a second person in initiating the decision to seek help was significant.[45] I know of no tested educational interventions to decrease delay time.

There is disagreement about the amount the patient can learn, about his use of denial, and the relationship between learning and denial once he is in the cardiac care unit (CCU).[120] Some suggest that the only outcome of teaching in the CCU will be to decrease the patient's anxiety and that the majority of patients need a complete review after learning the CCU.[24] Table 11 is a description of hypothesized behavioral stages of adaptation to myocardial infarction, with suggested nursing intervention, including teaching.[109]

Some very interesting reports deal with what the patient learns while in the CCU, as in witnessing the resuscitation of another patient. Increase in systolic blood pressure, psychologic symptoms of anxiety,[16] and increase in premature ventricular contractions[114] have been reported, as has significant and prolonged increase in heart rates.

The period after discharge has been described as difficult for patient and family.[120,137] Difficulties included recurrence of chest pain, of which the seriousness was not clear to wives,[119] belief that the weakness they felt was a harbinger of cardiac decline, sleep disturbances often related to nocturnal preoccupation with

Table 11. Behavioral response patterns commonly observed in cardiac patients*

Phase	Timing and duration	Behavioral responses
I. Shock and disbelief	Immediately following heart attack, to 48 hours	Anxiety and denial; occasionally aggressive sexual behavior
II. Developing awareness	After first 48 hours	Depression and anger
III. Resolution	After discharge	All behavioral responses of earlier phases

Manifestations, primary causes, and nursing interventions

I. Anxiety
  A. *Manifestations*
    1. Increased verbalization.
    2. Inability to concentrate, understand, or retain information.
    3. Restlessness or insomnia.
    4. Muscular rigidity.
    5. Palmar sweating.
    6. Tremulousness.
    7. Tachycardia.
  B. *Primary causes*
    1. Fear of death or chronic disability.
    2. Uncertainty of etiology of illness and prognosis.
    3. Being subjected to the "strange" complex environment and frightening procedures of a CCU.
    4. Development of complications (arrhythmias and cardiac arrest) in self or others.
    5. Threat to self-image.
    6. Misinterpretation of information and misconception of experience (i.e., perceiving the general physical weakness as proof of irreversible heart damage).
  C. *Nursing intervention*
    1. During periods of severe anxiety, maintain consistent, continuous nurse-patient contact; consistent personnel assists development of patient trust and facilitates an accurate assessment.
    2. Give initial and repeated orientation to CCU routines, equipment, and procedures to patient and family.
    3. Assess the patient's prior experience with illness, hospitalization, and severe stress and how it relates to current condition.
    4. Solicit expressions of concern and questions from patient and family.
    5. Prepare patient and family for each change or move in the patient's physical environment (transfers from the CCU to a convalescent unit or to home).

II. Denial
  A. *Manifestations*
    1. History of ignoring symptoms prior to admission.
    2. Avoids discussing the heart attack and/or its significance.
    3. Minimizes the severity of his condition and its consequences.
    4. Describes his condition by quoting others (the doctor says . . .).

*From Scalzi, C. C.: Nursing management of behavioral responses following an acute myocardial infarction, Heart Lung **2:**62-69, 1973.

Continued.

Table 11. Behavioral response patterns commonly observed in cardiac patients—cont'd

---

  II. Denial—cont'd

      5. May verbally acknowledge having had a heart attack but disregards activity and diet restrictions.

      6. Tries to keep interactions on a social humorous level, may seem overly cheerful.

      7. Asks the same questions of different staff members, as if "shopping around" for the answer he wants.

   B. *Primary causes*

      1. Inability to control the medical events; focuses on parts of existence that he can control; copes with anxiety or threatening situations by ignoring, rejecting, or refusing to believe that they exist.

   C. *Nursing intervention*

      1. Assess whether denial is inhibiting the treatment plan; is it verbal or active denial?

      2. If verbal, listen but do not reinforce the denial or force acceptance of a fact he is not ready to cope with.

      3. If active (for example, disregards activity restrictions), assess the consequences of his actions. Are they detrimental? Conveying concern and allowing more control of his environment are more successful than "threats."

      4. Assess "threat" producing the need for denial. What does this illness mean to this patient?

  III. Depression

   A. *Manifestations*

      1. Sad look, listlessness, and disinterest.

      2. Expressions of pessimism or hopelessness.

      3. Talks with short verbal responses.

      4. Slowness in movement and speech.

      5. Withdrawn (appears to sleep more, wants curtains to remain drawn).

      6. Loss of appetite.

      7. Crying.

      8. Expressions of direct or projected anger.

   B. *Primary causes*

      1. Patient becomes less able to maintain denial, becomes more aware of what has happened to him, and begins to think about how it will affect his future.

      2. May feel powerless, hopeless, or helpless.

      3. Thought content is centered on injury to self-esteem, particularly loss of job, independence, and fears of sexual impotence, invalidism, and premature old age.

   C. *Nursing intervention*

      1. Verbally reflect your observations (i.e., "you look really down," or "you seem to be depressed").

      2. Let patient know that it is normal to feel this way and that many patients become depressed when they are in the hospital.

      3. Solicit and listen to the patient's feelings; assess how he perceives his illness.

      4. Allow and encourage tearfulness or crying; can be done either verbally or nonverbally, through your presence and/or use of touch.

      5. Be "matter of fact" about patient's expressions of anger to prevent him from feeling guilty for being angry (depression results from internalized anger; thus it may be beneficial to have the anger expressed).

      6. If patient becomes extremely hostile or angry, do not try to clarify or reason with him at that time.

Table 11. Behavioral response patterns commonly observed in cardiac patients—cont'd

III. **Depression—cont'd**

    7. Manipulate environment (radio, television, reading material, increase the number of visitors, and so forth).

IV. **Aggressive sexual behavior**

  A. *Manifestations*

    1. Frequent seductive comments (i.e., overt bids for posthospital dates).

    2. Flirtatious compliments, frequently accompanied by attempts to hold, fondle, or kiss parts of the nurse's body.

    3. Deliberate exposure of genitals while being assisted with bath, use of urinal, linen change, and so forth.

    4. Frequently boasts about past sexual interests and prowess.

  B. *Primary cause*

    1. Threatened by fear of sexual inadequacy or impotence compounded by "forced" position of dependency, loss of self-sufficiency, and loss of physical strength; the perceived threat produces anxiety; the aggressive sexual behavior attempts to counteract the anxiety.

  C. *Nursing intervention*

    1. Assess what the patient is seeking by this behavior.

    2. If the patient's sexual behavior makes you uncomfortable and is unacceptable by your standards, be very honest and simply tell him that.

    3. Ask the patient if there was something that you (the nurse) might have done to stimulate his behavior.

    4. Realize that flirtatious compliments are attempts to bolster the patient's male ego and acknowledge politely by simple acceptance.

    5. Discuss sexual relations with the patient and spouse prior to discharge (the physician usually assumes this responsibility, but the nurse should verify that it has been done and be prepared to clarify or answer additional questions).

---

heart function, and irritability. In all of the 18 families studied by Wishnie, there was a steady, eroding conflict; in 11 families there was marked controversy over the specific meaning of the physician's instructions, which often hinged on misunderstanding the nature of coronary disease. Patients were slow to complain about symptoms during office visits; the excuse given was that the doctor failed to ask the specific question. Wishnie questions if this much difficulty is warranted.[137]

There is fair agreement on the content of patient education programs for myocardial infarction, although far less clarity about the actual behavioral goals desired for patients and the ability of the program to produce them. Areas of content include (1) nutrition (restriction of calories, fats, and, if necessary, sodium); (2) physical activity, including rationale for early restriction related to healing process, concept of gradually progressing in activity, magnitude and type of exercise prescribed, and advantages of enhancing and maintaining fitness; (3) specific counseling about resumption of sexual activity; (4) cessation of smoking advised, methods suggested, and rationale explained; (5) general information about normal heart function, then about coronary atherosclerotic disease and myocardial infarction, emphasizing structural changes that occur during infarction and healing; (6) understanding of information about all prescribed medications—name, purpose, dosage, detailed instructions for use, desired effects, and possible untoward effects; and

(7) importance of control of associated diseases and, particularly, coronary risk factors. Patient should be instructed how to respond to new or recurrent symptoms, particularly chest pain or arrhythmia; he and his family should know early warning signs of infarction and be taught to seek immediate medical care.

Education of the general public, employers, unions, insurance carriers, workmen's compensation boards, and so forth should include (1) early warning signs of heart attack, (2) detection and modification of coronary risk factors, and (3) emphasis that most patients can and should return rapidly to work and to their habitual life style after myocardial infarction.[133]

Hemophilia. Home transfusion of the hemophiliac was done in 11 centers in 1972 and seems to be most successful. Home transfusion is most important when the transfusion requirements are frequent, prophylactic transfusions are indicated, or the patient lives in a geographic area where good emergency care is not readily available. Programs with paients on home care require close follow-up. In one situation, the patient mails his self-kept report to the physician; a new supply of concentrate is sent by return mail if records were satisfactory.[66] In another, a regulated supply of antihistamines and steroids, given to decrease joint inflammation and to treat minor transfusion reactions, can be self-administered after phone consultation with the physician. Programs of home care can cut the overall cost of the patient's care in half.[115] Other reports of home care programs indicate that the interval between onset of hemorrhage and treatment decreased as did pain and disability; fewer serious orthopedic problems and days lost from school or work occurred[98]; and inhospital and outpatient department visits decreased.[66]

Chronic obstructive pulmonary disease (COPD)

Training, rehabilitation, or ambulatory care programs for persons with COPD commonly include learning an effective method of bronchial hygiene, breathing retraining that stresses abdominal-diaphragmatic control, physical reconditioning with simple daily exercises to improve exercise ability, use of oxygen and medications, and attention to life style. After such a program, it was reported that ventilatory function abnormalities did not change significantly but that for 2 years patients did not physiologically deteriorate at the expected rate. Patients' subjective feelings of well-being were reported as greatly improved.[90]

Genetic counseling

Available studies of genetic counseling consistently show less than desirable understanding on the part of the patients. It is suspected that contributing to this situation is a low level of public knowledge or even awareness of genetics, although no comprehensive study of this is available.[21] There is consistent evidence that people with higher formal education have better knowledge of biology and better understanding of such elements as the probability statements; however, understanding does not necessarily follow through to action.[64,71] Consider the mother who understood that the risks were statistical and who thus concluded that, unless she were planning to have a family of hundreds, the genetic risk figures were of no relevance to her.[64] The studies are consistently at fault for an almost total lack of description of the teaching done and often for very inadequate descriptions of the bases for concluding that knowledge was poor.

One study of parents with children with phenylketonuria (PKU) found that less than 20% of the parents had an adequate understanding of questions believed to be basic, such as cause, potential consequences, symptoms, and dietary treatment of the disease.[117] Of a group whose children had cystic fibrosis, PKU, Down's syndrome, or connective tissue disease, about half were judged to have the kind of comprehension that could make the information helpful to them; for one fourth of them the genetic counseling served little purpose.[64] A study of a group of parents from Scotland and Northern Ireland (total number, 189) whose children had cystic fibrosis found that only 20% had an excellent understanding of the disease ("excellent" meant full appreciation of the recessive nature of the inheritance, that their affected sons were probably sterile, their affected daughters had an increased chance of bearing an affected child, and that phenotypically well children could be carriers of cystic fibrosis). Others had grasped some but not all of the information. In 55% of the Scots and 20% of the North Irish studied, understanding was rated poor: parents knew simply that their child's illness had been inherited and that there was some chance that any other child conceived in the future might also be affected. Many of the parents indicated that they had no wish to look at the future in these terms. Feelings of guilt were much less evident among those parents who had a sound understanding of genetics.[71]

The information parents need in order to make rational decisions about further reproduction has been described to include: the origin of the disease in mutant genes or chromosomes, the risk of repetition, and the probability of carrier states among unaffected siblings and of carrier states in the population.[64] Beyond such factual knowledge, there are no clear answers to such value questions as: How severe must a disease be before it becomes too serious for parents to risk? How large a risk should parents be willing to take? Is the disease so bad that after amniocentesis the affected fetus should be aborted? Since there is a lack of a cultural blueprint suggesting appropriate decisions on genetic matters, counselors will very infrequently give direct advice. Besides factual information, parents often seek information about the range of decisions that other couples in their situation have made—the social comparison that would be present in the cultural blueprint.[121]

Recent laws about sickle cell anemia raise significant questions about public and individual rights. Thirteen states have laws about screening, but only three make provision for counseling persons screened, and only one of these and one other state provide for education of the public about sickle cell anemia. Subjects are not protected by confidentiality of test results in all states. However, even when such protection is given, subjects can still suffer from a sense of stigmatization or from personal anxieties stemming from their carrier status.[100,101]

Getting at-risk populations to screening is another educational task. Screening is sometimes hampered by the health care personnel's lack of knowledge about the disease and its genetic pattern, as Beck and co-workers found with Tay-Sachs gene screening in one study.[10] Another mode of delivery, of course, is as part of routine inpatient care. A retrospective record audit of 1,633 patients, with ten categories of genetic or congenital disorders, served in a children's hospital found genetic counseling given five times and "offered only" twice. It seems very infrequent that the genetic nature of a child's disorder is reflected in his inpatient management.[105]

Physical or mental handicap

Encompassing this broad group of disorders is a common threat of difficulty in getting information and of major learning tasks in the social role.[39,131] Barnard and Powell's book is an excellent resource for the nurse teaching a mentally retarded child.[9] Typically, the parent of a retarded child does not know which tasks the child will be able to master, approximately when, or how to stimulate his development. An area of particular concern now is sex ecudation for retarded children and their parents. Methods of communicating constructively in this area are aimed in part at the children's social and marital potentials and limitations.

Spina bifida represents a handicap with particularly severe learning and teaching problems. One study found that at the operative decision time most of the parents had never heard of spina bifida and had no appreciation of its complications and that at least some gained the impression that operation would restore the child to normal function. After the operation, many mothers first handled their baby on the day they took it home, and they were given no special instructions. Furthermore, this study found that the family's general practitioner and health visitor knew less about the problems of spina bifida than the parents knew.[131]

The intense social implications of a handicap can be illustrated by blindness. There is a large, multimillion dollar national network of organizations for whose services people are eligible when they meet the legal definition of blindness. Socialization to that system's definition of blindness as a disability is strong, and its services are limited if one is not educable for employment. However, most blind persons do not have resources to "buck the system" if they should disagree with its social definition of their handicap.[113]

Sexuality, pregnancy, parenting

These topics represent normal life experiences. Prenatal preparation gets the most medical attention, and increasing attention is being paid to the range of family-planning alternatives available. More infrequent educational roles include helping the transsexual patient to alter his gender after surgery by learning a new role: for example, learning to urinate, walk, and put on makeup as a female.[126] In some instances, strategies for delivering education about venereal disease, such as requiring attendance at an education session before receiving birth control devices, may be somewhat coercive.[99] Other strategies have made use of the social patterns of the patients, such as providing education and screening through a gay bar when venereal disease rates in homosexuals were found to have risen.[106] The level of sexual knowledge in certain populations continues to shock: one practitioner describes patients on a postpartum unit

who could not identify their sexual organs anatomically, thought they could get pregnant whenever they had intercourse, did not understand the purpose of menstruation,[28] or believed that one must have intercourse "often" in order to become pregnant.[94]

Achieving desired family planning depends on knowledge of contraceptives. In this area there have been some recent improvements. Studies between 1965 and 1970 showed that the historic socioeconomic differences in patterns of contraceptive use were considerably reduced, that nearly three in five couples who practice contraception now employ the most effective methods (pills, IUD, or sterilization), and that the incidence of unwanted pregnancies declined 36% between the first and second half of the 1960's.[55] A group of unmarried, poor adolescents was found to be most aware of those forms of contraception to which they had least access, such as the pill, whereas few had knowledge or experience with the nonprescriptive methods for women.[35] A 1-hour class on family planning held in 1966 at Harlem Hospital showed that before the class those attending had high knowledge about how the condom prevented pregnancy but changes in knowledge took place in the following items: knew how foam prevented pregnancy (61% to 86%), knew how diaphragm prevented pregnancy (58% to 87%), knew how tubal ligation prevented pregnancy (49% to 81%), knew how rhythm prevented pregnancy (29% to 62%), knew how IUD prevented pregnancy (15% to 42%), knew how pills prevented pregnancy (14% to 45%), and could correctly answer what time of the month a woman is most likely to get pregnant (40% to 80%). The answers on the family-planning quiz did not predict those who would accept or reject contraception. Common misconceptions were that the IUD creates a physical barrier to keep sperm and egg apart and that the pills prevent the sperm from fertilizing the egg when they meet.[32]

Stages of psychologic vulnerability to unwanted pregnancy have been outlined; the implied purpose of knowledge of these vulnerable periods is to help the patient anticipate them. The first vulnerable stage occurs during early adolescence when fecundity is absent or low but increasing and, as a consequence, contraceptive vigilance is incompletely developed. The second occurs at the start of the sexual career until the woman acknowledges that she has started her sexual career. The third is in relation to a stable sexual partner: before a stable sexual and contraceptive pattern has been established, during conflict or separation when patterns of communication and cooperation are disrupted, and after breakup with a partner when exposed to the old or a new partner. After each pregnancy, when the decision to stop having children is being dealt with, and during menopause are other times of vulnerability.[81]

Abortion counseling typically includes: orienting the client to the procedure, possible sequelae, and postabortion care; giving information on contraception and assistance in meeting the woman's individual birth control needs; assisting the client through the admission procedure; and offering emotional support during and after the procedure. There is less consensus on exploring the client's sexual and psychosocial development, which may have contributed to the unwanted pregnancy and to subsequent ones. The patient undergoing abortion has been described as undergoing a process of decision making: moving from acknowledging the pregnancy, formulating alternatives, selecting one with a tentative "trying it on" (or rehearsing that decision or several possible decisions), making a commitment to one decision with a recognition of fresh outcomes in favor of the decision, to adhering to the decision.[15] The quality of this process is, of course, of concern to health personnel. To take into account only a few factors or to experience restriction of choice is believed to adversely affect the quality of the outcome.

Parent education involves assistance in optimizing development of both child and parent. Some evidence indicates that typical behaviors related to a child's stage of development are misinterpreted by parents and thus cause conflicts and concerns.[20] The 2-year-old's negativism and 4-year-old's talk-back and sass need to be understood intellectually for what they are, as well as tolerated emotionally. Socioeconomic class differences in maternal expectations for child development have been found. In one study, 50% of lower-class mothers expected that toilet training should be completed by 2 years, whereas 16% of the middle-class mothers held this belief.[19] The obvious question is whether or not the physiologic readiness for training exists by 2 years or whether these differences in expectations represent only cultural differences.

Anticipatory guidance and primary prevention are common themes in parent education. One study used kindergarten entry (a natural crisis) as a time for education of middle class suburban parents, who at other times were found to be hard to reach. Sessions were held a week before and the evening after school began and included content on normal separation of children and parents, with small groups working through their fears and mother-teacher rivalry (teachers attended the second session).[118]

Helping parents with personality and social difficulties requires techniques beyond teaching but often incorporates teaching into the "treatment." In cognitive-intellectual functioning, a grossly immature personality reflects an absence of fine distinctions among ideas, a concreteness, an impaired reality testing, a limited ability to integrate and solve problems, and an inability to see things from the point of view of others and take their needs into consideration when responding to a conflict. Such patterns combined with a pattern of apathy-futility can be a way of life learned from one generation to the next.[93]

Concern has been expressed about the ability of health care professionals to assist parents, especially about behavior problems of children. The content of visits with medical personnel has been found in some studies to be predominantly concerned with physical needs, even though mothers were known to have behavioral concern[34,122]; there were no differences between physicians and nurses in the content included.[34] In visits where there were many blocks in communication (being vague, interrupting questions, talking in jargon), clients showed more dissatisfaction and lower compliance; this response was more common among lower-class patients.[41] In one study, almost half of the parents were still wondering, when they left the physician, what had caused the child's illness.[57] Since no comprehensive survey of practice exists, one wonders how representative such findings are. Clearly, health professionals in the above studies were not using well-advocated interpersonal techniques that focus on the parents' feelings and concerns and obtain their perceptions through such simple questions as, "Why did you bring Johnny to the clinic today?" "What worried you the most about him?" "Why did that worry you?" Preoccupation with unanswered concerns may make the parent unable to respond to the physician's questions and advice.[58]

Pre- and postoperative teaching

The operative experience, perhaps because it is stressful and occurs at a time when patients are in contact with health professionals, has been the focus of considerable patient education activity. Research studies on the operative experience are fairly plentiful in contrast to those available in other areas of patient education. A number of studies, however, are difficult to translate into practice because they lack explicit, operational definitions of both the experimental treatment and "usual care," which is often given to the control group. If "usual care" is given to the experimental group as part of care in addition to the experimental treatment, the study may be contaminated. Notice

that there is an implicit assumption that "usual care" is poor, since it is expected to provide a contrast with an ideal treatment.

Perhaps one can generalize from these studies that active learning of coping skills, in addition to learning of basic information, is necessary in order to acquire the desired effects. A single visit by an operating room nurse, which attempted to influence the emotional response of the patient, did not yield the desired effect.[67] The coping devices found effective in the research studies have included structured instruction in turning, coughing, and deep breathing[68]; exercise of cognitive selective attention to the more favorable aspects of the situation whenever the patient anticipated or experienced discomfort, calming self-talk, and cognitive reappraisal of anxiety-provoking events[60]; and a more general group discussion of fears, which includes information about what patients could expect and how they could aid in their recuperation, with practice encouraged.[111] Effects studied have included lung ventilation, degree of urinary retention, amount of postoperative vomiting, amount of anesthesia and pain medication required, rapidity of return to oral intake, patient reports of quality of sleep and anxiety, fearfulness of their recollections around the operative event, and length of hospital stay.

Special organizational mechanisms to accomplish the teaching include a preoperative admission unit,[95] biweekly preadmission patient-teaching clinic offered at the same time as other preoperative care,[70] and classes held between 4 and 5 P.M. Sunday through Thursday.[78]

Medication compliance

It is well known that errors in taking or not taking prescribed medications are widespread. In most studies at least one third of the patients failed to comply with instructions, and in some studies the rate of failure is 50% or higher. The type of action most commonly identified as noncompliance is omission of doses, although taking a medication for the wrong purpose and errors in dosage and in time of administration also occur. Failure to have the prescription filled and premature discontinuation of the medication by the patient are special patterns of noncompliance. Contrary to expectations, noncompliance can also be a problem in patients who are hospitalized or under close supervision. The full effect of these facts is probably not known. It has been said that failure to take the medication is probably the leading cause for failure of chemotherapy for patients with tuberculosis.[124]

Clinical judgment is often unreliable for identifying the noncomplier, although one investigator found that patients who said they were not complying usually were not.[108] Monitoring of medication compliance is easier if it can be done by a noninvasive measure. An example is monitoring salivary instead of serum theophylline levels in patients.[30] A difficulty remains in that a biologic base may not be available for selecting a cutoff point for defining noncompliance. Some patients who are unreliable in one situation may not be so in another. Although it has not proved possible to identify an uncooperative type, increases in noncompliance are found more commonly in patients who have prolonged conditions (especially when the treatment is prophylactic or suppressive), extremes of age, language difficulties, and multiple medications and frequent doses or in those who are less well educated and poorer.[53] Additional reviews of compliance studies have been done, showing many methodologic difficulties. One such review found that:

1. With the exception of patients with psychiatric labels, one cannot identify a noncomplier by his diagnosis.
2. The degree of behavioral change the regimen requires of the patient is important: positive cooperation for therapies administered by others is easiest, whereas breaking of personal habits such as smoking is more difficult. Complexity of the

regimen and its duration are also important.
3. Continuity of care in a convenient clinic, with sufficient supervision and satisfaction on the part of the client, is important.
4. Influence of the family appears to be considerable: stability and support for the patient are important.[49]

Factors contributing to noncompliance include failure to comprehend the importance of therapy and poor understanding of the instructions. A classic example of the latter is the prescription, ''Furosemide, 40 mg. as needed for fluid retention''; more than half of the patients on a medical ward thought the pill would help them retain fluid.[77]

A summary of studies of patient drug education does show increased compliance as compared with control groups; the amount of increase is variable, and, as usual, descriptions of the educational interventions are sketchy.[132] The extent of lack of understanding of the conditions and medications is indeed instructive. A recent study found many physicians unclear in communicating to patients what they expected them to do. High use of clear, specific written instruction with motivative strategies was associated with a higher rate of compliance.[127] Among poor patients receiving digoxin, 57% did not understand congestive heart failure, and reliability of medication taking was found related to understanding the pathologic process.[75] A study of 267 outpatients and inpatients receiving digitoxin, nitroglycerin, and anticoagulants showed that 72% did not know any side-effects; they did better in knowledge of action, dosage, and timing.[62] Cost, fear of becoming drug dependent, and unpleasantness of side-effects are additional factors affecting compliance. Interestingly enough, the number of dropouts from a hypertension clinic was reduced from 42% to 8% when an appointment system and better physician-patient relationships were instituted. Previously, patients had to wait 2.5 hours for an examination by a physician, which lasted 7.5 minutes, and 1.8 hours in the pharmacy.[31]

The pharmacist's role in educating patients about medications is becoming more formalized; a recent regulation adopted in the state of Washington required a pharmacist, when dispensing a prescription, to "explain to the patient or the patient's agent the directions for use and any additional information, in writing if necessary, to assure the proper utilization of the medication or device prescribed."[53] The profession's own definition of its clinical role, described in an earlier section of this chapter, clearly includes educating patients about medications as a major responsibility, both in institutions and in the community, and in some definitions the pharmacist's responsibility extends to visiting homes to assess compliance and encourage proper medication therapy in the home environment.[26] There are several reports of pharmacists serving as the primary caregiver with patients who have certain stable, medication-controlled chronic illnesses.[29] The chronic illnesses have included hypertension[72] and tuberculosis, the latter on an Indian reservation where compliance and economic savings were apparently considerably improved compared with the previous treatment of hospitalization.[79]

Suggestions for intervention with the medication compliance problem include simplifying dosage regimens to less frequent administration, using pills that do not look alike, and manufacturing combination medications. Suggestions for patient education are many. Standards for what the patient ought to know about a medication are: its name, general purpose, route and means of administration, the amount to be taken as a single dose; timing and frequency of administration; maximum amount that can be used in 1 day; how long it can be used; pertinent adverse effects; proper storage and handling; renewal instructions; and need to avoid other medications, foods, or activities.[53] Some suggestions can be made simply in a conversation that links the taking of the medication

with the outcome; for example, one might say, "Your blood pressure is being well controlled by your medicine at this time," as opposed to "Your blood pressure is normal."[43] Priorities used by the pharmacist result directly from what is known to be related to poor compliance: first teach those patients with the more complicated and confusing regimens and those with regimens offering the greatest potential for adverse effects if not taken properly.[44] A lack of knowledge and beliefs can be altered by an educational approach; whereas coping mechanisms are best instilled by an accommodative approach. The extremely anxious patient should be reassured; the autonomous, independent patient should be made to feel he is a partner in planning and carrying out his therapy.[40]

The use of self-medication programs for hospitalized patients is believed to be an educational strategy to aid the patient in compliance after hospitalization. According to medication standards from the Joint Commission on Accreditation of Hospitals, self-administration of medications shall be permitted only when specifically ordered by house staff or physicians.[129] When diligently taught, patients can self-administer medications at error rates lower than or comparable with those found in many traditional medication distribution and administration systems. For patients of average intelligence, it is suggested that medications be stabilized so that the patient can learn to self-administer them by repetition. It is sometimes easier to teach a patient one medication dosage and regimen at a time until he is self-administering the entire prescribed regimen.[107] It is my opinion that the evidence on teaching effectiveness of medication self-administration programs is not complete.

The problem-solving, teaching-learning complexities of medicine taking can be illustrated by one study of 100 children, ages 1 to 2 years, with acute otitis media, seen in an outpatient department.[76] Only five were found to be in full compliance. Some difficulties occurred at the local pharmacy, where all but two of the families went to get the medicines. There, 15% of antibiotic prescriptions were underfilled, and in seven instances labels were incorrect. At home, 20 of the families waited 1 to 2 hours before giving their child a second medicine because they were afraid to give more than one at a time; thus they could not administer the prescribed doses of each during the child's waking hours. They did not give the curative antibiotic medicines more reliably than medicines for symptomatic relief. Only four families could identify medicines completely and state their purposes. Many thought one or both of the medicines should relieve fever and pain directly in the first day and did not give aspirin once the prescription medicines had been started. Medicine spilled, was not refrigerated, or was taken by a sibling. A second group of 33 children received the medication from the hospital pharmacy, with verbal and written instructions, a graduated medicine tube to administer the doses, an illustrated calendar, with much of this material to be taped to the refrigerator where the antibiotic was stored. Full compliance rate was judged to be 51%. One wonders if this was determined by an external evaluator!

In general, combination approaches with heavy emphasis on behavioral approaches (not simply gaining of knowledge) seem to work best. For hypertension, these include having the patient measure and record blood pressure and medication daily, tailoring the regimen to his habits and rituals, and scheduling closer supervision.[108] In another study, the combination of exit interview for reinforcement of instructions, home visit to increase family support, and small group sessions to increase patient understanding and feeling of self-confidence about his problem was more effective than combinations of only two of these interventions.[95] The design and completeness of the intervention do appear to be important; one study found that screening for hypertension, telling those who had it and giving them a fact-oriented educational pro-

gram, was associated with increased absenteeism from work, compared with those workers' own previous records.[50] One might hypothesize that the educational treatment was incomplete in assisting patients with changing self-concepts and coping behaviors.

PROTOCOLS FOR IMPLEMENTATION OF PATIENT EDUCATION

As institutions have had more experience in developing and implementing patient education, useful materials have been produced, describing the institutions' educational processes and structures and making their actual teaching plans and guidelines available.

Development of teaching plans and guidelines at Tufts–New England Medical Center Hospital utilized a format and protocol that would provide a reference for the content knowledge the nurses need and a documentation tool to provide adequate data for audit.[138] Although individual agencies have developed many such materials and forms, there has been no central source of access to them. The American Hospital Association materials do provide useful examples.[4]

SUMMARY

Considerable experience has been accumulated in designing and implementing delivery systems for patient education for institutions and for patient groups, usually defined by disease entity. Coordinated planning at suprainstitutional levels is less visible, with the possible exception of scattered initiatives in legislation.

STUDY QUESTIONS

1. In 1967, a study was done by Bergman and Stamm to describe the amount of cardiac "nondisease" that existed in children. Of 20,500 school children of junior high school age, 93 were reported by parents to have had heart disease or rheumatic fever at one time. Heart disease was found to be present in 18% of the 93. Thirty (40%) were judged to be restricted in some way; six were severely restricted. The amount of disability from cardiac nondisease in children was estimated to be

Selected findings[12]	Educational reason and/or intervention
A. Confusion among parents about heart disease, especially heart attacks from overexertion, played a major contributing part.	A.
B. Children were particularly susceptible if there were close relatives with heart disease.	B.
C. If the parent recalled specific instructions from the physician, either for or against restriction, they tended to be followed. In cases in which they perceived that no strong statement about activity was made, restriction was apt to occur on the basis of the parents' own instincts. A high percentage of parents in the cardiac nondisease, restricted group still had doubts about what was supposed to be wrong with the child's heart.	C.

greater than that due to actual heart disease.[12] In the box above are selected findings from this study. Identify an educational reason and/or intervention that might be used with each.

2. Oremband and Oremband report a 1970 survey of 20 Bay Area hospitals, which include the leading pediatric facilities of the area. Eight hospitals had no plan for preparation of children for hospitalization. The remaining 12 had a broad spectrum of practices. Sometimes the program required referral by private physicians; therefore some patients were excluded. In some hospitals the program was offered to all by the hospital. In others there were different programs for different treatments or disease entities; these were only for a few, such as those patients who were scheduled for tonsillectomies and adenoidectomies or who had cardiac problems. Out of these 20 hospitals, only one had a comprehensive preparation program, including both prehospital and inpatient preparation.[88] How typical would you predict this situation to be?

3. A small hospital established a new education department. Also established was an educational advisory committee composed of department heads. The committee established the following goals for the educational services department:

1. To meet the expectations of the public for quality health care.
2. To maximize the utilization of resources, such as personnel, equipment, and facilities.
3. To assist personnel to adapt to the changing health care scene.
4. To relate attainment of employees' personal goals to quality care.
5. To recognize and preserve the human dignity of all patients and employees.
6. To assist in coordinating interdepartmental operations.
7. To provide a mechanism for conflict resolution within the hospital.
8. To preserve and maintain the hospital in its goal of meeting the health needs of patients and the personal goals of employees.
9. To centralize all training resources, such as materials, equipment, and personnel, into one department.*

How realistic are the goals?

4. How would you respond to a physician who is concerned that patient education in general might keep patients dependent?

5. In a large survey about the public's knowledge about high blood pressure, only 39% saw nurses as sources of information.[96] Does that surprise you? Why or why not?

---

*Kohles, Sr. M. T.: Education and training support quality assurance. Reprinted with permission from Hospitals, J. Am. Hosp. Assoc. **48:**(19):149-153, Oct. 1, 1974.

REFERENCES

1. Abercrombie, M. L. J.: Working with groups. In Health education theory and practice in cancer control, Geneva, 1974, International Union Against Cancer, pp. 28-36.

2. Albert, S.: Storefront converted to health education center, Hospitals **49:**57-59, Feb. 16, 1975.

3. Alderman, M. H., and Schoenbaum, E. E.: Detection and treatment of hypertension at the work site, New Engl. J. Med. **293:**65-68, 1975.

4. American Hospital Association: Implementing patient education in the hospital, Chicago, 1979, The Association.

5. American Hospital Association: Professional accreditation and legal statements supporting patient education, Chicago, 1979, The Association.

6. American Hospital Association: Statement on the role and responsibilities of hospitals and other health care institutions in personal and community health education, Chicago, 1974, The Association.

7. Antonovsky, A., and Hartman, H.: Delay in the detection of cancer; a review of the literature, Health Educ. Monogr. **2:**98-128, 1974.

8. Aufhauser, T. R., and Lesh, D.: Parents need t.l.c., too, Hospitals **47:**88-91, April 16, 1973.

9. Barnard, K. E., and Powell, M. L.: Teaching children with developmental problems; a family care approach, ed. 2, St. Louis, 1976, The C. V. Mosby Co.

10. Beck, E., and others: Advocacy and compliance in genetic screening, N. Engl. J. Med. **291:**1166-1170, 1974.

11. Beloff, J. S., and Korper, M.: The health team model and medical care utilization, J.A.M.A. **219:**359-366, 1972.

12. Bergman, A. B., and Stamm, S. J.: The morbidity of cardiac nondisease in schoolchildren, N. Engl. J. Med. **276:**1008-1013, 1967.

13. Blackwell, B.: Drug therapy; patient compliance, New Engl. J. Med. **289:**249-252, 1973.

14. Blue Cross now ready to reimburse patients for health education, Am. J. Nurs. **75:**216-218, 1975.

15. Bracken, M. B., and Kasl, S. V.: Delay in seeking induced abortion; a review and theoretical analysis, Am. J. Obstet. Gynecol. **121:**1008-1019, 1975.

16. Bruhn, J. G., and others: Patients' reactions to death in a coronary care unit, J. Psychosom. Res. **14:**65-70, 1970.

17. Bryant, D. and others: Computerized surveillance of diabetic patient/health care delivery system interfaces, Diabetes Care **1:**141-145, 1978.

18. Carlson, C. E., and Vernon, D. T. A.: Measurement of informativeness of hospital staff members, Nurs. Res. **22:**198-206, 1973.

19. Carlson, S. S., and Asnes, R. S.: Maternal expectations and attitudes toward toilet training; a comparison between clinic mothers and private practice mothers, J. Pediatr. **84:**148-151, 1974.

20. Chamberlin, R. W.: Management of preschool behavior problems, Pediatr. Clin. North Am. **21:**33-47, 1974.

21. Childs, B.: A place for genetics in health education, and vice versa, Am. J. Hum. Genet. **26:**120-135, 1974.

22. De-Nour, A. K., and others: A study of chronic hemodialysis teams—differences in opinions and expectations, J. Chronic Dis. **25:**441-448, 1972.

23. Diabetes educators organize, Am. J. Nurs. **74:**930, 1974.

24. Duncan, J. M., and others: A program for the teaching of cardiovascular patients, Heart Lung **2:**508-511, 1973.

25. Easson, E. C.: The role of the doctor in public education. In Health education theory and practice in cancer control, Geneva, 1974, International Union Against Cancer, pp. 14-20.

26. Eckel, F. M.: Community-oriented pharmacy services, Am. J. Hosp. Pharm. **30:**425-427, 1973.

27. The educated patient; a new health care resource, Hospitals **48:**88-90, Sept. 1, 1974.

28. Elder, M.-S.:Nurse counseling on sexuality, Nurs. Outlook **18:**38-40, Nov. 1970.

29. Ellinoy, B. J., and others: A pharmacy outpatient monitoring program providing primary medical care to selected patients, Am. J. Hosp. Pharm. **30:**593-598, 1973.

30. Eney, R. D., and Goldstein, E. O.: Compliance of chronic asthmatics with oral administration of theophylline as measured by serum and salivary levels, Pediatrics **57:**513-517, 1976.

31. Finnerty, F. A., Jr., and others: Hypertension in the inner city. I. Analysis of clinic dropouts, Circulation **47:**73-78, 1973.

32. Fischman, S. H., and others: The impact of family planning classes on contraceptive knowledge, acceptance, and use, Health Educ. Monogr. **2:**246-259, 1974.

33. Fletcher, S. W., and others: Improving emergency-room patient follow-up in a metropolitan teaching hospital, N. Engl. J. Med. **291:**385-388, 1974.

34. Freemon, B. L., and others: How do nurses expand their roles in well child care? Am. J. Nurs. **72:**1866-1871, 1972.

35. Furstenberg, F. F., Jr.: Birth control experience among pregnant adolescents; the process of unplanned parenthood, Soc. Probs. **19:**192-203, 1971.

36. Fylling, C. P., and Etzwiler, D. D.: Health education, Hospitals **49:**95-98, April 1, 1975.

37. Garfield, S. R.: The delivery of medical care, Sci. Am. **222:**15-23, April 1970.
38. Gargaro, W. J., Jr., Esq.: Cancer nursing and the law; informed consent (part 3), Cancer Nurs. **1:**249-250, 1978.
39. Gayton, W. F., and Waler, L.: Down syndrome; informing the parents, Am. J. Dis. Child. **127:**510-512, 1974.
40. Gillum, R. F., and Barsky, A. J.: Diagnosis and management of patient noncompliance, J.A.M.A. **228:** 1563-1567, 1974.
41. Gozzi, E. K., and others: Gaps in doctor-patient communication, Am. J. Nurs. **69:**529-533, 1969.
42. Green, L. W.: Evaluation and measurement; some dilemmas for health education, Am. J. Public Health **67:**155-161, 1977.
43. Griffith, E. W., and Madero, B.: Primary hypertension; patients' learning needs, Am. J. Nurs. **73:**624-627, 1973.
44. Grissinger, S. E., and others: A protocol for consultation with discharged patients about their medications, Hosp. Pharm. **8:**175-183, 1973.
45. Hackett, T. P., and Cassem, N. J.: Factors contributing to delay in responding to the signs and symptoms of acute myocardial infarction, Am. J. Cardiol. **24:** 651-658, 1969.
46. Hackett, T. P., and others: Patient delay in cancer, N. Engl. J. Med. **289:**14-20, 1973.
47. Harris, B. G.: Private practice in childbirth education. In Hall, J. E., and Weaver, B. R., editors: Distributive nursing practice; a systems approach to community health, Philadelphia, 1977, J. B. Lippincott Co.
48. Hart, L. K., and Frantz, R. A.: Characteristics of postoperative patient-education programs for open-heart surgery patients in the United States, Heart Lung **6:**137-142, 1977.
49. Haynes, R. B.: A critical review of the "determinants" of patient compliance with therapeutic regimens. In Sackett, D. L., and Haynes, R. B., editors: Compliance with therapeutic regimens, Baltimore, 1976, The Johns Hopkins University Press.
50. Haynes, R. B., and others: Increased absenteeism from work after detection and labeling of hypertensive patients, New Engl. J. Med. **299:**741-744, 1978.
51. Hemelt, M. D., and Macker, M. E.: Dynamics of law in nursing and health care, Reston, Virginia, 1978, Reston Publishing Co.
52. Holleb, A. I.: Status of knowledge about cancer relevant to public education, Health Educ. Monogr. **36:**3-10, 1973.
53. Hussar, D. A.: Patient noncompliance, J. Am. Pharm. Assoc. **15:**183-201, 1975.
54. Hypertension Detection and Follow-up Program Cooperative Group: Patient participation in a hypertension control program, J.A.M.A. **239:**1507-1514, 1978.
55. Jaffe, F. S.: Public policy on fertility control, Sci. Am. **229:**17-23, July 1973.
56. Kohles, M. T., Sr.: Education and training support quality assurance, Hospitals **48:**149-153, Oct. 1, 1974.
57. Korsch, B. M., and Negrete, V. F.: Doctor-patient communication, Sci. Am. **227:**66-75, Aug. 1972.
58. Korsch, B. M., and others: Practical implications of doctor-patient interaction analysis for pediatric practice, Am. J. Dis. Child. **121:**110-124, 1971.
59. Kos, B., and Culbert, P.: Teaching patients about pacemakers, Am. J. Nurs. **71:**523-527, 1971.
60. Langer, E. J., and others: Reduction of psychological stress in surgical patients, J. Exp. Soc. Psychol. **11:** 155-165, 1975.
61. Lansky, S. B., and others: School phobia in children with malignant neoplasms, Am. J. Dis. Child. **129:**42-46, 1975.
62. Leary, J. A., and others: Self-administered medications, Am. J. Nurs. **71:**1193-1194, 1971.
63. Lehmann, J. F., and others: Cancer rehabilitation; assessment of need, development and evaluation of a model of care, Arch. Phys. Med. Rehabil. **59:**410-419, 1978.
64. Leonard, C. O., and others: Genetic counseling; a consumer's view, N. Engl. J. Med. **287:**433-439, 1972.
65. Levine, D. M., and others: Health education for hypertensive patients, J.A.M.A. **241:**1700-1703, 1979.
66. Levine, P. H., and Britten, A. F. H.: Supervised patient-management of hemophilia, Ann. Intern. Med. **78:**195-201, 1973.
67. Lindeman, C. A., and Stetzer, S. L.: Effect of preoperative visits by operating room nurses, Nurs. Res. **22:**4-16, 1973.
68. Lindeman, C. A., and VanAernam, B.: Nursing intervention with the presurgical patient—the effects of structured and unstructured preoperative teaching, Nurs. Res. **20:**319-332, 1971.
69. Little, Arthur D., Inc.: A survey of consumer health education programs, Contract DHEW 100-75-0082, Washington, D.C., 1976, Department of Health, Education and Welfare.
70. McCone, C.: Preadmission patient teaching clinic, Can. Nurse **69:**39, Sept. 1973.
71. McCrae, W. M., and Cull, A. M.: Cystic fibrosis; parents' response to the genetic basis of the disease, Lancet, July 21, 1973, pp. 141-143.
72. McKenney, J. M., and others: The effect of clinical pharmacy services on patients with essential hypertension, Circulation **48:**1104-1111, 1973.

73. McKinlay, J. B., editor: Politics and law in health care policy, New York, 1973, Neale Watson Academic Publications, Inc.

74. Mackie, M.: Lay perception of heart disease in an Alberta community, Can. J. Public Health **64:**445-454, 1973.

75. Marsh, W. W., and Perlman, L. V.: Understanding congestive heart failure and self-administration of digoxin, Geriatrics **27:**65-70, July 1972.

76. Mattar, M. E., and others: Pharmaceutic factors affecting pediatric compliance, Pediatrics **55:**101-108, 1975.

77. Mazzullo, J. M., and others: Variations in interpretation of prescription instructions, J.A.M.A. **227:**929-931, 1974.

78. Meserko, V.: Preoperative classes for cardiac patients, Am. J. Nurs. **73:**665, 1973.

79. Mikkelson, M. K., and others: Ambulatory tuberculosis chemotherapy on an Indian reservation, Chest **64:**570-573, 1973.

80. Miller, L. V., and Goldstein, J.: More efficient care of diabetic patients in county-hospital setting, N. Engl. J. Med. **286:**1388-1391, 1972.

81. Miller, W. B.: Psychological vulnerability to unwanted pregnancy, Fam. Plann. Perspect. **5:**199-201, 1973.

82. Millis, J. S.: Looking ahead—the report of the Study Commission in Pharmacy, Am. J. Hosp. Pharm. **33:**134-138, 1976.

83. National high blood pressure education program; executive summary of the Task Force reports to the Hypertension Information and Education Advisory Committee, Washington, D.C., 1973, Department of Health, Education and Welfare.

84. National high blood pressure education program; report to the Hypertension Information and Education Advisory Committee, Task Force III—community education, Washington, D.C., 1973, Department of Health, Education and Welfare.

85. Nemchik, R.: Developing an education program. In Guthrie, D. W., and Guthrie, R. A., editors: Nursing management of diabetes mellitus, St. Louis, 1977, The C. V. Mosby Co.

86. Nordberg, T.: Third-party payment for patient education, Am. J. Nurs. **76:**1269-1271, 1976.

87. Nordberg, T.: Qualifying for third party reimbursement; two case histories, Diabetes Educator **3**(2):21-22, 1977.

88. Oremband, E. K., and Oremband, J. D., editors: The effects of hospitalization on children; models for their care, Springfield, Ill., 1973, Charles C Thomas, Publisher.

89. Organizing and implementing an inpatient education program, Lutherville, Md., 1977, Maryland Hospital Education Institute.

90. Petty, T. L.: Ambulatory care for emphysema and chronic bronchitis, Chest **58:**441-448, 1970.

91. Phillips, H. T., and Larkin, M. C.: Staff education for continuity of care, Hospitals **46:**54-57, 106, Feb. 16, 1972.

92. Pless, I. B., and Satterwhite, B.: Chronic illness in childhood; selection, activities and evaluation of nonprofessional family counselors, Clin. Pediatr. **11:**403-410, 1972.

93. Polansky, N. A., and others: Roots of futility, San Francisco, 1972, Jossey-Bass, Inc., Publishers.

94. Presser, H. B.: Early motherhood; ignorance or bliss? Fam. Plann. Perspect. **6:**8-14, 1974.

95. Prsala, H.: Admission unit dispels fear of surgery, Can. Nurse **70:**24-26, Dec. 1974.

96. The public and high blood pressure; a survey conducted for the National Heart and Lung Institute, Washington, D.C., 1973, Department of Health, Education and Welfare.

97. The public's awareness and use of cancer detection tests; conducted for The American Cancer Society, Princeton, N.J., 1974, The Gallup Organization, Inc.

98. Rabiner, S. F., and Fajardo, R.: Home transfusions of hemophiliacs, J.A.M.A. **221:**885-887, 1972.

99. Reichelt, P. A., and Werley, H. H.: A sex information program for sexually active teenagers, J. Sch. Health **45:**100-107, 1975.

100. Reilly, P.: Sickle cell anemia legislation, J. Legal Med. **1:**39-48, Sept.-Oct. 1973.

101. Reilly, P.: Sickle cell anemia legislation, J. Legal Med. **1:**36-40, Nov.-Dec. 1973.

102. Report of the Joint Committee for Stroke Facilities. IV. Guidelines for the nursing care of stroke patients, Stroke **3:**632-681, 1972.

103. The Report of the President's Committee on Health Education, New York, 1971.

104. Report of task force on the pharmacist's clinical role, J. Am. Pharm. Assoc. **11:**482-485, 1971.

105. Riccardi, V. M., and others: Genetic counseling as part of hospital care, Am. J. Public Health **68:**652-655, 1978.

106. Ritchey, M. G., and Leff, A. M.: Venereal disease control among homosexuals; an outreach program, J.A.M.A. **232:**509-510, 1975.

107. Roberts, C. J., and Miller, W. A.: Clinical pharmacy, self-administration, and technician drug administration services in a 72-bed hospital, Drug Intell. Clin. Pharm. **6:**408-415, 1972.

108. Sackett, D. L., and others: Patient compliance with antihypertensive regimens, Patient Counsell. Health Educ. **1**(1):18-21, 1978.

109. Scalzi, C. C.: Nursing management of behavioral responses following an acute myocardial infarction, Heart Lung **2:**62-69, 1973.

110. Schechter, D. S.: Hospital trainers tell problems, needs, Hospitals **48**:65-78, May 16, 1974.

111. Schmitt, F. E., and Woolridge, P. J.: Psychological preparation of surgical patients, Nurs. Res. **22**:108-116, 1973.

112. Schropp, M. L.: Patient education; brink of a boom, Group Practice, Sept.-Oct. 1974, pp. 8-11.

113. Scott, R. A.: The making of blind men; a study of adult socialization, New York, 1969, Russell Sage Foundation.

114. Sczekalla, R. M.: Stress reactions of CCU patients to resuscitation procedures on other patients, Nurs. Res. **22**:65-72, 1973.

115. Sergis, E., and Hilgartner, M. W.: Hemophilia, Am. J. Nurs. **72**:2011-2020, 1972.

116. Shapiro, M. I., and others: Community health services for stroke, Stroke **5**:115-144, 1974.

117. Sibinga, M. S., and Friedman, C. J.: Complexities of parental understanding of phenylketonuria, Pediatrics **48**:216-224, 1971.

118. Signell, K. A.: Kindergarten entry; a preventive approach to community mental health, Community Ment. Health J. **8**:60-70, 1972.

119. Skelton, M., and Dominian, J.: Psychological stress in wives of patients with myocardial infarction, Br. Med. J., April 14, 1973, pp. 101-103.

120. Sobel, D. E.: Personalization on the coronary care unit, Am. J. Nurs. **69**:1439-1442, 1969.

121. Sorenson, J. R.: Biomedical innovation, uncertainty, and doctor-patient interaction, J. Health Soc. Behav. **15**:366-374, 1974.

122. Starfield, B., and Borkowf, S.: Physicians' recognition of complaints made by parents about their children's health, Pediatrics **43**:168-172, 1969.

123. Statement on pharmacist-conducted patient counseling, Am. J. Hosp. Pharm. **33**:644-645, 1976.

124. Stead, W. W.: Patient education, the key to success in modern chemotherapy of tuberculosis, Chest **57**:3-4, 1970.

125. Stokes, J. B., III, and Ward, G.: The national high blood pressure education program, Urban Health **3**:56-57, 62, June 1974.

126. Strait, J.: The transsexual patient after surgery, Am. J. Nurs. **73**:462-463, 1973.

127. Svarstad, B. L.: Doctor-patient communication. In Patient education in the primary care setting, Madison, 1978, University of Wisconsin.

128. Tjoe, S. L., and Luria, M. H.: Delays in reaching the cardiac care unit; an analysis, Chest **61**:617-621, 1972.

129. Tousignaut, D. R.: New JCAH standards and modern hospital pharmacy practice, Am. J. Hosp. Pharm. **28**:178-183, 1971.

130. Ulrich, M. R., and Kelley, K. M.: Patient care includes teaching, Hospitals **46**:59-65, April 16, 1972.

131. Walker, J. H., and others: Spina bifida—and the parents, Dev. Med. Child Neurol. **13**:462-476, 1971.

132. Weibert, R. T.: Patient drug education; why, what and how, Minn. Pharmacist **28**:9-11, Aug. 1974.

133. Wenger, N. K.: Benefits of a rehabilitation program following myocardial infarction, Geriatrics **28**:64-67, July 1973.

134. Weingarten, V.: Report of findings and recommendations of the President's Committee on Health Education, Health Educ. Monogr. **2**(Suppl.):11-19, 1974.

135. Werlin, S. H., and Schauffler, H. H.: Structuring policy development for consumer health education, Am. J. Public Health **68**:596-597, 1978.

136. Wesenberg, C.: Consumer health education: steps in planning and developing a hospital based program, J. Cont. Educ. Nurs. **8**:32-34, 1977.

137. Wishnie, H. A., and others: Psychological hazards of convalescence following myocardial infarction, J.A.M.A. **215**:1292-1296, 1971.

138. Zander, K. S., and others: Practical manual for patient teaching, St. Louis, 1978, The C. V. Mosby Co.

CHAPTER 11

Directions and development in delivery of patient education

■ During the past few years, sufficient activity and interest in the delivery of patient education have developed that policy issues have been identified and for some issues programs undertaken. In general, these issues reflect concerns in the broader health field—costs and outcomes, often interacting with a self-care philosophy. There is also more than peripheral interest in "mining" the behavioral sciences generally for their usefulness for health care. Dissemination of materials and expertise has been a major activity by organizations interested in developing patient education.

This chapter focuses on these directions in development of patient education, which are for the most part just beginning, with little information available about the eventual pay-off. As the first two sections indicate, present practice still is not very supportive of patient education. In addition, since there is no coordinated, comprehensive development of patient education, it is likely that the development done by an individual profession can affect both the overall course of patient education and the place of that profession in patient education activity.

BARRIERS TO PRACTICE

Every professional who tries to implement patient education will encounter many barriers to its actualization. Following are some of the major barriers.

Medical versus educational models

Medicine has utilized the disease model to such an extent that it has become known as the medical model. It focuses on identification and cure of pathologic conditions, with the patient as passive recipient of treatment. The educational model focuses on changing the patient's behavior, which is not a cure in the usual sense, and requires the patient to be active in order to learn. Because the dominance of the disease model has not satisfactorily met needs, these two models now coexist in some settings, especially in programs for mental retardation, rehabilitation, and psychiatry. However, the two can compete in an unsatisfactory way, especially in the behavior each requires of the client.[20]

The only reasonable way to deal with the question of admissibility or growth of educational services in a particular setting is to examine data about benefits to patients. Although such data are sometimes available in the literature, the research in most areas of patient education is not sufficient to allow for generalizations. However, case studies or demonstration models may have been reported in a rigorous enough way to serve as an example to be tried in a particular setting. Such models should always be evaluated in the new setting to see if they are working satisfactorily. Another approach, the results of which are often more believable to local practitioners, is to gather data on a group of patients in one's own setting before education and after. Such data can be used during the development period as formative evaluation, to identify weaknesses in the program and correct them, and after development, as a basis for deciding whether a program should continue.

Sharing information seen as threat

The professional-client relationship depends on a differential in skills and knowledge between client and professional, and teaching is an attempt to alter this differential. How much information one should share with the client requires a difficult judgment and must be approached with a conscious rationale and with the patient's welfare as the ultimate criterion. Although probably not well appreciated, withholding information or educational-supportive therapy can be as devastating to the client as withholding other treatment, such as medications. Sharing information can be a tool in building a trusting relationship as well as a means for a client to maintain a medical regimen and a meaningful existence. The patients' rights statement mentioned earlier is based on the premise that the physician and other medical personnel are not always the most competent parties to make certain health-related judgments.[20]

Uncertainty regarding proper content, behavior, and means to obtain it

It is difficult to predict whether teaching will move a client toward desired behavior; moreover, there is often doubt about what behavior would be useful. This uncertainty not only reflects the freedom of both client and professional to hold various values but also indicates a lack of empirical data about the outcomes of particular kinds of behavior that affect health. For example, the relationship between particular kinds of parenting and children's behavior is not clear. One's impulse is to suspect the value of teaching if it lacks such clarity, particularly if one is accustomed to the clarity of a procedure

manual. In view of the potential benefits of therapy, however, the more useful approach is to use a teaching program with corrective feedback and expect that one will not always be successful.[20]

There are several useful responses to the issue of uncertainty. Many staff members will function more comfortably if institutional guidelines are available. Guidelines can take such forms as: a clarifying policy statement about the role of the nurse in patient education; instructional packages with lists of potential objectives, teaching materials, and evaluation tools, from which a nurse can choose those appropriate to a particular client; or inservice education opportunities in patient education. Pressure for conformity or for agreement on teaching methodologies and other approaches to the patient is not useful. There is more than a little evidence that, outside of certain basic guidelines, teaching methodologies are somewhat interchangeable, and strategies of approach often represent varying styles in the helping relationship. It is perhaps best to view the details of patient education as matters of professional judgment delegated to a professional who has at least minimal competency as a helping person and knowledge of the skills the patient must obtain.

Deficient delivery structure

A segmented, incomplete health care delivery structure severely impedes education as therapy. It works against learning as a continuous process and precludes continuous interpretation and support over time. Patient education may not be available in otherwise comprehensive health care institutions. Such systems provide attention to the patient when he is physically ill and not necessarily when he is ready to learn.

Physician dominance

Physicians are the only health professionals with unlimited license to practice; yet their use of educational therapy has been limited. Because of the natural dominance of this group in the fields of health and disease, it is difficult for an approach with which they are not familiar to gain legitimacy. Nurses, whose license may more or less explicitly include health teaching, are thus placed in a difficult position. Physicians rightfully control the prerogative to share information, at least initial information, in such key areas as diagnosis, prognosis, and often treatment plan. This information is often a prerequisite to independent or follow-up teaching by the nurse. The teaching roles of the two professions could be clarified not only by a definition of standards of practice for both but also through standing orders for educational therapy or educational experiences (such as cardiac rehabilitation classes), which physicians could order for their patients, often jointly planned and implemented by the two (and more) professions.[20]

Perhaps the nurse is in a more ambiguous position regarding patient education than are other professionals whose areas of expertise are more sharply defined and perhaps better understood by physicians. Nutritionists deal with diet, pharmacists with medications, physical therapists with physical training. Teaching by nurses focuses on support of activities for daily living, on integration of the patient's and family's experiences in the health situation, and often on coordination and reinforcement of teaching with other disciplines so that the patient finds a feasible way to change his life. Looked at from another point of view, society and physicians have implicitly, but often not explicitly, delegated a great deal of the personal support roles to other health workers, who give much of the direct care to patients. It is mandatory for such professions giving direct care to demand explicit clarity about their role and responsibilities.

Nursing support

Theoretically, nursing has long been committed to an instructional role with clients; however, available evidence (as presented in several portions of this book) does not strongly indicate that this commitment has always been actualized. Since many nurses have largely followed medical thought and practice, which may not have been supportive of patient education, they may feel a lack of confidence in their teaching skills. Indeed, nurses have not been accountable for teaching as a part of nursing care, although instruction in communication skills and in elements of a helping relationship, which are basic to teaching, has undergone considerable change in nursing education in recent years. Nevertheless, in view of the ambiguity of standards and predictability of outcomes, nurses need the support of colleagues in their teaching efforts.

TASKS BEFORE NURSING

Nursing is moving to implement a total person, or a holistic, approach to practice in health as well as illness. It is clear that the need for assistance in learning about health may be the primary need of many clients at a particular time. Thus nursing must make certain that its practitioners are organized and able to provide the public with care that meets minimum standards.

Definition of standards of practice

Standards should define as malpractice not only the omission of teaching when it could reasonably be expected to be therapeutic but also the production of incapacitating confusion or the forcing of values on the patient when it could reasonably have been avoided.[20] Meanwhile, process criteria seem useful, at least as a focus, for describing the full range of patients' needs that an institution serves and for setting priorities for practice. The following guidelines are suggested[21]:

1. Document the need for teaching for all rational patients and for families of nonrational patients.
2. Develop a priority system for meeting patient education needs.
3. Ensure that all patients or their agents

have adequate understanding and skill to carry out prescribed treatments safely, including medications that will be self-administered. Medical regimens often introduce powerful therapeutic agents that are new to patients. Many patients have no reasonable way of learning how to avoid the dangers of such agents, unless they are provided with instruction (not just information).

4. Ensure adequate skill in and understanding of self-care activities, to the extent that the contract with the patient requires. Adults are largely responsible for the health aspects of their daily living functions. During illness they often need help with those functions. However, the goal is to return that responsibility to these individuals. They retain the right to perform those functions as they wish, unless affected by law or by a contract with a health professional for services.

5. Demonstrate evidence of adequate skill in the process of teaching. Obtain and use assessment of client readiness (motivation and already existing skills and knowledge). Articulate clearly goals that reflect client readiness and desired medical outcomes. Develop facility with a range of instructional methodologies and be able to match them to the kind of learning to be accomplished. Obtain and interpret evaluative data and be able to correct the teaching process as suggested by the data.

A priority system for meeting patients' needs for education (the second standard) might be developed in the following way:

1. *Acute* educational needs exist when a lack of understanding is causing psychosocial anguish, physical danger, or both.

2. *Preventive* educational needs exist when a condition of some threat is likely to occur to an individual or group that has little skill for handling it. The seriousness of the threat and the probability of its occurring both vary.

3. *Maintenance* educational needs exist for those who are living with medically derived alterations in their living patterns and will need more or less frequent reteaching and for those whose deficit of understanding and skill is causing difficulty with normal developmental tasks.

Although not inclusive, two brief examples of patients and families with acute educational needs may help to clarify this category system. Psychosocial anguish is seen in the explosive tension that builds up in the family of a patient who is at home after myocardial infarction, if neither the patient nor the family understands the nature of the disease or the physician's instructions. Physical danger is present when a patient who is taking anticoagulants has a serious bleeding episode and does not know how to handle it or how to distinguish it from minor bleeding episodes.

Preventive needs vary in their predictability, but obvious examples include patients who rate very high on risk factors for cardiovascular disease or diabetes and who could be taught to reduce these risks and to recognize the disease in its early stages.

The maintenance category of educational needs recognizes that many persons with chronic disease, who are on a long-term medical regimen, will decrease their degree of compliance. Reteaching, usually combined with screening for complications, can boost that compliance. A person whose social competency and understanding is minimal (such as a mentally retarded adult) may well need periodic education in times of change and stress, such as when he or she becomes a parent.

These categories are quite fluid and sometimes not mutually exclusive. However, such a system allows for setting priorities according to an estimate of the seriousness of the difficulty. It should also allow for analysis of the nurse's pattern of responding to needs. For example, are maintenance and preventive needs too often allowed to become acute?

Core of nurses able to practice according to standards

Evidence of a body of nurses able to practice patient education according to clearly defined standards of practice is most essential. It is not now clear how large a core exists, but models of practice should be made available to the community of practitioners. For example, Marcella Davis has suggested that psychologic monitoring be practiced in the coronary care unit.[9] Such practice could be demonstrated and thus emulated by others through a videotaped or filmed presentation of Ms. Davis's practice. My experience is that practitioners are highly criticial of the teaching shown on videotapes; paradoxically, they also affirm that if the amount of teaching observed would occur in their own settings, it would be a distinct improvement. If such teaching models are made available to nurses, conformity should not be demanded, particularly when teaching still requires an element of art.[20]

Excellence in the teaching-supportive aspects of care is central to expanded nursing roles. Moreover, we need to provide nurses wishing to improve their teaching skills with the same conditions that patients need: that is, an open, warm relationship with someone whose behavior they can use as a model and who can help them to analyze their own. This might be done by assigning a nurse to a teaching team or to a mentor who would aid in developing increasingly complex teaching skills.[20]

Almost nothing is reported on staff development for patient education. One is forced, therefore, to fall back on more general research and limited findings in order to construct what might be a reasonable approach to it.

Basic helping skills

In his book *Helping and Human Relations,* Robert Carkhuff summarized a great deal of research that is central to this topic.[6] The effectiveness of counseling and psychotherapy, education, supervision, and parenting, all of which are seen as helping processes, depends on certain characteristics and skills of the helper. To be minimally helpful, one must be functioning at a particular level of empathy, concreteness, genuineness, and self-disclosure and communicate respect and immediacy in the relationship. These behaviors allow one to be facilitative. The second characteristic of effective helpers is that they stimulate action or direction-oriented work in the relationship with the client. Several things must be noted about present training programs for professionals. They concentrate on discriminative learning of theory and not on the skills of helping, apparently not relating the two elements. One needs practice in a helping role, but teaching of discrimination about theories does not translate itself readily into functioning in this role. It is indeed possible to become a less effective helper, or at least not to improve one's skills, through one's experiences in a professional school. There is not much evidence that use of one theory is superior to use of another.[6,7]

How do nurses rate in helping skills? A single study, focusing on how the patient perceived the relationship, found nurses to be lowest of all professionals (educators, lawyers, clergy, mental health professionals) tested.[28]

Knowledge of content

Another difficulty with the teaching role is the possibility of insufficient knowledge of the subject matter to be taught; a study of venereal disease knowledge of junior and senior high school nurses in Massachusetts found this to be true.[17] Related to this may be the difficulty of projecting what behavior will need to develop, unless one has had experience (often as part of public health nursing) in making such a judgment.

Summary

I know of no comprehensive studies of nurses' helping skills or their knowledge of content to be taught. Compounding the problem is the lack of clarity about standards: what is adequate in terms of patient outcomes, and how do you know good patient education if you see it?

Perhaps a program for staff development might be as follows. Theory of patient education can be learned by reading about it. One might next have groups of nurses view videotapes of nurses doing good patient education, so that they can define for themselves what makes quality care and can retain a mental image of the quality performance. Screening for basic helping skills, perhaps using the Carkhuff scales, may be a useful procedure; but certainly critical would be an assessment of a nurse's actual practice skills in patient education. If they are deficient, a kind of internship with a nurse whose skills are good would be the next step. This should provide practice with feedback, essential to any skill development, and the use of video or audio recordings can provide an accurate account of that practice for later feedback. Work on audit standards can also stimulate staff development.

It should be expected that development of teaching skills will not be valued by and may well constitute a threat for some nurses. Change of focus from direct care to teaching others to give their own care and perceived alteration in balance of power with the patient are factors in the threat.

In providing for high-quality services, we should guard against the nurse's becoming unnecessarily helpful; we should also prevent the isolation and despair that can occur in a patient when instructional programs are not available. Nursing needs to take responsibility for research that will guide patient education in practice. Especially needed are studies showing ways in which combinations of interventions, including teaching, can be employed and how they affect patient welfare.[20]

To take the initiative in providing truly comprehensive care requires initiating effective programs for a full range of socioeconomic and educational backgrounds, regional planning for efficient use of resources, and the use of educational resources as part of continuous care.

CONCEPTUAL, PHILOSOPHICAL, AND PRACTICAL DEVELOPMENTS

A number of developments relating to patient education have emerged relatively recently. One is further concentration of interest in the behavioral aspects of health. Some have described the increased attention to use of behavioral science in health as behavioral medicine, which is an emerging field. It is a field of study, rather than a discipline, and was stimulated by the recognition that life style and behaviors are important determinants of health and illness. Risk modification efforts in behavioral medicine utilize health education, behavioral analysis and control, pain control, biofeedback, relaxation training, and other approaches.[15]

Self-care

Self-care is developing in two ways: (1) as a philosophical position aimed at giving the individual more tools to manage his health, regulate bodily processes, and direct his use of the system and (2) as the delegation of responsibility to patients and families for kinds of medical care formerly provided by health professionals.

Some advocates of self-care see patient education as dominated by professionals' definitions of what patients should learn and too heavily focused on compliance and cooperation. The self-care philosophy aims at improvement of the imbalance in the physician-patient relationship, moving from a dependent one on the part of the patient to more of a contractual one. Although little is known about the amount and kind of self-care given daily by the population, such practices are often ignored by health practitioners as "not real medicine," patients' skills in self-care are not supported, and their definition of the problem not accepted as important.

Self-care may be viewed as involving both the continuous substrate of behavior (custom, life style) and discrete or episodic actions such as self-diagnosis and self-treatment. Self-care practices are particularly prominent at the level of primary care, both in terms of health practices and health judgments. Some functions are complementary to those of a health care practitioner, some substitutive.[16] Some authors have felt that the legal base for self-care is not clear and that laws governing licensing of professionals and delivery of health care reflect the common assumption that medical care is synonymous with health professions. Medical practice acts not uncommonly define practice of medicine and then limit that practice to licensed individuals, overlooking the option of self-care.[1]

A number of educational programs for self-care have developed, as have mutual aid groups. Examples include a program of the Maternity Center Association, in which some of the routine prenatal care was carried out by the couples themselves (urine analyses; checking of blood pressure, weight, height of fundus, and fetal heart tones).[18] The Course for Activated Patients teaches participants use of medical equipment in order to become better observers of common problems, emphasizing the role of life style and use of the health care system, and is estimated to be useful to about one third of the population. The Health Activation Network helps interested individuals to start and evaluate similar programs.[23]

A great deal of work remains to be done in study of and responsible support for self-care. Just as we need to know the effective limits of professional care, the individual self-care model will have limitations for some individuals in some instances, which should be recognized. Tools for self-care also need to be tested. Study of a self-care algorithm that had enjoyed wide distribution raised questions about its effects in overutilization of physicians.[3]

Examples of self-administration and shared management of medically prescribed treatments have been cited in Chapter 10. Dialysis and total parenteral nutrition have successfully been carried out at home. There continues to be experimentation with patient management of still other procedures, testing of the support systems and the technology needed, and comparison of outcomes with professionally provided care in terms of quality and cost. A study of intravenous antibiotic therapy at home found: quality of care as good as that usually provided in the hospital; cost of $40 for home treatment as opposed to $137 had the patients remained in hospital; most patients able to resume normal activities while receiving the home therapy. Patients completed a 1- to 3-day in-hospital training program and could call a nurse for information and assistance if necessary.[25]

Improvement of technology for ease of home use and accuracy is important. For example, a recent study tested glucose and nitrite detection methods for home follow-up of children with recurrent urinary tract infections in an effort for improvement over home culture methods.[27] Home monitoring can have very useful effects on patient motivation, as, for example, with some diabetic patients who began home blood glucose monitoring.[24] The symbolic significance or the timing of the feedback to them of information about the effects of their diet actions may have been the cause.

Cost

Cost has become an increasingly important element in decisions about all of health care, including education. Costs of patient education programs include materials and equipment and staff time for developing, delivering, and evaluating patient education, including associated administrative costs. One must also consider opportunity costs—those of forgoing the activity that would have probably been chosen if the decision had been made not to develop patient education. Benefits from patient education can be medical, social, and administrative and have been suggested throughout this book. They include patient satisfaction, persistence and compliance with regimens, public support, appropriate utilization of health services, and others.[11]

Cost-benefit analysis involves enumerating costs and benefits of each alternative action, whereas cost-effectiveness analysis aims to identify the alternative action with the lowest cost that meets a predetermined standard. Each is useful to assist in decision making.

Such analysis can be done for particular programs and, based on evidence from literature, an estimate made of the potential cost-benefit of paticular health education strategies and particular benefits. For some behaviors, such as increased seat belt usage, health education did not seem to be cost-effective; therefore, an alternate, such as legislation, would need to be used. Improvements in the cost-benefit ratio may be obtained by improved administrative relationships (to make the program function better) and alteration of the degree of coercion of the intervention strategy. Attention also needs to be paid to the point of diminishing returns (when further investment no longer yields increased returns) and the ceiling effect (the largest effect that a particular educational intervention can have, because it misses the unique motives of other individuals, often 50% of them.[11] The length of time the effect holds is also important; some outcomes can be sustained with small, intermittent interventions. This offers the opportunity of continuing benefits with little additional cost.

Long-term studies are important in understanding patterns of morbidity and mortality but often also suffer from inability to separate the effects of various elements in the patients' lives. One such retrospective study was done in a large hospital in Copenhagen; it tried to ascertain the cost-benefit ratio for outpatient supervision for 20 years after diagnosis, on survival of persons with juvenile diabetes mellitus.[10] Presumably, the outpatient supervision included patient instruction, including information about the patient's physiologic condition. With an average of 4.4 annual outpatient follow-up visits, the duration of diabetes (survival) was prolonged by nearly 12 years. The benefit of this prolongation was ten times the cost of the follow-up.

Green has described use of a cost-benefit index that can be used to make comparisons between programs, places, and times.[11] It utilizes notions of potential benefits, the portion of the target population that responded to the program, and the total cost.

Individuals wishing to start patient education programs (or to defend old ones) often are required to provide evidence that the venture can be successful. It is commonplace to cite five or six widely known studies that have shown considerable cost savings and benefits. One must be clear that those studies simply demonstrate that such effects are possible and will not necessarily occur in the new program. It is expected that information about the outcomes of new programs should be obtained regularly and used solely for the purpose of improving them, to obtain the maximum benefits. Such studies should also be done intermittently for older programs, since multiple conditions may change, causing them to lose effectiveness.

Standards

Process standards have probably been most discussed in patient education, although they still appear to be commonly violated in practice. Much of this book is about process standards—reasonable ways of going about teaching patients, which hopefully are backed up with research findings.

The paucity of research findings about the outcomes of patient education has made it difficult to develop standards. Efforts are presently being made to define outcome standards, usually short-term, by the judgments of expert panels, using what literature exists. Some such efforts are part of the definition of all outcomes of care for treatment of a particular disease entity, of which patient knowledge and skills are a part.[2] Some are more completely developed for outcomes from patient education, for example, the efforts of the Working Group to Define Critical Patient Behaviors in High Blood Pressure Control.[30] This group defined four critical behaviors, with further detailed definition of

DISCHARGE PLANNING TOOL

Patient_____ Birth date_____ Discharge date_____
Parents' names_____ Phone #_____
Primary nurse_____ Discharging nurse_____
Follow-up after discharge_____ Appointment date_____
PKU_____ Hct. _____Head circ. _____ Ht._____ Wt._____Eye exam._____

DISCHARGE CRITERIA	YES	NO	COMMENTS
1. Parent knows phone numbers of SCN, Totline, and for source of follow-up			
2. Parent demonstrates bathing baby			
3. Parent demonstrates cord care			
4. Parent demonstrates care of circumcision			
5. Parent demonstrates diapering of baby			
6. Parent is able to take infant's rectal temperature and accurately read thermometer			
7. Parent discusses action and side effects of prescribed medication			
8. Parent administers medication to baby and verbalizes medication schedule			
9. Parent satisfactorily completes any special treatment or procedure to be done upon discharge			
10. Parent has decided whether to breast or bottle feed			
11. Parent discusses frequency and amount of feeding			
12. Parent demonstrates feeding baby			
13. The mother who is breast feeding discusses breast care, milk expression, diet, and identifies a source of support after discharge			
14. Parent discusses formula preparation/sterilization if bottle feeding			
15. Parent discusses conditions of home and defines a plan for integrating the baby into the family			
16. Parent verbalizes expectations for infant's development and plans for appropriate stimulation			
17. Parent discusses when baby may be taken out of the house			
18. Parent demonstrates appropriate bonding behaviors			
19. Parent verbalizes time and place for follow-up care (name of clinic or pediatrician)			
20. Visiting nurse has spoken with parent(s)			
21. Social work referral has been made (if indicated)			

SUMMARY AND FOLLOW-UP PLANS:

Fig. 16. Implicit outcome standards, from discharge planning tool. (From Cagan, J., and Meier, P.: A discharge planning tool for use with families of high risk infants, J. Obstet. Gynecol. Neonat. Nurs. **9**(3):146-148, 1979.)

knowledge, attitudes, and skills. The four critical behaviors are: makes the decision to control blood pressure, takes medication as prescribed, monitors progress toward the blood pressure goal, and resolves problems that block achieving control.[30]

Of course, such standards must be validated in practice in a couple of ways. They must eventually be shown to relate to other desired health goals, such as decrease in morbidity or a feeling of well-being. And they must be attainable. A number of these efforts on the part of expert panels seem to me to be very optimistic for certain subgroups of patients.

Of course, more or less explicit outcome standards are followed every day in practice. An example is given in Fig. 16, in the form of a discharge planning tool for parents of high-risk infants. It serves not only to consolidate previously scattered information about the parents' skills but also defines those behaviors that must be obtained.

DEVELOPMENT AND RESEARCH IN PATIENT EDUCATION

Quality control methods, already known in the field of education, must be instituted in patient education as a routine part of practice. At the same time, well-designed research on important questions needs to be done to determine and optimize the therapeutic value of patient education.

Development

Two deficits stand out glaringly when one looks at the field of practice: lack of tested teaching tools and lack of evaluative instruments. It is difficult to think of significant advancement in the field without basic development work in these areas.

Educational product development techniques typically require setting a standard of desired learning (criterion), developing the product and trying it with a few learners, interviewing and testing them to obtain feedback on the quality of the educational program, revising, trying the product with learners again, and revising until the criterion is met or no further learning gains can be obtained, in which case the criterion may need to be altered. A variety of educational products, reflective of the range of learning goals commonly desired for patients needing education in an area and ranging in abstractness-concreteness to fit different learning abilities, need to be systematically developed for each area of patient education.

In 1976, the Office of Cancer Communications, National Cancer Institute, and the National High Blood Pressure Education Program, National Heart, Lung, and Blood Institute, began working to develop the Health Message Testing Service. The service seeks to provide a standardized testing technique and a bank of normative test data to interpret response to messages.[26] This kind of service should be of great value not only in the specific messages it tests, but also in demonstrating commitment to the concept that a message can be judged and improved.

Test development really should not take the verbal emphasis that it has in schools; instead, it should focus on the real situation in which patients will have to function or on audiovisual simulations of that situation. Such simulations are excellent teaching tools, but their use (and use of a range of tools) in evaluation should provide a basis for more accurate prediction than is now available. These tools should indicate the way in which the patient will assume the behaviors required by the learning goals.

The national survey of evaluation efforts in health education (see Chapter 10) recommends high priority on the long-term impact of programs; study of the intensity and duration of educational intervention required to produce and sustain appropriate impact; development of standard measurement instruments; evaluation of impact on costs, utilization of services, and manpower; and use of prospective instead of retrospective studies to improve the quality of data.

Research

Basic to research are appropriate questions that can be studied, theoretic frameworks, and tools of research methodology. Perhaps most critical is description of questions to which research should be addressed in order to assist development of the field. One such question inquires about the kind and amount of patient learning that occurs in health care institutions: how much of it is intended and how much is nonbeneficial to patients? A second question seeks to find out the limits of power of patient education therapy: given optimal teaching conditions, how much of a problem can be reduced? Compliance with medication regimens provides an example. Given adequate labels on medications, written and verbal explanations of why the medications should be taken, teaching calendars necessary to serve as memory aids, adequate description (written, audiovisual, or both) about intended effects and side-effects, practice to criterion on all major learning goals, easy availability of advice by telephone (should the patient have problems), and persuasion to commitment on the part of the patient and his significant others, how much of the compliance problem could be eliminated? Such a system is not necessarily difficult to provide, and it is superior to using one small portion of a potential educational intervention and judging the potential of patient education by it. A third question aims at the interface between education and health care management: what learning goals or systems of treatment are obtainable? For example, can the exchange diet be learned by most diabetic patients? The answer provides an important complement to the question: how good is the system for controlling the disease?

Since both instructional and nursing theory are just beginning to be developed, patient education research will often use eclectic conceptual frameworks based on learning principles or theories on influence from the social sciences. Research tools developed specifically for patient education are almost unknown, and in addition there are few, if any, consistent behavioral measures in medical records.

A compilation and review of tools related to health behavior may be found in the handbook by Reeder and co-workers.[22] A very few instruments have been developed to measure elements directly related to patient instruction; they are, for the most part, in the early stages of development. Carlson and Vernon have developed a measure of informativeness of hospital staff members, first used to assess the amount of information surgeons, anesthetists, and nurses routinely give preoperatively to their patients.[8] One of the factors in a related tool, the Hospital Stress Rating Scale, is "lack of information." In some initial research with the tool, medical patients indicated more stress than did surgical patients, related to this factor, perhaps because procedures and outcomes are likely to be more clear-cut for surgical patients.[29]

Interaction analysis tools have also been developed to describe conversation between patients and staff. An example of such a tool is that developed by Klinzing and associates for use in a pediatric hospital. It includes coding categories such as "gives the patient directions, orders," and "gives information to the patient."[14] Experience with such tools in the field of education has found that enormous numbers of categories can be generated, describing content, affect, interaction processes, and so on. A very complex system of categorizing the events is often necessary to capture the reality of the situation being described.

Some examples of verbal achievement tests do occur in the literature, but rarely is information about their validity available. When published, they are sources of items; however, they have all the limitations of highly verbal testing methods, usually testing in the cognitive domain only and also usually at lower levels of that domain.[4,19]

In research in patient education, it is especially crucial to describe the independent variable and to determine that it clearly differs from the control condition. It is indeed possible to end up appraising nonevents! Description should take place at several levels: (1) institutional commitment—as found in the program's description, pronouncements, and statements of intention; (2) structural context—managerial acts such as hiring people, forming committees, scheduling classes, and purchasing instructional materials; (3) role performance—the behavior patterns of teachers observed to change or to conform with the role performance required by the innovation; and (4) learning activities—those required in the treatment that the student is actually doing.

Green and Figa-Talamanca have suggested several experimental designs for evaluation of patient education programs.[12] The more experimental designs, with random assignment of subjects to treatments, the more desirable; this is true for experimental designs for research. To avoid ethical problems of withholding treatment, control groups can receive education at the conclusion of the treatment. Several of the recommended designs incorporate multiple observation points over time in order to study sustained or diminished effects of the educational program. Such effects include delayed impact, decay, or forgetting. An example may be found in a study done by Green and co-workers on the impact of aides on homemakers' improvements in nutrition. The impact diminished after a year, suggesting that a shift in the educational treatment would be necessary if criterion goals had still not been met.[13]

REFERENCES

1. Andrews, L. B., and Levin, L. S.: Self-care and the law, Social Policy **9**(4):44-49, 1979.
2. Avery, A. D., and others: Quality of medical care assessment using outcome measures; eight disease-specific applications, Santa Monica, Calif., 1976, The Rand Corporation (R-2021 DHEW).
3. Berg, A. O., and LoGerfo, J. P.: Potential effect of self-care algorithms on the number of physician visits, N. Engl. J. Med. **300**:535-537, 1979.
4. Black, L. F., and Mitchell, M. M.: Evaluation of a patient education program for chronic obstructive pul-

monary disease, Mayo Clin. Proc. **52**:106-111, 1977.
5. Cagan, J., and Meier, P.: A discharge planning tool for use with families of high risk infants, J. Obstet. Gynecol. Neonat. Nurs. **9**(3):146-148, 1979.
6. Carkhuff, R. R.: Helping and human relations, New York, 1969, Holt, Rinehart & Winston, Inc., Vols. 1 and 2.
7. Carkhuff, R. R.: The development of human resources; education, psychology and social change, New York, 1971, Holt, Rinehart & Winston, Inc.
8. Carlson, C. E., and Vernon, D. T. A.: Measurement of informativeness of hospital staff members, Nurs. Res. **22**:198-206, 1973.
9. Davis, M. A.: Socioemotional component of coronary care, Am. J. Nurs. **72**:705-709, 1972.
10. Deckert, T., and others: Importance of outpatient supervision in the prognosis of juvenile diabetes mellitus; a cost/benefit analysis, Diabetes Care **1**:281-284, 1978.
11. Green, L. W.: Toward cost-benefit evaluations of health education; some concepts, methods and examples, Health Educ. Monogr. **2**(Suppl.):34-64, 1974.
12. Green, L. W., and Figa-Talamanca, I.: Suggested designs for evaluation of patient education programs, Health Educ. Monogr. **2**:54-71, 1974.
13. Green, L. W., and others: A 3-year, longitudinal study of the impact of nutrition aides on the knowledge, attitudes, and practices of rural poor homemakers, Am. J. Public Health **64**:722-724, 1974.
14. Klinzing, D. R., and others: A preliminary report of a methodology to assess the communicative interaction between hospital personnel and hospitalized children, Am. J. Public Health **67**:670-672, 1977.
15. Laman, C., and Evans, R.: Behavioral medicine; an emerging field, Health Values: Achieving High Level Wellness **2**:287-290, 1978.
16. Levin, L. S., and others: Self-care; lay initiatives in health, New York, 1976, Prodist.
17. McGrath, P., and Laliberte, E. B.: Level of basic venereal disease knowledge among junior and senior high school nurses in Massachusetts; a survey, Nurs. Res. **23**:31-37, 1974.
18. Parents; do it yourself, Am. J. Nurs. **78**:1206, 1978.
19. Rahe, R. N., and others: A teaching evaluation questionnaire for postmyocardial infarction patients, Heart Lung **4**:759-769, 1975.
20. Redman, B. K.: Client education therapy in treatment and prevention of cardiovascular diseases, Cardiovasc. Nurs. **10**(1):1-6, 1974.
21. Redman, B. K.: Guidelines for quality of care in patient education, Can. Nurse **71**:19-21, Feb. 1975.
22. Reeder, L. G., and others: Handbook of scales and indices of health behavior, Pacific Palisades, Calif., 1976, Goodyear Publishing Co., Inc.

23. Sehnert, K. W.: A course for activated patients, Social Policy **8**(3):40-46, 1977.
24. Skyler, J. S., and others: Home blood glucose monitoring as an aid in diabetes management, Diabetes Care **1**:150-157, 1978.
25. Stiver, H. G., and others: Intravenous antibiotic at home, Ann. Intern. Med. **89**:690-693, 1978.
26. Testing television messages about health, Public Health Rep. **92**:392, 1977.
27. Todd, J. K.: Home follow-up of urinary tract infection, Am. J. Dis. Child. **131**:860-861, 1977.
28. Truax, C. B., and others: Therapeutic relationships provided by various professionals, J. Community Psychol. **2**:33-36, 1974.
29. Volicer, V. J., and others: Medical-surgical differences in hospital stress factors, J. Hum. Stress **3**(2):3-13, June 1977.
30. Working Group to Define Critical Patient Behaviors in High Blood Pressure Control: Patient behavior for blood pressure control, J.A.M.A. **241**:2534-2537, 1979.

APPENDIX A

Suggested answers to study questions

Chapter 1. The place of teaching in nursing

1. The head nurse's request is open to several interpretations and needs to be clarified with her. The composition of her staff may be such that many members need assistance in carrying out teaching because they lack skills or orientation to the station. The head nurse may see her role as a coordinating one in which she will decrease inconsistencies, misinformation, and omissions in the teaching; this may or may not be the most effective method of achieving the coordination needed for good teaching. Her request does overlook the fact that a nurse cannot always predict when a patient will indicate a need that may best be met by doing the teaching naturally, without hesitation, as care is given. One also wonders whether or not the head nurse has taken into account the teaching that occurs as a result of the general interpersonal environment of the station. Nurses functioning in a truly professional role would rightfully resent the controls this head nurse is placing on their practice.

2. The statement means that there is potential need for behavior change in persons with all disease conditions. Teaching is one means by which behavior change (learning) might be effected.

Chapter 2. Overview of the teaching-learning process

1. Assessing readiness for learning: Sending questionnaires and invitations to parents, as well as hearing their comments about the program for girls, helped to assess their readiness. Reports of teachers seeing evidence of curiosity about sex and of knowledge of normal growth and development indicated readiness on the part of the boys.

2. Objectives are stated in the article as follows:
   a. To establish an intellectually permissive atmosphere in which to discuss relatively simple information about sexual development.
   b. To encourage closer father-son relationships and provide fathers with a starting point for offering further guidance and counsel.

3. Preparing teaching materials and a plan for teaching: Planning included acceptance of the idea by the PTA committee and the principal, sending invitations, preparing a list of teaching materials, deciding to use a speaker who was not a physician, and having the PTA mothers prepare drawings.

4. Carrying out the teaching: The speaker gave a 40-minute talk with slides and conducted a question-and-answer period, which yielded information about readiness of the students for further classes. Content of the classes included functions of reproductive organs and social and psychologic aspects of puberty in boys.

5. Evaluating in terms of the desired learning: A questionnaire indicated a favorable response to the session. When observed for a short period of time, three sixth-grade children seemed to show a lack of embarrassment in discussing the content of the class. One would hope for further evidence of success, particularly on the second objective.

Chapter 3. Readiness for health education

1. Topics for some major lead questions are suggested. They can be followed up to obtain more specific information.
   a. General hygiene—rest, activity, elimination, and nutrition patterns that the individual now follows.
   b. Level of understanding and feelings of the patient about suspected or actual illness; motor skills for self-care, if pertinent.
   c. Understanding and feelings of the patient about the health agency and his role in it.
2. Evidence of wanting to learn is important for situations *a* to *d*.
   a. Your questions should determine the patient's previous experience with catheterization, including her understanding of the purposes for doing it and her general understanding of anatomy of the bladder and urethra.
   b. Your questions should determine the mother's understanding of the purpose of forcing fluids and of how much fluid is necessary and her skills in persuading the child to drink or helping him to drink.
   c. Your questions should determine the women's understanding and feelings about cancer, about preventive care in general, about manipulating their own breasts, and about the meaning of finding a lump. Some may have had instruction in the procedure and will be able to do some or all of it correctly.
   d. Some of your questions should enable you to discover how retarded the boy is. Can he understand language, and, if so, what words? How well can he grasp things and move his arms in a feeling motion? Other questions will deal with his independence and his mother's ability to cooperate in the training program. Do he, his mother, and the rest of the family want him to be independent? Is the mother patient yet precise enough to carry out a training program? Could she interpret his behavior in terms of progress toward the goal?
3. Before his visit home, Mike seemed to be in disbelief and developing awareness stages (or transition from health to illness). On readmission, he seemed to have entered the reorganization and resolution and identity change phases (beginning convalescence).

4. This statement may be true if understanding can be equated with ability to predict behavior—empathy. Most people do not use these terms synonymously. Also, the statement smacks of unquestioned superiority of the nurse's judgment and seems to slight the value of shared goals.
5. Yes and no. Some people will not be receptive to early education. Analyzing the situation in terms of the Health Belief Model, one would conclude that they do not feel any threat—not even susceptibility. The hypertension cannot be seen (it may have no symptoms); therefore, the patient's ways of checking reality are very limited.

Chapter 4. Objectives of health teaching in nursing

1. a. Teaching is an important means of helping the patient to achieve independence.
   b. This statement reflects the philosophy that patients try to explain what is happening to them during illness. Teaching helps the patient to meet this goal.
   c. This statement has multiple meanings for nursing practice, including patient teaching. Perhaps foremost is the responsibility to provide opportunity for each patient, including the opportunity to learn. Related to this is his right to expect consideration of his cultural background, native ability, and his individual feelings in making plans for learning.
   d. The maintenance of health requires knowledge of how this can be done. In planning what the objectives are to be, the patient and his family are the only persons who have access to certain information that is necessary to planning realistically. This includes information about the physical and social setting in which they live, their goals in life, what they feel is important to learn, how they and the patient view illness, and so forth.
2. a. Main objective: To take routine care of his wife's indwelling urinary catheter.
   Subobjectives:
   *(1) To compare the character and amount of urine collecting in the bag with the acceptable norms for this patient (Cognitive, comprehension)
   *(2) To report to the public health nurse or physician evidence of complications (Cognitive, comprehension)

*(3) To maintain a system free of infection from extracorporeal sources (Cognitive, comprehension)

(4) To cleanse the genitals around the catheter daily, leaving no detectable odor (Psychomotor; cognitive, comprehension)

(5) To irrigate gently with aseptic technique if the catheter appears to be plugged (Psychomotor; cognitive, comprehension)

b. The subobjectives are numbered in order of sequence. Subobjective 4 can be taught any time. Subobjective 2 depends on the understanding of subobjective 1, and subobjective 5 requires more complex skills than do the other four subobjectives. The sequential arrangement also takes into consideration priority; that is, the skills in subobjectives 1, 2, and 3 that are starred (*) are essential for the husband to safely care for his wife.

c. The subobjectives are at a common level of difficulty. In view of their focus, it does not seem crucial for the husband to know even the general anatomy of the urinary system. However, this can be explained to him in uncomplicated terms. Probably more important is the checking of his understanding of cleanliness, basic to asepsis, and of his manipulative skills.

3. Cognitive, knowing: To describe the way an ileostomy bag is used.

Cognitive, application: To apply principles of physics in determining characteristics that a good ileostomy bag should have.

Affective, valuing: To try to devise a more adequate design for an ileostomy bag.

4. Certain missing pieces of information from the study would greatly enhance the accuracy of the judgment to be made. These include how many patients were involved in the study and how many responded; if not all responded, how those who did were different from or like those who did not; what kinds of deviations were reported and to what degree they were serious; and to what extent the mothers knew how to deal adequately with the deviations they found. Depending on the answers to these questions, it may be necessary to see that they have good access to medical care and that there is a teaching objective regarding recognition of deviancy and some simple treatment measures to be taught while the mother is in the hospital or during early follow-up. If such an objective already exists, what evaluative data are there that indicate its effectiveness? Resources needed for the task can be estimated from the size of the group that seems to need help.

5. If he can raise the question, one would judge that he could understand a simple explanation about the difference in desired effects of the two medications. Some understanding of why the effects are not contradictory is important, since it is difficult to anticipate twists of logic patients are likely to make and the actions they will take based on these twists if they lack some basic understanding.

6. a. "As instructed" leaves lack of clarity regarding what is to be measured and the degree of accuracy desired.

b. This is explicit if there is a clear definition of "low-sodium diet."

c. This is a good objective—one assumes that the list of foods consists of those that are part of the general diet.

d. The most obvious concern about this set of objectives is the assumption that after instruction the patient will comply. It would be more realistic to specify a percentage of a group of patients or degrees of compliance for individual patients and to project a reasonable increase over the degree to which these patients or others like them are presently complying. A second point is that "will know," in objective 1, is not behavioral. "Will explain" or "will state" would be a better choice. Subobjective 1e contains two content areas—the side-effects could more probably be placed with 1f.

Chapter 5. Learning

1. a. Knowledge of the adequacy of one's behavior helps one to maintain or attain such desirable behavior.

Many persons are motivated by a sense of control over their destiny.

One would hope that the preparation the patient has had for this role would have included practice of the necessary behaviors, thus aiding complete learning, so that she could successfully execute the behaviors under stress.

b. Learning principles give little explicit information that helps to set the limits. The most relevant learning principle in this situation is that a person learns best that which he is ready to learn, but a decision about how much information to give always rests on a judgment as to the actual readiness of a particular patient to utilize the information in a positive manner.

2.

Behavior	Possible rationale
A first response to this illness was anxiety and a frantic search for a "cause" of the illness, as a way to control the disease by excluding this activity.	This may be part of the disbelief stage, depicting a lack of readiness to accept oneself as vulnerable to the illness.
Some patients had an urgent need for rigid definition by the physicians about the correct way and extent of exerting themselves during convalescence and later, which is a kind of bargaining for control of the symptoms.	Learners will seek resolution of ambiguity. This may also reflect anxiety accompanying convalescent phase of adaptation.
Some patients wished to remain confused about their understanding of the illness.	This may be indicative of disbelief or a way to maintain power over one's illness.
Other patients sought to identify with others whom they knew had suffered a coronary occlusion. This helped to decrease the ambiguity they experienced in the early stages of the illness because, by following the pattern of convalescence of their colleagues, they were able to structure some expectations for their own future.[2]	A model to imitate is a powerful learning tool. In addition, learners will try to structure and attach meaning to their experiences.

3. There is an assumption here that parents are ready to and interested in taking this approach. If this is not so, parents may not feel success from such an approach. Even if there is some readiness for this objective of self-determined and self-evaluated parenthood, one has to be careful not to deprive people of the support of standards defined by groups of people.

4. a. Everyone hunts for a reason or an explanation for what is happening to him, and, in the absence of one based on "scientific" evidence, an explanation is "made up." The emotional, vague assumption of wrongdoing is sometimes the only alternative that can be concocted if alternatives are not known.

   b. This finding should be used as an interesting early hypothesis to which new evidence can be added through research and clinical experience.

Chapter 6. Teaching: definition, theory, and interpersonal techniques

1. a. The terms and concepts suggest that the learner would need at least a high school education with a science background and a familiarity with anatomic terms.

   b. Saran Wrap sticks together and pleura should not; therefore, the analogy can create confusion. The comparison of a leaky valve to a warped door seems less confusing since it does portray the concept of a flat piece of material covering an opening in which the fit is more or less perfect, the moving of the piece occurring only by means of force. The analogy breaks down in obvious ways: The door can be opened from both sides, whereas the valves cannot; there is no corollary in the valve to the latch mechanism present on most doors; and the amount of warping occurring on most doors would seem to have considerably less effect on their fit than would the damage on the diseased heart valves. If the learner can be told in what ways the valve is like the door, the analogy is not so likely to be overinterpreted.

2. It could be true, depending on the quality of the helping skills and the expertise with the content that each individual member has. Other patients sometimes already enjoy an advantage over staff in credibility, which is important in learning.

3. Clearly, a combination of didactic and group interaction strategies is necessary. The didactic provides information in efficient form. The parents' needs, to personalize the information to their child and to work through the feelings that arise as the topic forces them to face the whole pattern of adjustment to the retardation itself, are permitted and sustained in the group by the leader.

4. How about, "Have you ever had a doctor or nurse drain urine from your bladder with a tube?"

Chapter 7. Teaching tools: printed and nonprinted materials

1. Objectives to which the pamphlet on chronic cough may contribute:

   a. To define the characteristics of the chronic cough in terms of length of time present, frequency of coughing, and the relationship of the cough to smoking.

b. To list four diseases that are the most likely causes of chronic cough.

c. To seek medical aid for a chronic cough that is accompanied by pain and bloody phlegm; or, more likely (depending on the learner's state of readiness), to agree that medical care may be necessary for a cough that continues for more than 1 month and that produces pain or bloody phlegm.

d. To state that cough medicine only relieves the cough without removing the cause.

e. To agree that only a physician can determine the cause of the cough.

2. Terms and suggested alternative terms:
Maternity care
a. Menstruation—period, monthly
b. Father's role—how father feels or fits in
c. Adjustment to parenthood—how it feels to be a parent
d. Uterus—womb
e. Episiotomy care—care of stitches
f. Signs of illness in pregnancy—list of symptoms for each illness
g. Fetal growth—growth of baby before birth
h. Conception—how pregnancy occurs
i. Antepartum—before the baby comes
j. Postpartum—after the baby comes
k. Mood swing—how your feelings change
l. Anesthesia—medications during labor and delivery

Infant care
a. Layette—clothing and supplies for the baby
b. Genitals—baby's bottom or private part
c. Weaning—weaning from breast or bottle
d. Immunizations—baby shots
e. Growth and development—what to expect

Child care
a. Sibling rivalry—jealousy between brothers and sisters
b. Enuresis—bed wetting or night bed wetting
c. Communicable disease—childhood disease
d. Peer relationships—relationships with other children
e. Socialization—how your child is with other children and adults

Family planning
a. Birth control—family planning
b. How to control pregnancy—planning your pregnancy
c. IUD—coil

d. Condom—rubbers
e. Anatomy and physiology—how men and women are built, inside and out[6]

3. Readability is seventh grade, which is one grade above recommended level for handout material. The explanation about why the patient feels better but must continue to take the medicine is likely to be plausible to patients. This information sheet covers only some of the standard points for teaching about medications. Very important, it leaves out mention of possible side-effects, as well as how to store the medicine and how to take it. If other directions (such as the label) are not clear, the patient may still take the medicine wrong. The study that used this sheet did find differences between use of the sheet (experimental group) and no sheet (control group) in compliance (measured as physical count of the remaining dosagae units at time of the interview), significant at .05 level. The single-impact message may well have been best, although the study did not measure other aspects of compliance.[5]

4. a. Children demonstrated diabetic procedures in the morning. Group teaching included daily use of skits, films, songs, plays, puppet shows, and rhymes the children composed on diabetes. There was a group of physicians, nurses, and adolescents meeting daily. During Parents' Day, slides and films, question-and-answer periods, and individual parent-staff conferences were held.

b. Almost impossible to answer because of lack of norm data: precamp behavior of these children or comparison behavior on other children like them.[2]

Note: This article depicts excellent use of the teaching process: assessment of need and readiness; development of behavioral objectives, which were sharpened as the instruction progressed; use of a variety of instructional procedures clearly oriented to the attitude and technical skill goals but also individualized for a particular child's need (see discussion of Scott); team planning; involvement of family, including goals set for the future; provision for follow-up by a public health nurse; and evaluation.

5. Other possible reasons for no improvement in learning with the cartoons include: (1) the cartoons did not add any information or at least did not add to the information tested; (2) the cartoons

did add information, but these patients were of the educational level to learn from text alone; (3) everybody knew all the material before reading the booklet—no pretest was given to check this possibility; (4) other?

Chapter 8. Teaching: planning and implementing

1. More investigation is, of course, in order as to why Mrs. Paganelli does not take her pills. Does she live alone? Can she count on the aid of a friend or relative if necessary? How bad is her eyesight? Does she become confused? If these problems are not great, perhaps the nurse can motivate and teach her how to take the medications. She takes her digitalis every morning and her diuretic on Monday, Wednesday, and Friday mornings, one tablet of each medicine. She can be taught to feel the differences in shape and size of the tablets. As an extra aid, a large red cardboard heart may be attached to the digitalis bottle (not the cap) so that its outline can be felt and the color seen. A separate problem may be remembering which days are Monday, Wednesday, and Friday. A very large calendar can be obtained or made, requiring Mrs. Paganelli to cross off the number ''1'' or ''2'' on every day, thus reminding her to take one or two pills. If that fails, a friend could call her to remind her on Mondays, Wednesdays, and Fridays.

2. All these goals may be met by nurse participation with the patient in taking the health action and interpreting the meaning of various situations to him in several visits over a period of time. For the patient with more learning resources, a single teaching episode that is verbal as well as audiovisual (using demonstration-redemonstration tools) could be used. These two teaching approaches, based on patient readiness, represent ends of a continuum from more abstract, short-term learning to concrete, prolonged learning.

3. The nurse can suggest that the mother place green peas, cereal bits, apple slices, and other similar foods on the baby's food tray to aid practice of skills he needs to develop. Explanation should also be given of the organizing idea, of which this action is a part—ways in which the mother can aid the baby's development. There are available from the United States Department of Agriculture sim-

ple large-print booklets on this subject, which can be read by mothers with limited literacy. The nurse can directly facilitate learning through modeling play and vocal games with the infant during visits and through her own expression of pleasure.[1] All three of these strategies are likely to be used. If this learning goal is needed by a number of mothers, consider development of a group teaching situation.

4. These are descriptions of real situations, and they do represent learning tasks that diabetic patients and their families need to master. At the Diabetes Education Center in Minneapolis, thse and other situations were used for group discussion after individuals had had sufficient instruction to be successful in tackling the problems. The groups might be formed so that all members are solving problems with which they now deal or with which they soon will be faced (homogeneous grouping), or they might be formed with a variety of age levels and learning tasks (heterogeneous grouping). In either case, they often gain from other group members' analyses of the problem and discussion of the way in which they have or would have handled it.

5. The format seems generally acceptable. The major concern would be with the plan—it is doubtful that a change in eating behavior can be brought about with such minimal intervention. It will probably be necessary to see her regularly after hospitalization for teaching. In many instances it would also be necessary to use some other approaches, such as peer group influence.

Chapter 9. Evaluation of health teaching

1. To comprehend the means of attaining asepsis in giving an injection.

2. a. The following methods of measurement might be used to evaluate the learning:

   Subobjective A: Written or oral questions with use of photographs for color and response to massage.

   Subobjective B: Observation of behavior when turning, for alignment and body mechanics of the turner. If possible, nurses should observe whether turning is carried out every 2 hours, although they will usually have to rely on questioning and evidence of skin breakdown. Persons doing the turning should be questioned orally as to the schedule of turning, why it must be done, and so forth.

Subobjective C: Observation of behavior, written or oral questioning regarding the importance of this measure and regarding ways to keep linen wrinkle free.

Subobjective D: Observation of massaging. The nurse has to rely to some extent on oral questioning and evidence that skin breakdown is not occurring to assess the adequacy of massage.

Subobjective E: The action required by this objective may occur with varying frequency. Oral questioning plus observation of the skin to determine whether action was taken when it was appropriate are probably the best measures.

b. Instruction for subobjective A appears to have been remiss if the teacher expected the goal to have been met by viewing photographs without using real skin. Even if she did include instruction on real skin, it apparently was not effective, and since this subobjective is a crucial item, it must be retaught. Observation of the skin is in order, as is further questioning about how often and why the patient complains about being turned. The suggested evaluation for other subobjectives should be carried out, since some are crucial to the main objective, which in turn is crucial to the welfare of the patient.

3. Transfer is involved every time the evaluation task is different from the learning tasks, which is the case with all levels of the taxonomy with the possible exception of knowledge. It is possible to index the degree of transfer of which the learner is capable by systematic testing of a wide variety of situations that require varying degrees of transfer (on a continuum from those tasks that are very much like the original learning task to those that are very little like it).

4. Possible factors causing inattentiveness and rebelliousness	Nurse action
The complexity of the tasks the nurse was teaching might have been too great for the learner's ability, thus yielding failure or even lack of willingness to begin learning.	Do a more careful analysis of prerequisite skills the learner possesses. If the goals are found to be too complex, breaking the skills into smaller units and/or teaching the last part of the skill first (so that the learner experiences success) would have merit.
The individual may be preoccupied with other life problems and therefore may not feel motivated to develop this new behavior.	Assess the accuracy of this hypothesis by talking with him and others who know him and by watching his behavior. It may be possible to create motivation by persuading him that solving of his other problem can be aided by learning the dressing skills. Another alternative is to wait a few weeks and try again.
This may be the individual's usual response to many things.	Assess the validity of this statement. If true, it may be possible to do some teaching in spite of the inattentiveness and rebelliousness. The success of learning may alter these responses. Another alternative is teaching aimed first at alteration of these attitudes.

5. a. This person may not understand how blood sugar is measured—a certain amount per standard volume of blood. Check this out.

b. This is likely to be indicative of affective rather than cognitive learning. Because she is in the somewhat ambiguous situation of not being insulin dependent, she is not motivated to move beyond the lower levels of the affective domain. It is also possible that she has not progressed beyond the denial or disbelief stage of psychosocial adaptation to illness.

c. This comment may be evaluative of either cognitive objectives, affective objectives, or both. See if the rest of the conversation provides a more specific clue, and, if not, question the father yourself. The comment may mean that the man has not understood how diabetic patients accommodate to such activities as hunting trips, or it may represent a seeking of verification from an experienced person that diabetic patients really can hunt and that his son can paticipate in such manly activities.

6. The statement of need occurs primarily on pp. 1497 and 1498 before and after the outline of goals. Level of readiness is not completely described, although the account of the living situation implies a particular level. A more explicit

statement of the patients' perception of their motivation and the goals they would like to reach would have been helpful. The goals include a number that will be implemented by teaching, including demonstration by the nurse; there are other goals in which the nurse's support is aimed at freeing the patients for learning. The article contains only anecdotes from the implementation of the teaching program, which occurred over a 2½-month period of time, but it does seem to be built on principles of learning appropriate to the readiness and goal statements: teaching by action in the home setting, providing a model for the mother to imitate and a series of success and nurse reinforcement to stimulate learning. This is particularly clear in the sections on nutritional status on p. 1500 and child guidance on pp. 1498 and 1499. The evaluation section on p. 1502 is oriented to the general goals outlined earlier in the article and primarily uses the approach that the status of the family and actions they have taken are evaluative of the intervention. Data on understanding and attitude changes, not necessarily always displayed overtly, would help in evaluation. Note that evaluation guided the teaching while it was in process—in Mrs. G.'s handling of the children, including Tiny, in feeding of the family, and in acknowledgment of lack of attention to the father's role in the changes.

7. A number of the questions are in poor form. For example, question 1 asks only what a diuretic is, not what it is used for; however, the latter is expected in the answer. Most of the rest of the questions really require only a yes or no answer; however, a substantive answer is expected. Question 3 is quite misleading in that the patient could name *any* side-effect; but hypokalemia is the answer desired.

It is excellent to have preferred answers written out. In addition, it would have been desirable to indicate a scheme for scoring and deciding when a reply is close enough to the preferred answer. The patient will probably remember the questions from the pretest, which may well have served as a teaching tool. However, it will be difficult to know how much of the pre-to-post change is due to instruction and how much to the instructive effect of the pretest.

This test generally requires recall, not recognition, which is consistent with what the patient will have to do at home. However, it would have been wise to include some items that give a problem situation and require the patient to figure out what to do, since this kind of response will also be required of him after discharge.

8. The authors state one limitation—that the test measures only knowledge of information. This limitation, however, was not reflected in the title of the article.

The judges in the validity study were all pediatricians—why not some mothers or other professionals, since the tool is to measure maternal competence? Such a procedure might have changed the inclusion of items. For example, how important is it for mothers to be able to answer *vitamins A, C, and D* (1d) to the question, "If vitamins are not already in infant's diet, which ones should be added"? Would it not have been sufficient if the mother obtained and gave the vitamins prescribed by the physician? How is she to judge if sufficient vitamins are not in the infant's diet?

It was known that some women in the target population could not read; yet one of the statements, "A baby should get most of his primary immunizations by the time he is a year old,"[4] contains language probably too difficult for those who could not read.

The norm-referenced approach to elimination of test items seems a poor choice. Rather, the criterion-referenced approach of maintaining those that are important items for a domain of knowledge would have been better. One should be concerned if mothers do not know when their babies should hold up their heads or stand alone. In addition, items not homogeneous with the total score may still reflect maternal competence (which may not be a homogeneous skill); yet such items were eliminated. The higher scores by multiparas do provide some weak evidence of validity.

Chapter 10. Present delivery of patient education

1. Educational reason and/or intervention:
   a. Education could very likely have cured this problem since it is a factual, conceptual one.
   b. Increase in susceptibility (see Health Belief Model) is a potent motivator.
   c. People will not remember instructions. They

must be written so that they can be reviewed over and over again when people are not anxious. In the absence of clear information, people will improvise their own instructions.

2. Very typical. For comparison, look at the evidence in the Report of the President's Committee on Health Education. Perhaps this situation in the Bay Area has changed by now.

3. Goals 1, 5, 6, 7, and 8 are very global, and goal 2 is quite global. Although the Education Department could reasonably be expected to have some impact on each one of these global goals, there is the danger of not being specific about goals. The danger is a setup for failure since no education department can measure up to these goals. Such expectations can also mean that the members of the committee are not knowledgeable about education and therefore will have difficulty advising about it.

4. Of course, you need to clarify with the physician if there is a specific reason why he has this concern or holds this view. It is true that one of the potential "side-effects" of patient education can be undesirable patient dependence. However, patients are often kept more dependent by *not* having learned the knowledge and skills to become independent. One does need to be certain that the program does not foster undesirable dependence; this can be accomplished by defining objectives at an appropriate level, by making a contract with the learner if you are concerned that dependence may occur, and by making clear and frequent evaluations to ascertain if the desired progress in learning is occurring.

5. There is no "right" answer to this question. Thirty-nine percent does not surprise me, although I think it a bit high. Although it seems to nurses that they are always being consulted by neighbors and family regarding health information, their formal role has not included authoritative dispensing of information.

References

1. Honig, A.: The role of the nurse in stimulating early learning, J. Nurs. Educ. **9**:11-16, Jan. 1970.
2. McFarlane, J., and Hames, C. C.: Children with diabetes; learning self-care in camp, Am. J. Nurs. **73:** 1362-1365, 1973.
3. Martin, H. L.: The significance of discussion with patients about their diagnosis and its implications, Br. J. Med. Psychol. **40:**232-242, 1967.
4. Peters, E. N., and Hoekelman, R. A.: A measure of maternal competence, Health Serv. Rep. **88:**523-526, 1973.
5. Sharpe, T. R., and Mikeal, R. L.: Patient compliance with antibiotic regimens, Am. J. Hosp. Pharm. **31:**479-484, 1974.
6. Tiede, J., and others: Report of the evaluation of "A community nurse's catalogue," Minneapolis, 1970, Combined Nursing Service.

APPENDIX B

Case studies*

The following are patient problems that were written by graduate nurses. Indicate how the teaching problem might be approached.

Case 1

A 71-year-old woman presented herself at the emergency room with the statement, "I'm a clinic patient and I'm sick." She mentioned that she lived alone and was short of cash. The intern described her as "saucy and sassy." Her chief complaint was abdominal pain. After a physical examination that included rectal and pelvic examinations, the physician wanted a clean voided urine specimen. The patient, when asked, said she had never had to obtain a clean voided specimen before. She was instructed on how to obtain a specimen. After the nurse finished the explanation, the patient was asked to repeat the steps and then was asked whether she had any question, which she did not. How can the nurse be sure that the patient obtained the urine specimen correctly and did not contaminate it?

Case 2

A 20-year-old man was admitted to the hospital with a diagnosis of renal shutdown, comminuted fractures of the right tibia and fibula, comminuted fracture of the right femur, right acetabular fracture with separation of the symphysis pubis, comminuted fracture of the right elbow, and possible brain damage. The patient had frequently suffered from mental agitation in the past and had a very low pain threshold. Mental retardation or a low IQ was suspected.

---

*These cases were developed by nursing staff of the University Hospital, University of Washington.

The patient worked occasionally as a farmhand. He had no insurance coverage and his parents refused to be responsible for him.

The teaching problems in this case centered around the fact that the patient was unaware of proper personal hygiene. For example, he had never brushed his teeth in his life or seen a dentist, although he had extensive dental caries. The patient refused to let nurses brush his teeth, assist him, or teach him to brush them himself. The teaching goals for this patient, as written by the nursing staff, were as follows:

1. Teach patient principles of good oral hygiene.
2. Get patient to brush his teeth.
3. Teach patient the fundamentals of a nutritious diet.
4. Encourage patient to seek dental attention.

Success in teaching the patient the principles and practice of good oral hygiene was limited. A toothbrush was procured for him and its use demonstrated, but the nurse was unable to get him to use it. She was, however, able to get him to eat apples between meals, although he refused to eat any other hard vegetables or fruits that might mechanically clean his teeth.

As for good nutrition, the patient ate an adequate diet while in the hospital, but the nurse did not succeed in teaching him the concept of balanced meals.

In view of these limited accomplishments with the patient, how ought the teaching to have been improved?

Case 3

The patient was a 64-year-old woman, well developed and well nourished, who appeared younger than her stated age. She was apprehensive on admission to the hospital. This patient was admitted to the hospital for a permanent colostomy because of cancer of the rectum. There was no evidence of metastasis at the time of surgery. The patient had led a very active life, and there was no reason why she should not continue to do so.

In this case the problem of the nurse was to teach the patient to accept the colostomy and to be independent in caring for it. While the patient was in the hospital, the colon was irrigated at the same time every day, according to her normal rising time at home, and was quite well regulated by the time she was discharged. The patient was encouraged to perform the irrigation procedure for herself when she was feeling better and did so under supervision, reluctantly. She was given an irrigating set and bags and told where she could buy new ones when she needed to. She was instructed thoroughly in the care of the stoma and of the skin. She was told about the Colostomy Club. She was given free samples of colostomy pads and a belt that we happened to have on hand. She was also given a booklet, *Care of Your Colostomy.* Her teaching was reinforced many times.

The patient continued to lean toward dependence and talked about having relatives care for her at home. She was told that she really should not need this and should be and was capable of caring for herself. The patient asked for and received a public health referral when she was discharged. The public health nurse was told that the patient needed reinforced teaching and encouragement toward independence.

This patient was still apprehensive when she went home; thus the nurses felt that they did not solve this problem of dependence. The patient also had a drain-ing perineal wound at the time of discharge. She had been taking sitz baths for this and was told to continue doing so at home. She was also given a small sample sitz pan to use on the toilet if she wished. She was told that the perineal wound would heal quite slowly and that this was normal in a colostomy. She did not appear too worried about the wound. The public health nurse was also informed about the wound.

Case 4

Mrs. E., who was admitted to the hospital for the birth of her third baby, had breast fed her previous two children. The teaching problem with Mrs. E. involved assisting her in breast feeding and trying to bring about some changes in her method of breast feeding. Mrs. E. insisted on lying down for feeding. She was used to being flat in bed for 10 days following delivery and then on continued bed rest for several more days. She had difficulty in accepting the policy of early ambulation. While breast feeding, Mrs. E. did not cuddle and hold the baby lovingly. The baby was fussy following feeding.

The following goals were made part of the teaching plan for Mrs. E. The nurse-teacher would:

1. Try to have Mrs. E. sit up while breast feeding in order to enhance the flow of milk.
2. Emphasize that Mrs. E. had to be relaxed while feeding the baby, not involved in making phone calls, so as to increase milk flow.

Mrs. E. showed some change even after the few times that she breast fed while in the hospital. She did not breast feed long enough to give the nurse any indication of definite change in her attitude. She was then discharged from the hospital.

APPENDIX C

Illustrious teaching examples

The process of teaching has necessarily been segmented into chapters in this book. This appendix cites ''whole'' teaching examples that I believe to be illustrious and explains why they represent good practice.

Example 1

Bergner, M., and Hutelmyer, C.: Teaching kids how to live with their allergies, Nursing 76, Aug. 1976, p. 11. Read especially the section on food allergens.

Rationale: The objective is realistic and practical—one the patient will need daily. Teaching tools are the kind children will like. The evaluation situation is realistic and not just verbal.

Example 2

Jones, P.: Patient education—yes, no, Supervisor Nurse **8**(5):35-43, May 1977.

Rationale: The approach to the innovation was positive—involvement of those to use it. There is a clear focus to the learning activities and support for those who needed to learn.

Example 3

Pepper, G. A.: Bedside report—would it work for you? Nursing 78 **8**(6):73-74, June 1978.

Rationale: This approach thoroughly integrates teaching into nursing and provides a natural check on patient understanding and involvement in planning his own care.

Example 4

Schmidt, J.: Using a teaching guide for better post-partum and infant care, J. Obstet. Gynecol. Neonat. Nurs. **7**(3):23-25, May/June, 1978.

Rationale: This example shows how organization in providing patient education can assist with general development of the patient, as well as provide efficient service in teaching particular skills.

Example 5

Verso, M. A.: This is how we do it at . . . diabetic day care; a method for diabetic education and control, Diabetes Educator **4**(1):16-17, Spring 1978.

Rationale: The patient is followed through until he is controlled. The delivery method apparently results in considerable cost savings.

APPENDIX D

Questions on patient teaching

1. The nurse-teacher must understand the impact of the health crisis on the receptivity of the learner because:
    a. A health crisis can provide motivation for learning.
    b. Much health teaching occurs around the time of health crisis.
    c. Learning helps the patient adjust to his health crisis.
    d. All of the above.
2. T F Research has now shown that fear is not effective as a motivator in health education.
3. The principle that too great anxiety interferes with learning has pertinence for which of the stages of psychosocial adaptation to illness?
    a. Transition to illness.
    b. Acceptance of illness.
    c. Convalescence.
    d. *a, b,* and *c.*
    e. *a* and *c.*
4. T F Research has provided clear answers to times during the psychosocial stages of illness in which the most efficient learning occurs.
5. What is wrong with this objective: To develop critical thinking?
    a. Learners whom nurses teach will not develop to this level of complexity.
    b. Critical thinking is a vague term.
    c. No content is specified.
    d. *b* and *c.*
    e. *a, b,* and *c.*
6. In applying this principle of learning—Learning takes place more effectively in situations from which the student derives feelings of satisfaction —which teaching action would be most effective?
    a. Do not ask the learner to learn anything he does not think he is capable of learning.
    b. Structure the learning so that the learner will be able to accomplish the goals.
    c. Evaluate only the things the learner is doing well.
    d. Allow the learner to define the objectives.
7. Providing a baby bath demonstration utilizes primarily which principle of motivation?
    a. Provide for realistic goal setting.
    b. Aid your patient in making and evaluating progress toward goals.
    c. Focus learner attention toward desired learning outcomes.
    d. Provide concrete and symbolic incentives if necessary.
8. Which principle of attitude teaching is most specifically involved in the practice of using a particular nursing "approach" to a patient?
    a. Provide for pleasant emotional experiences.
    b. Provide appropriate context for practice of the attitudes.
    c. Extend informative experiences about the attitude.
    d. Provide desirable identifying figures for the learners.
9. The following principle of motivation—Aid your patient in making and evaluating progress toward goals—is most directly related to which principle of learning?
    a. Learning takes place more effectively when a patient is ready to learn.
    b. Active participation by a learner is preferable to passive reception when learning.
    c. Learning takes place more effectively in situations from which the student derives feelings of satisfaction.
10. On the basis of the following principle of learning—Recognition of similarities and dissimi-

larities between past experience and the present situation facilitates the transfer of learning—the nurse-teacher would:

a. Show the patient how the handwashing procedure he is learning before changing dressings is like the handwashing he has always done.

b. Not teach two skills at the same time.

c. Show a patient who has never given himself injections and is now learning to give insulin the similarities between an insulin syringe and a 2-ml. syringe.

d. Recognize that this principle does not operate in the learning of attitudes.

11. Writing lesson plans in column form is suggested because:

a. The teacher should make certain that there is a teaching action for every entry in the content column.

b. The contiguity is helpful in assessing the appropriateness of teaching actions for particular content.

c. Some form of organization helps the teacher present the material in a logical sequence.

d. This form can be most easily adapted to more or less detailed lesson plans.

e. *a* and *b*.

12. Which principle related to instructional outcomes can be implemented *least* well through the use of teaching machines?

a. Practice and review until facts are firmly established.

b. Provision for sequential, cumulative learning.

c. Reinforcement of correct responses and overcoming of errors immediately.

d. Provision of opportunities for stating and testing hypotheses.

13. The only objective for a particular lesson is: to brush his own teeth effectively. In planning the lesson the teacher plans to include a discussion of the incidence of dental disease among natives of Africa. This is not useful because:

a. It does not relate to meeting the objective.

b. The dental problems of the natives of Africa are known to be unlike the dental problems in the United States.

c. The learner is probably not motivated to learn about the dental problems of African natives.

d. The learner may not have the experiential

readiness to learn about dental problems of African natives.

14. T F Selecting or preparing audiovisual aids before identifying the objective for the lesson will assure the clarity of the objective.

15. If teachers have clues or ambiguity in their test items and test trivia, they are lowering:

a. Reliability   c. Reliability and validity

b. Validity   d. Comprehensiveness

16. Teachers can best judge the effectiveness of instructional materials through:

a. A thorough program of standardized testing.

b. A thorough program of informal testing at the end of each unit.

c. Systematic evaluation of the students' responses.

d. Asking other teachers to criticize the materials.

17. The nurse-teacher should use written tests when:

a. This method is easier than observing behavior.

b. Testing in the cognitive domain.

c. Testing individuals alone or in groups.

d. *a* and *b*.

e. *b* and *c*.

18. T F It is better to use untrained observers when evaluating learning because they are less likely to have preconceived ideas about what the behavior means.

19. Anecdotal records might be best used to evaluate progress of learning in which situation (or situations)?

a. A patient's progress in becoming more independent.

b. A mother learning to take her child's temperature.

c. Acceptance of need for seeking medical care when sick.

d. *b* and *c*.

e. *a* and *c*.

20. T F Tests of comprehension should be in language and context different from that originally learned.

Answers to questions

1. d	5. d	9. b	13. a	17. e
2. F	6. b	10. a	14. F	18. F
3. d	7. c	11. e	15. c	19. e
4. F	8. b	12. d	16. c	20. T

Index